Concepts of the Nursing Profession

Karin A. Polifko, PhD, RN, CNAA
Remington College
Orlando, Florida

THOMSON
DELMAR LEARNING

Australia Brazil Canada Mexico Singapore Spain United Kingdom United States

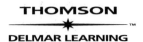

THOMSON

DELMAR LEARNING

Concepts of the Nursing Profession
By Karin A. Polifko, PhD, RN, CNAA

Vice President, Health Care Business Unit:
William Brottmiller

Director of Learning Solutions
Matthew Kane

Acquisitions Editor:
Tamara Caruso

Product Manager:
Elizabeth Howe

Editorial Assistant:
Chelsey Iaquinta

Marketing Director:
Jennifer McAvey

Marketing Manager:
Michele McTighe

Marketing Coordinator:
Danielle Pacella

Technology Director:
Laurie Davis

Technology Project Manager:
Carolyn Fox

Production Director:
Carolyn Miller

Senior Content Project Manager:
James Zayicek

Art Director:
Jack Pendleton

Library of Congress Cataloging-in-Publication Data

Polifko-Harris, Karin, 1958-
    Concepts of the nursing profession / by Karin Polifko-Harris.
        p. cm.
    Includes bibliographical references and index.
    ISBN-13: 978-1-4018-0886-0
    ISBN-10: 1-4018-0886-7
    1. Nursing—Philosophy. I. Title.
    [DNLM: 1. Nursing--United States. WY 16 P767c 2007]

RT63.P6544 2007
610.73—dc22

                                    2006029080

Notice to the Reader

Publisher does not warrant or guarantee any of the products described herein or perform any independent analysis in connection with any of the product information contained herein. Publisher does not assume, and expressly disclaims, any obligation to obtain and include information other than that provided to it by the manufacturer.

The reader is expressly warned to consider and adopt all safety precautions that might be indicated by the activities described herein and to avoid all potential hazards. By following the instructions contained herein, the reader willingly assumes all risks in connection with such instructions.

The publisher makes no representations or warranties of any kind, including but not limited to, the warranties of fitness for particular purpose or merchantability, nor are any such representations implied with respect to the material set forth herein, and the publisher takes no responsibility with respect to such material. The publisher shall not be liable for any special, consequential, or exemplary damages resulting, in whole or part, from the reader's use of, or reliance upon, this material.

To my Dad, who is missed daily.

CONTRIBUTORS

Lora Humphrey Beebe, PhD, APRN, BC
Associate Professor
College of Nursing
The University of Tennessee
Knoxville, Tennessee
*Chapter 2: History and Evolution of
Nursing*

Amy Barlow Britt, MS, RN, CEN
Riverside School of Health Careers
Newport News, Virginia
Chapter 18: Evaluator

Mary Ann Brown, BSN, JD
Assistant Legal Counsel
The Campania Group
Vienna, Virginia
*Chapter 12: Legal Accountabilities in
the Health Care Environment*

Theresa Perfetta Cappello, RN, PhD
Professor
School of Nursing
Dean
School of Health Professions
Marymount University
Arlington, Virginia
*Chapter 8: Health Services in the
United States*

Maureen C. Creegan, PhD, RN
Director
Division of Nursing
Dominican College
Orangeburg, New York
*Chapter 1: From Practice to Professionalism:
The Struggle Within*

Sheryl Curtis, MSN, ARNP
Clinical Assistant Professor
Department: Women, Children, and Family
College of Nursing
University of Florida
Gainesville, Florida
Chapter 21: Mentoring and the Profession

Sharon Guillet, RN, PhD
Associate Professor
School of Nursing
Chair
Baccalaureate Degree Program
School of Health Professions
Marymount University
Arlington, Virginia
Chapter 10: Health Care Policy Issues

Vicki P. Kent, PhD, RN
Clinical Associate Professor
Department of Nursing
Towson University
Towson, Maryland
*Chapter 6: Theoretical Basis for the Practice of
Nursing*

K. Alberta McCaleb, DSN, RN
Associate Professor
School of Nursing
University of Alabama
Birmingham, Alabama
*Chapter 20: Defining a Professional: Graduate
Education*

Nancy N. Menzel, PhD, RN, COHN-S
Associate Professor
Las Vegas School of Nursing
University of Nevada
Chapter 19: Manager of Information Systems

Mary Jo Regan-Kubinski, RN, PhD
Dean
Division of Nursing & Health Professions
Indiana University
South Bend, Indiana
Chapter 22: Responsibilites of the Profession

Pamela J. Sherwill-Navarro, AHIP
Health Science Center Libraries
University of Florida
Gainesville, Florida
Chapter 5: Seeking and Managing Information

Cathleen Shultz, PhD, RN, FAAN
Dean
College of Nursing
Harding University
Searcy, Arkansas
Chapter 14: Teacher/Learner

Linda M. Sigsby, MSN, RN
Assistant Professor
College of Nursing
University of Florida
Gainesville, Florida
*Chapter 13: Ethical Considerations in the
   Health Care Environment*

Amy Spurlock, PhD, RN
Associate Professor
Department of Nursing
Troy University
Troy, Alabama
*Chapter 9: Professional Accountability:
   Credentialing and Accreditation*

Sheila Cox Sullivan, PhD, RN
Associate Dean
College of Nursing
Harding University
Searcy, Arkansas
Chapter 7: Evidence-Based Practice

Angela S. Taylor, PhD, RN, BC
Associate Professor
Department of Nursing
The University of Virginia's College at Wise
Wise, Virginia
Chapter 3: Educating the Profession

Cesarina Thompson, PhD, RN
Chairperson & Professor
Department of Nursing
Southern Connecticut State University
New Haven, Connecticut
Chapter 15: Change Agent

Linda Wagner, EdD, MSN, RN
Associate Professor
Department of Nursing
Southern Connecticut State University
New Haven, Connecticut
Chapter 15: Change Agent

Lillian Wise, MSN, RN
Associate Professor
School of Nursing
Troy University
Troy, Alabama
*Chapter 9: Professional Accountability:
   Credentialing and Accreditation*

CONTENTS

PREFACE   viii

ACKNOWLEDGMENTS   x

REVIEWERS   xi

ABOUT THE AUTHOR   xii

U N I T
ONE
Foundations of the Profession / 1

CHAPTER 1   **From Practice to Professionalism: The Struggle Within**   3
             Maureen C. Creegan

CHAPTER 2   **History and Evolution of Nursing**   16
             Lora Humphrey Beebe

CHAPTER 3   **Educating the Profession**   30
             Angela S. Taylor

CHAPTER 4   **Finding and Maintaining Work/Life Harmony**   45
             Karin A. Polifko

CHAPTER 5   **Seeking and Managing Information**   64
             Pamela J. Sherwill-Navarro

CHAPTER 6   **Theoretical Basis for the Practice of Nursing**   78
             Vicky P. Kent

CHAPTER 7   **Evidence-Based Practice**   96
             Sheila Cox Sullivan

U N I T
TWO
Environment of the Profession / 111

CHAPTER 8   **Health Services in the United States**   113
             Theresa Perfetta Cappello

CHAPTER 9   **Professional Accountability: Credentialing and Accreditation** 137
             Lillian Wise and Amy Spurlock

CHAPTER 10   **Health Care Policy Issues**   **159**
              Sharon Guillet

CHAPTER 11   **Diversity**   **178**
              Karin A. Polifko

CHAPTER 12   **Legal Accountabilities in the Health Care Environment**   **197**
              Mary Ann Brown

CHAPTER 13   **Ethical Considerations in the Health Care Environment**   **215**
              Linda M. Sigsby

U N I T
THREE
Leading the Profession / 229

CHAPTER 14   **Teacher/Learner**   **231**
              Cathleen Schultz

CHAPTER 15   **Change Agent**   **266**
              Cesarina Thompson and Linda Wagner

CHAPTER 16   **Delegator and Decision Maker**   **279**
              Karin A. Polifko

CHAPTER 17   **Collaborator and Negotiator**   **294**
              Karin A. Polifko

CHAPTER 18   **Evaluator**   **312**
              Amy Barlow Britt

CHAPTER 19   **Manager of Information Systems**   **322**
              Nancy N. Menzel

U N I T
FOUR
Envisioning the Future of the Profession / 343

CHAPTER 20   **Defining a Professional: Graduate Education**   **345**
              K. Alberta McCaleb

CHAPTER 21   **Mentoring and the Profession**   **362**
              Sheryl Curtis

CHAPTER 22   **Responsibilities of the Profession**   **377**
              Mary Jo Regan-Kubinski and Karin A. Polifko

INDEX   **389**

PREFACE

Organization

The purpose of this book is to provide the introductory materials necessary for several nursing student audiences: the returning RN student enrolled in a transition course and both the second-degree nursing student and the generic baccalaureate student enrolled in an introductory concepts course. This book focuses on the skills needed in real-world applications.

Highlights

Concepts of the Nursing Profession is written in a manner that will encourage the student and the professor to become engaged in an active discussion, whether in a traditional classroom or via the Web, and is based upon many years of teaching concepts to a variety of nursing students. First and foremost, the book focuses on the skill sets necessary to be successful in the marketplace, whether it is in an acute-care setting or in a public health department. *Concepts of the Nursing Profession* offers skills that new graduates can immediately apply in their first professional role as a registered nurse. Here are some other points of interest:

- The book engages the reader rather than simply being a text to read.

- Each chapter contains case studies that may be used individually or as a group assignment.

- There is extensive use of application in the clinical settings, allowing a student to immediately visualize a variety of situations with nurses' potential responses.

- Guided questions are placed throughout the chapters to encourage continuing dialog, thoughtful discussion, and oftentimes classroom debate.

Features

Concepts of the Nursing Profession is divided into four primary sections, with the following headers:

- **Foundations of the Profession** includes the history of nursing, its educational system, and its theoretical basis; a brief discussion of evidence-based practice methods; and a chapter on how to achieve balance in a busy life.
    - One highlight of this section is a chapter written by a nursing librarian, who outlines numerous helpful strategies when initiating library research.

- **Environment of the Profession** discusses the current issues surrounding health care in general, and nursing in particular, including legal and ethical issues, licensure, the policy arena, and the impact that our diversity has on health care delivery and the nursing profession.
    - One highlight of this section differentiates and clearly explains accreditation, state-approval processes, and credentialing.

- **Leading the Profession** offers actual skills that will enable both the neophyte and the experienced nurse to be successful, regardless of the setting. These skills include teaching, delegation, decision making, collaboration, negotiation, and evaluation.
    - One highlight of this section is a clear, concise discussion on information technology. It is especially helpful for the novice computer user.

- **Envisioning the Future of the Profession** asks, "What does the future of nursing hold?" This section offers a review of the current literature and predictions for the largest health care profession in the United States.

■ One highlight of this section is a complete explaination of mentoring, from the perspective both of the mentor and the person being mentored.

Each chapter contains the same focus areas to enhance learning in a variety of methods:

■ *Learning Objectives*

■ *Key Terms,* which are defined throughout the chapter.

■ *Written Exercises,* which directly guide the student to critically think and problem solve scenarios in the health care setting. Many of these written exercises can be used for classroom discussion and debate, as a writing exercise, or as part of an examination.

■ *Case Scenarios* offer the student the ability to practice decision-making skills with real-life situations. Like the written exercises, these scenarios can be used for classroom discussion and debate, as a writing exercise, or as evaluation of subject comprehension.

■ *Research Application Article* reviews current nursing research as it applies to each specific chapter.

ACKNOWLEDGMENTS

The completion of this project could not have been successful without the many friends and colleagues who so willingly agreed to contribute their expertise. While many will not be adequately recognized by their organizations for their writing, they all have talents to share so that others can learn. I appreciate everyone who took time out of busy schedules and lives to help write this book.

Special thanks goes to Elizabeth "Libby" Howe, my Product Manager at Thomson Delmar Learning, who was absolutely wonderful to work with, regardless of the deadline or the problem.

A final thank you goes to my husband Jay, who is always supportive of my pursuits and aspirations, and to my two China princesses, Jilaina and Calissa.

REVIEWERS

The author would like to thank the following reviewers:

Cynthia Archibald, PhD, ARNP
Professor
College of Nursing
Florida Atlantic University
Davie, Florida

Mary Bell Braxton, MSN, RN
Nursing Resource Center Coordinator
Nursing Department
University of West Georgia
Carrollton, Georgia

Harlene Caroline, RN, BSN, MS
Professor
Department of Nursing
Curry College
Milton, Massachusetts

Charles Dykes, RN, MSN
Instructor
School of Nursing
Southeastern Louisiana University
Hammond, Louisiana

Jo Ann Eckhardt, BS, MS, PhD
Associate Professor
Nursing Department
The College of Saint Catherine
St. Paul, Minnesota

Carol Elliott, PhD, RN, CS
Assistant Professor
Department of Nursing
University of New England
Westbrook, Maine

Marcia Hobbs, RN, MS, DSN
Professor
Department of Nursing
Murray State University
Murray, Kentucky

Dana Manley, RN, ARNP, MSN
Lecturer
Department of Nursing
Murray State University
Murray, Kentucky

Susan Rieck, PhD, RN
Assistant Professor
School of Nursing
Northern Arizona University
Flagstaff, Arizona

Cheryl Ross, MS, RN
Associate Professor
School of Nursing
Oklahoma City University
Oklahoma City, Oklahoma

Rebecca Whiffen, ADN, BSN, MSN, ANCC
Lecturer
Department of Nursing
Murray State University
Murray, Kentucky

Anne White, DSN, RN
Associate Professor
School of Nursing
Kennesaw State University
Kennesaw, Georgia

ABOUT THE AUTHOR

Karin Polifko's career has spanned both the academic and service fields of health care. Along with teaching appointments and experience at the undergraduate, graduate, and doctoral levels, Dr. Polifko has held academic positions as the Associate Dean for Academic and Student Affairs at the University of Florida's College of Nursing, and Chair of Nursing and Graduate Director at Christopher Newport University in Virginia. She has extensive administrative experience in a variety of health care settings, in the roles of Vice President of System Development and Research, Administrative Director, Director of Nursing, Nurse Manager, and Clinical Nurse Specialist. Recent consulting projects include nursing program development, accreditation preparation, organizational change assessment and evaluation, outcomes systems management, and leadership assessment. Her first textbook, *Case Applications in Nursing Leadership and Management*, was published in 2004. She is the author of numerous book chapters that focus on leadership and management topics and has lectured extensively on these topics.

Dr. Polifko received her Bachelor of Science in Nursing from the University of North Carolina, Charlotte; her Master of Science in Nursing from the University of Pennsylvania; and her Doctorate in Public Administration with a certificate in Advanced Policy Analysis from Old Dominion University. She is nationally certified as a Nurse Administrator, Advanced, by the American Nurses Credentialing Center. Further, Dr. Polifko is a Certified Family Mediator for the State of Florida.

Foundations
of the Profession

CHAPTER 1

From Practice to Professionalism: The Struggle Within

Maureen C. Creegan

"It was the best of times, it was the worst of times . . ."
—Charles Dickens

CHAPTER OBJECTIVES

At the completion of the chapter, the learner should be able to do the following:

1. Describe the ambiguities and opportunities in our current health care and educational systems.
2. Identify nursing opportunities afforded by multiple entry and exit points and their utility in shaping the future nursing workforce.
3. Provide a forum for discussion about our roots and identity as professionals.
4. Identify, describe, and make recommendations for collaboration, communication, and quality improvement processes that ensure positive patient-centered care and population-based outcomes.

KEY TERMS

Collaboration	Nursing professional identity	Patient-centered care
Communication	Nursing professionalism	Professional roots
Nursing in changing times	Nursing workforce	Quality improvement

We live in a time of acceleration. Ambiguity and "an earthquake of system instability" (Kirkman-Liff, 2002) mark the current time, yet the time has never been better for growth and change. Forces that drive organizations and academic institutions outpace our very thought processes, and keeping up means keeping pace with advances in technology, market economies, expansive new knowledge, and increasing diversity (Lindeman, 2000; Larsen, McGill, & Palmer, 2003; Institute of Medicine, 2003). The public demands accountability from health professions, seeks participation in shared decision making, and expects culture-conscious care. In addition, a rapidly growing elder population, an increase in the prevalence of chronic disease, increased survival rates among individuals with acute illnesses, and emphasis on population-based, and **patient-centered care** are providing the momentum that ultimately will shape the composition and profile of the future **nursing workforce** (Lindeman, 2000; Kirkman-Liff, 2002; Larsen, McGill, & Palmer, 2003; Institute of Medicine, 2003). The health care system has been slow to change, and understanding its evolution helps formulate an interdisciplinary agenda worth effort and action.

NURSING IN CHANGING TIMES

As a nation we engaged in fee-for-service health care and improved preventive care from 1965 to 1982 (Barger, 2004; Etheredge, 2001). During this time of Reorganizing Care, calls for more nurses escalated as hospitals expanded to deliver what was known as Progressive Patient Care (PPC), which apportioned care according to acuity (Lynaugh & Brush, 1996). The rise of intensive care units is a clear example of the PPC concept, because the sickest patients were concentrated in areas where highly skilled personnel delivered highly skilled care. The concept of primary nursing evolved and redefined nursing, leaving team nursing behind. One nurse became primary caregiver to a set group of patients, and 24-hour responsibility was expected.

Although nursing numbers continued to expand in the mid-60s, turnover among registered nurses rose to 67% at a time when turnover among factory workers was approximating 40% (Lynaugh & Brush, 1996 p. 30). Also noteworthy was physician presence in the hospital. Characterized as absent more than present, physicians were responsible for day-to-day care, while nurses, a constant presence, were directly responsible for clinical decision making, yet powerless to make decisions (Anderson, 1968).

Also noted were nurses' increasing focus on diagnosis and therapy and diminished attention to the provision of nursing comfort care. "Nurses and physicians who were closest to patient care rather quickly realized that close collaboration and shared decision-making were crucial to success in patient care." (Lynaugh & Brush, 1996, p. 34). Nurses soon found their ambiguous position intolerable and were advised to "become bold, show initiative, and be responsible for making timely and important recommendations . . ." (Stein, 1967).

In 1972 the National Joint Practice Commission (NJPC) was formed to discuss and plan interdisciplinary education between medicine and nursing. The Commission was composed of members from the American Medical Association, the American Nurses Association, and the W. K. Kellogg Foundation. The Commission debated issues that resonate today. "The basic issue . . . concerns the problem of underutilization of the professional competence of registered nurses in this country . . ." (Lynaugh & Brush, 1996, p. 40). Given the expansion of their responsibilities, nurses pressed to broaden their scope of practice and practice settings. Expanding the scope of nursing practice supported need for more education. "The poor fit of nursing education and nursing practice required nurses to constantly retrain [and] one out of every ten nurses engaged in formal retraining" (Lynaugh & Brush, 1996, p. 29). In 1965 the American Nurses Association (ANA) issued its seminal work, the ANA Position Paper, which demanded that "education for those who are licensed to practice nursing should take place in institutions of higher education" (ANA, 1965). Nursing education, fragmented and lacking standardization, began to shed the apprenticeship model and moved to four-year academic institutions and two-year community colleges. Three separate educational systems emerged: the traditional hospital-based apprenticeship diploma program, offering three years of training; four-year college programs, which emphasized liberal arts and sciences, typically during the first two years, followed by two years of nursing studies; and the associate degree, which offered a year of arts and sciences and a year of nursing studies. The debate over educational preparation and standardized curricula for levels of nursing practice intensified during this era and continues today.

From 1983 to 1992 the nation moved to a system of government-set rates and widespread adoption of Diagnostic Related Groupings (DRGs). Entitlement programs for women and children expanded to rural areas, with emphasis shifting to primary care. As the federal government increasingly focused on Medicare and Medicaid reform, and as state regulations changed, employers developed their own cost control measures and health insurance solutions. During the period from 1993 to 2000, a doomed comprehensive health proposal followed, ending the traditional fee-for-service structure and opening the gates to managed care, which was touted as the remedy for spiraling costs. It became evident that projected cost savings of managed care superseded quality. Public outcry grew, and calls for accountability and quality led to the development of practice guidelines and **quality improvement** initiatives. During this period the emphasis on primary care shifted educational priorities to community-based curricula and the education of nurse practitioners as primary care providers (Barger, 2004; Etheredge, 2001). Also known as the Relocating Care era, nursing care moved from the hospital to the home, as previously delivered in the early 1800s (Lynaugh & Brush, 1996). The sickest patients were still confined to the hospitals, requiring even more sophisticated nursing care. As a matter of fact, in the early 1980s, turnover rates for hospital nurses reduced to approximately 30% from previous skyrocketing levels, and disputed claims that nurses left positions to find other types of work. In contrast to the Reorganizing Care era (1965–1982), 76% of nurses were actively practicing, and those who were not working engaged in personal and family activities. For the 24% who were dissatisfied with nursing work, the primary reasons for turnover were hospital climate, mental and physical fatigue, and limits to the scope of practice (Bleich, Hewlett, Santos,

Rice, Cox, & Richmeier, 2003; Institute of Medicine, 1983; Lynaugh & Brush; 1996; Laschinger, Finegan, Shamian, & Wilk, 2001).

THE ERA OF AMBIGUITY AND OPPORTUNITY 2001–?

As the twenty-first century opened, the United States entered a period of ambiguity, a turning point, inviting change in structures and infrastructures, changes in the way we conduct ourselves and do business with others, and changes in professional preparation for the future. The aging of the nursing workforce and a trend among women to seek other career opportunities were widely reported (Bednash, 2000; Bleich, et al., 2003; Brewer, 1996; Buerhaus, Staiger, & Averbach, 2000; Needleman & Buerhaus, 2003; Dworkin, 2002). The market-driven economy and highly competitive healthcare system called for a savvy nurse, one who uses technology, is cognizant of shifting demographics, adapts to change with fluidity, and keeps pace with accelerating scientific knowledge (Aiken, Clarke, Sloane, & Sochalski, 2002; Buerhaus, 1994; Institute of Medicine, 2000, 2001, 2003).

The explosion in technology has enhanced and revitalized **communication.** Computer networks enable us to record changes in patient status while in the field and provide distance education so that larger numbers of students can be taught without ever entering a classroom. Information is collected and stored in computerized medical records. Health care providers have access to these records and because of information sharing, possible medical error may be reduced (Institute of Medicine, 2003; Whitis, 2001). Through sophisticated telemedicine, health care providers can diagnose and treat patients who may never enter an office. Providing the computing infrastructure necessary for communication among health care professionals remains a challenge, because it requires knowledgeable people who can design the processes and evaluation methods as well as record and take corrective action to improve outcomes of care (Institute of Medicine, 2003). Educating the next generation of computer-savvy health professionals is an immediate need. Academe and the health care industry are playing catch-up, as the corporate world moves forward rapidly to assemble information and conduct global communication (Whitis, 2001).

Rapid-fire communication means accelerated knowledge development. Conventional ways of teaching and learning—listening to lectures and formulating facts—will become obsolete. We must abandon content-laden curricula and develop nurses who think analytically, discuss issues, write clearly and succinctly, synthesize data, and translate into practice the best evidence that guides action and enhances decision making.

Knowledge of shifting demographics enables nurses to provide culture-conscious care. The most rapidly growing sector of the population, elders over 85 years, are living longer with chronic diseases and taking multiple medications. Some will need custodial care, and many will require social support. As the face of the nation changes, people of color and multiple ethnicities will expect care to be tailored with respect for their values and belief systems. New students entering the field will also be part of this profile and will come with diverse learning styles and goals, as well as values and belief systems. (Lindeman, 2000). Physically challenged individuals will also be integrated into the profession. Providing learning opportunities for these students will require faculty creativity. Practicing nurses must also find creative ways to use the talents of colleagues with disabilities (Carroll, 2004; Moore, 2004).

The purpose of a nurse to deliver timely, quality care to diverse populations has always been evident, yet it is overshadowed by the continuing struggle with definition and preparation. To this day the struggle continues. An understanding of practice and professionalism is rooted in history. Our **professional roots** define who we are and help us envision and plan the future.

ROOTS OF PROFESSIONALISM

Our history describes us as men and women who care for people as individuals and in aggregates long before client-centered and population-based care was in vogue. Linda Richards was one of those pioneers who served the sick during the Civil War because "there were not enough male nurses to care for mass casualties . . ." (Holder, 2004). In 1854 there were no female nurses in the United States, the Crimean War had just begun in southern Russia, and Florence Nightingale was embarking on her nursing career in the military. Intelligent, independent, and strong women like Richards took care of the wounded and sick in battlefield hospitals. "It is estimated that 10,000 women provided care to soldiers during the Civil War" (Holder, 2004). At the close of the war in 1865, military nurses went home and, in keeping with the social mores of the day, returned to the genteel life, because nursing was considered a job for men (Holder). As the social climate began to change, Richards continued her quest for acceptance as a nurse trainee. In 1870, at age 29, she went to Boston seeking work, but try as she might, male physicians refused to train a woman as a nurse (Holder, 2004). Finally, in 1872, Richards was interviewed by Susan Dimock, a female physician (a rarity at the time) at New England Deaconess Hospital, for the twelve-month nurses' training program. Working 16 hours a day, Richards performed routine care activities—checking pulse, respiration, and temperature; administering medications; and attending physician lectures—while maintaining 24-hour responsibility for assigned patients. The apprenticeship system began, and the services of female nurses were just starting to be valued, though little worth was assigned to formal education.

Lillian Wald, another pioneering nurse and suffragette, was dissatisfied with her meager nursing knowledge and enrolled in the Medical School at Women's Medical College in New York, where she developed and integrated business and clinical acumen (Simms, Price, & Ervin, 2000). Wald established the Henry Street Settlement House in 1909. She visited poverty stricken poor in tenements across the city, dressed wounds, taught nutrition and hygiene, and focused her energies on indigent women and children. Like Richards, Wald formed a social contract with the communities she served: she was proactive, outspoken, and determined.

As a heroine and a leader of nurses, much has been attributed to Florence Nightingale. She improved sanitary conditions as well as the lives of the sick, wounded, and traumatized and set the standard for education, practice, and research. Through her writings she revealed vision and determination: "[W]hat you want are facts and opinions . . . teach [nurses] what to observe—how to observe—what symptoms indicate improvement . . ." (Nightingale, 1859). Clearly the seeds of the evidence-based practice movement were planted in 1859.

All three pioneers, and many others who have followed, are models for those nurses who will meet the challenges of the twenty-first century: a workforce that has as its legacy integration of theory, research, and practice, as well as clinical skills, public-health knowledge, and ever-expanding means to enter and advance their formal education. Nurses need to liberate themselves by "develop[ing] an individual and collective positive self-esteem through a renewed appreciation for their own history and attributes . . ." (Roberts, 2000). Their quest to identify and image a professional and public identity is ongoing.

PROFESSIONAL IDENTITY

The dichotomous nature of nursing work as both clinical and social service contributes to the confusion surrounding nursing and nurses. In their Social Policy Statement (1995), the ANA specified this definition of modern nursing: "An important process in any profession is the development of **professional identity**. Fundamental to its formation are service to society, a distinct body of knowledge on which practice is based, self-regulation, adherence to a code of ethics, commitment to lifelong learning, and a unique subculture." The American Association of Colleges of Nursing (1998) noted that professionalism is transmitted through a liberal education, professional values, core competencies, core knowledge, and the development of professional nursing roles. The Nursing Social Policy Statement (1995) defined the core values of nursing as compassion, ethics, and intuitive knowledge as modeled by pioneers such as Wald and Nightingale.

The professional practice of nursing works to improve the health of communities through proactive participation in change as manifested by nurses dedicated to the betterment of society. Participation on local school boards, in health fairs, state and local health department activities, civic organizations, and local grassroots politics are indirect ways to practice **professionalism** and effect change. As the move to client-centered and population-based care forges ahead, new and different practice settings will demand professional competency, autonomy, and certification as well as differentiated professional identity. In an age of ambiguity, resourcefulness and fluidity will be necessary attributes of the twenty-first century professional.

Understanding and modeling professionalism for nurses begins upon entry into programs of study. Secrest, Norwood, and Keatley (2003) explored the development of professional identity in the United States. They described junior and senior nursing students' perceptions in three dimensions—belonging, knowing, and affirming—when working on medical and surgical units in different hospitals. The students defined belonging as being a valued member of the nursing team, of enjoying camaraderie and connection with colleagues, and subsequently experiencing an enriching clinical experience. Knowing facilitated a sense of competence, of being whole with the team. Knowing also provided an avenue for affirmation of one's professional status. In this group of nursing students, knowing was interconnected with personal learning. Affirmation took place when interacting with clients: making a difference in someone's life is affirming. Based on these findings, developing a sense of professionalism is just as important as development of knowledge and skills. "Feeling professional meant belonging, not feeling alienated; being affirmed, not feeling demeaned; and knowing, not feeling ignorant." (Secrest, Norwood, & Keatley, p. 81).

Professional identity underscores our myriad nursing roles, and because many initial educational experiences for students are in hospital settings, it is not surprising that professional identity develops through relationships with hospital RNs. "If you want to change the world, there is no time like the present." (Simms, et al., 2000, p. 394). Hospital RNs should affirm students' interactions with patients, mentor fledgling nurses, and provide colleagueship. Seasoned registered nurses are obliged to foster connections with novice nurses and contribute to the growth and development of the profession (Beck, 2000; Campbell, 2003). Knowing, affirming, and belonging are inextricable and build shared vision. When nurses talk to each other in the workplace, they should engage in brainstorming activities that stimulate discussion and action directed toward improving the lives of patients and the profession. Both novice and seasoned nurses should strengthen collegiality by calling on the collective support of all nursing professionals, whose knowledge, experience, intuitive sense to improve care, and ability to provide links to needed resources are invaluable.

Failure to utilize professional nurses according to their education and expertise is a malady of misuse. Education and expertise are intertwined and encompass knowing, belonging, and affirming. Nursing education emphasizes clinical training; integration of theory, research and practice; and carves out multiple nursing roles, which can be accessed through multiple routes. Nurses frequently champion the plight of patient access to care and are resolute in removing inherent barriers. In contrast, nurses have many ways to access education, and few barriers exist to career mobility. Many of the ways to access education are portrayed in a negative light, hence the profession misses the opportunity to celebrate nursing diversity and career mobility. Licensed practical nurses, associate degree registered nurses, and baccalaureate and higher degree registered nurses bring essential skills and knowledge to nursing practice. Integration of theory, research, and practice in our current educational system can be done only through recognition of all areas of expertise. Differentiation in the practice environment means capturing and using differing levels of nursing expertise appropriately in the various settings in which nurses practice. Temperament and expertise are equally important when nurses choose places to work.

According to a Canadian study, nursing attracts a "guardian" personality type, which is defined as a person who thrives in a structured, policy- and rule-bound climate (McPhail, 2002). Nurses' education, numbers of years in practice, where they'd worked, and their personality type were strongly correlated (McPhail, 2002, p. 2). Nurses with higher education had different personality types—intuitive, sensing—moved beyond direct care, and gravitated toward administration, teaching, and research. Although further research is needed to support these findings, it is interesting to make some projections about the use of variously prepared nurses in the twenty-first-century workforce. Perhaps guardian types would thrive in licensed practical and associate degree nurse roles, because these nurses function well in structured environments. The current and future health care environment needs various personalities who work in both structured and fluid environments. Curricula in baccalaureate and higher degree programs might well develop nurses who fit in less structured and more fluid environments where planning, decision making, and assessment of outcomes is expected. Skill mix takes on new meaning when personality fit is factored into the equation. Level of skill and complementary personality may characterize the future workforce and offer the personnel fit organizations need and want.

RESEARCH APPLICATION ARTICLE

Cook, T. H., Gilmer, M. J., Bess, C. J. (2003). Beginning students' definitions of nursing: An inductive framework of professional identity. *Journal of Nursing Education, 42*(7), 311–317.

Cook, Gilmer, and Bess produced a qualitative study that explored students' perceptions of professional nursing using the question, "What is your definition of nursing?" The purpose was to develop a framework to foster professional identity, which was defined as "an internal representation of people-environment interactions in the exploration of human responses to actual or potential health problems." Seventy-five percent of the sample was composed of students who held a baccalaureate degree in another discipline. Participants stated several personal definitions of nursing, such as caring for patients, a way of facilitating

care, a helping profession based on compassion and scientific application of the healing arts, helping patients recover from illness, and promotion of health. Caring, nurturing, treatment of illness, and promotion of health were most frequently described, whereas nurses as advocates, managers, and promoters of self-care were least described. Beginning students did not identify legal, ethical, cultural, and economic aspects of nursing as components of nursing identity.

This study has important implications for nurse educators. Advocating for and managing groups of patients and the promotion of patient-centered and population-based care define twenty-first-century nursing. Faculty must teach, model, and provide educational experiences to shape the future nursing workforce.

PUBLIC IDENTITY

Every nursing professional needs a grounding in managerial and leadership skills in order to participate in improving and changing the health care system. Nursing is more than clinical skills and expert knowledge: it is effecting large change through small change, not only at the bedside and in the clinic, but in the board room and in legislative chambers. The Nurses Strategic Action Team (N-STAT) is a national grassroots network of the American Nurses Association, whose primary function is to effect policy changes that influence health care and the delivery of nursing care. Calling and writing to legislators and informing nurses about bills under consideration by Congress are some of N-STAT's activities. Making sure that our message is heard by people who set policy that influences nursing jobs, salaries, and roles is critical to expanding the professional

identity of nurses (ANA, 1995; Des Jardin, 2001; Feldman & Lewenson, 2000). Nurses must learn to communicate comfortably on issues that affect the public, and because the public obtains most of its information primarily through media such as television, newspapers, radio, and magazines, these are the venues through which nurses can influence policymakers; but most legislators and public personalities rely on accurate information that will come from you: an impassioned, informed nurse.

Effecting change in nursing and health care also requires integrity. The ANA Code of Ethics (2001) stipulates that professional nurses engage in public discourse to help shape public policy. Efforts to promote health and reduce disparities are the responsibilities of all health professionals (U. S. Dept. of Health & Human Svcs, 2000; Dugas, 2005). Nurses' ethical responsibilities include seeking social justice as well as protecting and advocating for the vulnerable and disenfranchised. The Code also sets standards for relationships among colleagues and speaks about providing care that is

WRITING EXERCISE 1.1

Write a letter, or community viewpoint, to the editor of your local newspaper expressing your point of view on an issue that is pressing to nurses. The letter should be to the point, factual, and approximately 300 words long. It should state the issue in the first two or three sentences, be in language that is clear to lay readers, and stick to the facts. Steer clear of emotional statements. Here is an example of a Community View column that will help guide the development and expression of your ideas.

Creegan, M. C. (14 March 2002). "Not for the Warm and Fuzzy Guys," Community View, *Journal News, Gannett newspapers,* Rockland County, NY edition.

The shortage of nurses is real and near catastrophic. Bemoaned by all of us nurses at some point in time are salary issues, the work environment, and the downright difficult laborious work of the profession. More appealing to me is to read about approaches to the problem. In which directions should we head to confront this shortage of personnel? The current professional profile is one of the problems.

Those of us in the field spell out prerequisite qualities for entry: Courage, hearts, brains, and more recently diversity. When speaking about diversity, our efforts encompass recruiting and retaining a multiethnic student body that mirrors the population and allows us to render culture-appropriate care. Indeed, we should continue these efforts, but we are missing a major minority: male nurses.

Currently, the "maleness" of the profession is at an overall 5.4% of the nursing workforce, hardly an impressive figure. Why is this so? In interviews with male student nurses at Dominican College, as well as male nurse graduates of the program, they tell me about a number of persistent myths. Among them are statements like nursing is just not "macho": it's soft, warm and fuzzy stuff that keeps men away. Well, is that so? Let's talk a bit about the men in the business of caring.

Three of my students were police officers. As police officers, they worked with special victims, which means abused women and children. As male nurses, they currently work with children 6 to 10 years of age who have acute and chronic mental illnesses. Their responsibilities have shifted somewhat from apprehending criminals to caring for victims of crime. How's that for warm and fuzzy?

Another former student works as a traveling nurse. He likes that just fine, as he sees the world while doing what he likes best, biking across the country on a motorcycle. This fellow takes care of children in a pediatric intensive care unit. Rugged and real, I'd say.

I could give countless other examples, but I'd rather make some recommendations on where to begin to remedy the situation. Publishers: When laying out your newspaper copy, consider placing advertisements for nurses adjacent to sports stories or sporting events. Appeal to the male action image. Guidance counselors: Tell your male students, preferably the bright ones, that they're needed in emergency rooms, trauma centers, psychiatry, and obstetrics, too. (Why not? Male physicians dominate in women's health.)

And all you dads, how about admitting how much you nurture your children, how much a hug and a gentle, comforting word means to your distressed high-school-aged son or daughter? Give witness to the foolish testimony that nurturing is exclusively female. Nursing offers lots of excitement, lots of kindness, lots of intellect, and lots of humanity. Men, if this is what you want, go for it. In fact, what are you waiting for? (Creegan, 2002).

holistic and collaborative. All professional nurses must develop team-building skills and be comfortable in networking with multiple groups. "Preparation for leadership necessarily includes serious attention to the inextricable linkage between those whom we label leaders and those whom we label followers." (Dumas, 1986, p. 4). The multifaceted role of the nurse continues to evolve, take shape, and, out of necessity, raise the bar in education. To remain a practicing member of the profession, both formal and continuing education will be necessary to place nurses at the table as participants in health care redesign.

THE PROFESSIONAL WORKFORCE IN THE TWENTY-FIRST CENTURY

What will the professional workforce look like? What are the necessary competencies required to deliver quality care to a diverse society? A set of core competencies for health care professionals that crosses discipline boundaries is envisioned (Institute of Medicine, 2001). Patient-centered care, interdisciplinary work, provision of evidence-based practice, applying quality improvement procedures, and investing in informatics are the vital core competencies needed by all health professions to meet the health care needs of patients and populations in the twenty-first century, see Figure 1.1 (Institute of Medicine, 2003).

Patient-centered care takes into account the patient's needs, values, and beliefs as well as those of significant others and family members. Core competence in this area requires that nurses be culture conscious and versed in the family/human dynamics that affect the way people approach health care, seek services of health care, and obtain successful outcomes as a result of health care. Involving patients in health care decisions, promoting healthy lifestyles through education, and attending to end-of-life issues are areas ripe for nursing work. In addition, patients should be queried about their experiences with both students and health care facilities. "[R]esearch supports the view that . . . using patient focus groups to provide feedback on performance . . . greatly enhance[s] patient satisfaction and facilitate[s] better student performance with patients" (Institute of Medicine, 2003).

Collaboration among disciplines, a team approach, is not only cost-effective, but assures that patients get the consistent quality care that can be delivered only when health professionals communicate with each other. "Lack of understanding about what each profession does and absence of a common language . . . and turf battles remain the norm . . ." (Institute of Medicine, 2003, p. 79). Interdisciplinary education is far from the norm, though it has been encouraged for decades. Early introduction to interdisciplinary education among social workers, physical therapists, occupational therapists,

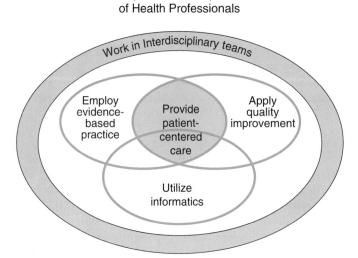

Overlap of Core Competencies
of Health Professionals

Figure 1.1 **Overlap of core competencies of health professionals.**

SOURCE: Reprinted with permission from *Health Professions Education: A Bridge to Quality* © 2003 by the National Academy of Sciences. Courtesy of the National Academies Press, Washington, DC.

speech and language therapists, medicine, nursing, and pharmacy would open the existent educational channels and encourage a free exchange of ideas and activities to the betterment of patients served by such teams (Institute of Medicine, 2001; 2003).

Commitment to lifelong learning is a professional mandate as vast amounts of knowledge continue to accumulate in the ever-changing health care scene. The rate of development of that knowledge outpaces human retention of facts! What is new today is old tomorrow, and "[I]f you read two articles every night, you're 500 years behind at the end of the first year . . ." (Stead, 2002). Systematic reviews of research by experts give health care professionals the best evidence on which to make practice decisions. The challenge for the future is to teach both faculty and students how to collect and use evidence to create uniform practice guidelines that everyone uses to improve patient care. In addition, how we evaluate our performance as well as outcomes of care are important action-oriented competencies that guarantee checks and balances in the system.

Are the persons delivering care doing the best possible job given the resources and technology available? How do we measure up? What do patients think about services provided? How do patients respond to interventions? Measuring outcomes encourages corrective action and improves safety. Recognizing and documenting "mistakes" then become part of quality improvement instead of grounds for fear of retaliation. Teaching students how to collect and act on information and how to perform as members of a project team are quality improvement activities that outmode lecture and rote memorization of procedures and facts. Communicating with one another in a consistent and accurate manner will bridge interdisciplinary differences and close gaps in information sharing. Advances in technology will also help achieve interdisciplinary communication. For example, many students in multiple disciplines have access to more resources through remote library access. Students currently use course management systems (CMS) to collect information in the field, send it to teaching faculty and classmates, and store data for future

CASE SCENARIO 1.1

Mr. Harrington is a 45-year-old male with diabetes and peripheral vascular disease. He is overweight and inactive, married with two high-school-aged children. Mrs. Harrington works full time and frequently visits her aging mother, who lives in an assisted-living facility nearby. You are the nurse assigned to her case. In light of the five competencies: patient-centered care, interdisciplinary involvement, evidence-based care, quality improvement, and informatics, answer the following questions:

1. Listing Mr. Harrington's health problems, where will you find the latest information about treatment?
2. With what members of the health care team will you meet to plan care?
3. What will you expect each team member to bring to the planning table?
4. Will you invite family members? Why?
5. What information will you want to know about the family?

discussions on campus (Hodson-Carlton, Siktberg, Flowers, & Scheibel, 2003, p. 180). In the clinical arena, computers enhance decision-making capability by rapidly providing relevant information. McHugh (2000, p. 452) noted that "the paper chart often acts as an impediment to quality improvement . . . [whereas] . . . a computer-based patient record . . . provides enormous opportunity to examine, analyze, and evaluate nursing care protocols and activities across many hundreds or thousands of patients." As technology expands, opportunities for information sharing will increase among disciplines. It is envisioned that quality and effectiveness of care will be the ultimate result.

Informatics is the fifth "vital sign" in the list of competencies. Computing infrastructures are not fully in place in academe, which has not kept pace with industry. Resistance on the part of old guard faculty to be informed and facile with computers and software has held back the introduction of learner-driven learning. Computer searches and downloading information are two ways to seek out interdisciplinary information. Links among hospitals, pharmacies, and health care agencies that serve patients will allow cost savings, sharing of information, and decreased margin for error. Robotic operations using high-tech surgical equipment are increasingly in use in medical centers, and virtual reality via telemedicine is here to stay and moving forward rapidly. One overarching problem is too few persons educated in informatics to provide the education that will improve patient-centered care. Inclusion of the five competencies in nursing education is a challenge and one that we must meet head-on to prepare the next generation of nurses.

CHAPTER SUMMARY

The health care system is changing. Out of ambiguity arises opportunities for nurses to show professionalism and professional identity by committing to patient-centered care, evidence-based practice, quality improvement, and better communication through technological savvy. The time is ripe to influence health policy through grassroots activism and to remember the legacy left to us by Richards, Wald, and Nightingale. The time is now to work in interdisciplinary teams and break open the educational silos that limit our vision. The time will never be better to recognize the diversity within the profession and put differentiated practice into action. The nursing workforce can provide cost-effective, quality care as it sheds the internal struggle and reshapes itself among colleagues. It is the best of times.

"There is nothing more difficult to take in hand, more perilous to conduct, or more uncertain in its success than to take the lead in the introduction of the new order of things."

—Machiavelli

REFERENCES

Aiken, L. H., Clarke, S. P., Sloane, D. M., & Sochalski, J. H. (2002). Hospital registered nurse staffing and patient mortality, nurse burnout, and job dissatisfaction. *The Journal of the American Medical Association, 288*, 1987–1993.

American Association of Colleges of Nursing (1998). *The essentials of baccalaureate education for professional nursing practice.* Washington, DC: Author.

American Nurses Association (2001). *ANA Code for Nurses with interpretive statements.* Washington, DC: Author.

American Nurses Association (1995). *ANA Social policy statement.* Washington, DC: Author.

American Nurses Association (1995). *Legislative action handbook.* Washington, DC: Author.

American Nurses Association (1965). *Educational preparation for nurse practitioners and assistants to nurses: A position paper.* Washington, DC: Author.

Anderson, O. (1968). Toward an unambiguous profession: A review of nursing (pamphlet) *Center for Health Administration Studies.* Chicago, IL: Author.

Barger, S. E. (2004). Academic nursing centers: The road from the past, the bridge to the future. *Journal of Nursing Education, 43*, 60–65.

Beck, C. T. (2000). The experience of choosing nursing as a career. *Journal of Nursing Education, 39*, 320–322.

Bednash, G. (2000). The decreasing supply of registered nurses: Inevitable future or call to action? *Journal of the American Medical Association, 283*, 2985–2987.

Bleich, M., Hewlett, P., Santos, S., Rice, R., Cox, K., & Richmeier, S. (2003). Analysis of the nursing workforce crisis: A call to action. *American Journal of Nursing, 103 (4)*, 66–74.

Brewer, C.S. (1996). Through the looking glass: The labor market for registered nurses in the 21st century. *Nursing Health Care Perspectives, 18*, 260–269.

Buerhaus, P. I. (1994). Price controls, healthcare reform, and new RN shortages. *Nursing Economics, 12*, 309–317.

Buerhaus, P. I., Staiger, D. O., & Averbach, D. I. (2000). Implications of an aging registered nurse workforce. *Journal of the American Medical Association, 283*, 2944–2954.

Campbell, S. L. (2003). Cultivating empowerment in nursing today for a strong profession tomorrow. *Journal of Nursing Education, 42*, 423–426.

Carroll, S. M. (2004). Inclusion of people with physical disabilities in nursing education. *Journal of Nursing Education, 43*, 207–212.

Cook, T. H., Gilmer, M. J., & Bess, C. J. (2003) Beginning students' definitions of nursing: An inductive framework of professional identity. *Journal of Nursing Education, 42(7)*, 311–317.

Creegan, M. C. (14 March 2002). "Not for the warm and fuzzy guys," Community View, *Journal News, Gannett newspapers,* Rockland County, NY edition.

Des Jardin, K. (2001). Political involvement in nursing—education and empowerment. *Journal Association Operating Room Nurses, 74*, 468–481.

Dugas, R. (2005). Nursing and genetics: Applying the American Nurses Association Code of Ethics. *Journal of Professional Nursing, 21*, 103–113.

Dumas, R. G. (1986). Preparing adults for leadership roles in the 1980's and 1990's. Presented at the University of Michigan National Nursing Conference on Leadership, Ann Arbor, September 17, 1986. In Simms, L. M., Price, S. A., & Ervin, N. E. (2000). *Professional practice of nursing administration* (3rd ed., p. 4). NY: Delmar.

Dworkin, R.W. (2002 Summer). Where have all the nurses gone? *The Public Interest, no. 148*, 23–36.

Etheredge, L. (2001). On the archeology of health care policy: Periods and paradigms. *Institute of Medicine Special Report.* Washington, DC: National Academy.

Feldman, H. R. & Lewenson, S. B. (2000). *Nurses in the political arena: The public face of nursing.* New York: Springer.

Hodson-Carlton, K. E., Siktberg, L. L., Flowers, J., & Scheibel, P. (2003). Overview of distance education in nursing: Where are we now and where are we going? In Oermann, M. H. & Heinrich, K. T. (eds.) *Annual review of nursing education* (Volume 1, p. 180). NY: Springer.

Holder, V. L. (2004). From handmaiden to right hand— the infancy of nursing. *Journal Association of Operating Room Nurses*, 79, 374–386.

Institute of Medicine (1983). *Committee on Nursing and Nursing Education: Public policies and private actions*. Washington, DC: National Academy.

Institute of Medicine (2000). *To err is human: Building a safer health system.* (L. Kohn, J. M. Corrigan, & M. S. Donaldson, eds.). Washington, DC: National Academy.

Institute of Medicine (2001). *Crossing the quality chasm: A new health system for the 21st century.* Washington, DC: National Academy.

Institute of Medicine (2003). *Health professionals education: A bridge to quality.* (A. C. Greiner & E. Kinebel, eds.). Washington, DC: National Academy.

Kirkman-Liff, B. (2002). Keeping an eye on a moving target: Quality changes and challenges for nurses. *Nursing Economics, 20,* 258–267.

Larsen, P. D., McGill, J. S., & Palmer, S. J. (2003). Factors influencing career decisions: Perspectives of nursing students in three types of programs. *Journal of Nursing Education, 42,* 168–173.

Laschinger, H. K. S., Finegan, J., Shamian, J., & Wilk, P. (2001). Impact of structural and psychological empowerment on job strain in nursing work settings: Expanding Kanter's model. *Journal of Nursing Administration, 31,* 260–272.

Lindeman, C. A. (2000). The future of nursing education. *Journal of Nursing Education, 39,* 5–12.

Lynaugh, J. E. & Brush, B. L. (1996). *American Nursing: From hospitals to health systems.* Cambridge, MA: Blackwell.

McHugh, M. (2000). Computer information systems and productivity management. In Simms, L. M., Price, S. A., & Ervin, N. (2000). *Professional practice of nursing administration* (3rd ed., p. 452). NY: Delmar.

McPhail, J. (2002). The nursing profession, personality types and leadership. *International Journal of Health Care Quality Assurance, 15,* 7–10.

Moore, C. A. (2004). Disability as difference and the nursing profession. *Journal of Nursing Education, 43,* 197–201.

Needleman, J. & Buerhaus, P. (2003). Nurse staffing and patient safety: Current knowledge and implications for action. *International Journal for Quality in Health Care, 15,* 275–277.

Nightingale, F. (1859; reprinted 1926). *Notes on nursing: What it is and what it is not.* New York: Appleton.

Roberts, S. J. (2000). Development of a positive professional identity: Liberating oneself from the oppressor within. *Advances in Nursing Science, 22,* 71–82.

Secrest, J. A., Norwood, B. R., & Keatley, V. M. (2003). "I was actually a nurse": The meaning of professionalism for baccalaureate nursing students. *Journal of Nursing Education, 42,* 77–82.

Simms, L. M., Price, S. A., & Ervin, N. E. (2000). *Professional practice of nursing administration.* 3rd ed., NY: Delmar.

Stead, W. (2001). Panel discussion. *In Crossing the quality chasm: A new health System for the 21st century.* Washington, DC: National Academy.

Stein, L. (1967). The Doctor-nurse game. *Archives of General Psychiatry 16,* 699–703.

U.S. Department of Health and Human Services, Public Health Services (2000). *Healthy People 2010.* Washington, DC: U.S. Government Printing Office.

Whitis, G. R. (2001). *A survey of technology-based distance education: Emerging issues and lessons learned.* Washington, DC: Association Academic Health Centers.

CHAPTER 2

History and Evolution of Nursing

Lora Humphrey Beebe

The knowledge of the past is desired only for the service of the future and the present.
—Fredrich Nietzsche

LEARNING OBJECTIVES

At the completion of the chapter, the learner should be able to do the following:

1. Describe the importance of the study of nursing history.
2. Analyze the influence of Christianity on nursing's history.
3. Synthesize the contributions of major nursing leaders to the history of the profession.
4. Discuss factors contributing to the feminization of nursing.
5. Articulate the roots of the entry-into-practice debate.
6. Describe the influences on the development of nurse practitioner and other advance practice programs.
7. Identify societal processes affecting the future of nursing.

KEY TERMS

Evidence-based nursing

Feminization

Industrial revolution

Nursing education model

Urbanization

The nursing profession has a rich history replete with drama, heroism, political intrigue, and fascinating personalities. Our nursing practice today was shaped by the profession's past. As Kalisch and Kalisch (1976) state, "insight into what nursing is and what nursing can be will come from the knowledge of what nursing has been" (p. 622).

Understanding nursing history can shed light on many issues the profession deals with in the present, including gender differences in the profession, the entry into practice debate, and relationships between nurses and other health care providers, to name a few. The current state of these issues involves complex social forces such as war, feminism, industrialization, technology, and politics. The study of nursing's history provides us with a sense of the past and an understanding of cultural history and influences. In addition, historical information puts problems and successes into context and helps us feel connected to earlier nurses, be they clinicians, educators, researchers, political activists or some combination of these. Finally, a historical perspective fosters a sense of pride and esteem for our forebears, which deepens our commitment to do our part to move the profession forward.

Thus, today's triumphs, struggles, and decisions will shape the nursing of the future. As we move into the future, not only do social and scientific changes affect nursing, conversely, nursing has the opportunity to affect society for the greater good. An understanding of nursing's history will clarify the values and goals that will guide us as we make the individual and collective decisions that will shape the future of nursing for those who follow.

NURSING IN ANTIQUITY

Primitive Societies

From ancient times, health beliefs have influenced the provision of care. Early man explained many events (including the presence of illness) by way of a belief in the supernatural. The earliest records indicate that medicine men (or women) possessed special curative, palliative, or healing powers that were accomplished through the use of herbs, heat, cold, touch, chanting, rituals, and even some primitive surgery (Nutting & Dock, 1935). The cures used by medicine men and women often were designed to drive evil spirits from the body by inducing unpleasant sensations through pummeling (possibly the forerunner of therapeutic massage), squeezing, beating, starving, noises, unpleasant smells, or nausea (Withington, 1894). While the evidence regarding primitive nursing is not conclusive (Kelly & Joel, 1999), authors assume that nursing care (distinct from medicine men and

women) was performed by family members (Joel & Kelly, 2002), and that particularly gifted caregivers probably taught nursing skills to others.

Greece and Rome

Like other ancient civilizations, those of ancient Greece believed in illness-related spirits in the form of gods, goddesses, and demons. The god of medicine, Asclepius, embodied the ideal of the ancient physician and is the patron saint of physicians to this day. While there is debate as to whether Asclepius was an actual person (Kelly & Joel, 1999), his influence was widespread. Temples for the sick were founded in his honor, where mineral baths, exercise, and other treatments were used to restore health. Early physicians were known as "asclepiads" or sons of Asclepius circa 500 BC. They prescribed such treatments as herbal medications, diet, exercise, bathing in warm or cold water, fasting, and various types of mental activity, including composing odes (Edelstein & Edelstein, 1975). Asclepius was depicted with a long staff in his left hand and his right hand over the head of a serpent. The staff may have been a walking stick, because he was said to wander far and wide in his healing role. On the other hand, the staff may have symbolized relief and support, indicated interventions to prevent the "fall" into ill health, or symbolized the difficulty of the healing arts. The serpent likewise has a number of interpretations, including rejuvenation (symbolized by the shedding of the skin), sharp-sightedness, vigilance, guardianship, and healing power (Edelstein & Edelstein, 1975). The staff and serpent of Asclepius are thought to be the basis of the modern caduceus (Joel & Kelly, 2002).

Hippocrates practiced medicine during Greece's golden age (about 400 BC). He developed systems for patient assessment and recording, established ethical standards, and rejected the supernatural explanation of disease (Kelly & Joel, 1999). Hippocrates was born on the island of Cos (western coast of Asia Minor) circa 460 BC. He wrote that medicine rests on observations and reason, and that observations are gathered through the senses of sight, hearing, smell, touch, and taste. He traveled through-out Greece practicing and teaching rational medicine, or the belief that health and disease are due to strictly natural phenomena, rather than supernatural events. He wrote detailed cases describing, among other ail-ments, puerperal fever, tetanus, malaria, and epilepsy. He advocated conservative treatments, including diet and exercise first and, only if these were ineffective, more invasive interventions such as drugs and sur-gery. In addition, Hippocrates was concerned with the physician/patient relationship and taught how to earn patients' confidence and cooperation. He insisted upon respect for patients and families and defined ethical practice standards (Adler, 2004). The Hippocratic oath, to "do no harm," is still taken in some medical schools (Nutting & Dock, 1935).

Unfortunately, there are no formal accounts of nurses in pre-Christian Greece. However, it is known that women of that time were considered inferior and denied educational opportunities, thus their options for work outside the home were in all likelihood extremely limited (Kelly & Joel, 1999).

Rome's most enduring health care contribution is likely the development of hospitals, which were originally used for the treatment of wounded sol-diers (Joel & Kelly, 2002). Excavations have uncov-ered hospitals that could treat up to 200 patients and were equipped with baths, pharmacies, and recreation areas (Kelly & Joel, 1999). Both men and women attendants watched over the sick (Kalisch & Kalisch, 1995; Nutting & Dock, 1935), performing some functions we think of today as nursing.

THE EARLY CHRISTIAN ERA, MIDDLE AGES, AND THE REFORMATION

Early Christian Era

Christianity was adopted as the official religion of Rome in 335 AD. This belief system placed great importance on the sanctity of life; and caring for widows, children, the poor, and the sick was viewed as one's Christian duty (Hood & Leddy, 2003). Although bishops were officially given the responsi-bility of caring for these vulnerable persons, deacons and deaconesses actually supervised and provided the services. Whereas their assignments varied according to location, deaconesses performed such duties as visiting ill female church members, the baptism of women, relaying messages, and visiting prisoners. Deaconesses were joined in their work by elderly widows and some virgins who chose to take vows of service (Kelly & Joel, 1999).

Phoebe was the first deaconess identified as pro-viding nursing care. She lived in Italy circa 60 AD and in Romans 16:1–2 (KJV) was referred to by Saint Paul as "a succorer of many and myself also." Nutting and Dock (1935) refer to Phoebe as the founder of visiting nursing.

Other women who contributed to the care of the sick during the Early Christian era were Olympias, Marcella, and Fabiola. Olympias was born in Con-stantinople in 368. After being widowed at a young age, this wealthy woman became a deaconess, erected a convent, and supervised 40 other deaconesses in caring for the elderly and orphans. Another wealthy Roman women, Marcella, converted her palace into a monastery. She is notable for instructing her associ-ates in the care of the sick. Fabiola was a Christian convert who was taught by Marcella (Joel & Kelly, 2002). She founded the first free hospital in Rome in about 390 and personally nursed those in need with such great compassion that she was beloved by all Romans (Kelly & Joel, 1999).

After the closing of the temples of Asclepius, "houses for the sick" replaced them. These early hos-pitals were supervised by bishops and managed by deacons to care for the poor, travelers, or others who could not be cared for at home (the most com-mon location for the provision of nursing care). In addition, the bishops founded shelters, hospices, and orphanages where both men and women pro-vided care. This lifestyle of service was an accept-able alternative for women from the social constraints of the day, including arranged marriages (Hood & Leddy, 2003).

Middle Ages

The Middle Ages were marked by political unrest, economic change, and the decline of the deaconesses. By the twelfth century, invasions against the Roman Empire had formed many smaller kingdoms, including England, France, Scotland, Sicily, and Spain (Kelly & Joel, 1999). Trade flourished between the larger cities, bringing change to economies as well as occupations. The feudal system in central Europe contributed to famine and disease, which were exacerbated by inadequate or unavailable medical and nursing care.

Because of church opposition, the deaconesses became nearly extinct during the Middle Ages. Three orders of caregivers replaced them: monastic, secular, and military. Monastic orders were composed of monks and nuns. Monks served as priests and cared for men, while nuns managed hospitals and cared for women (Nutting & Dock, 1935). One of the more prominent monastic orders was the Order of St. Benedict. Lay people formed secular orders to care for the poor and sick without taking the church vows (required of both men and women) of poverty, chastity, and obedience. One of the most important secular orders was the Beguines of Flanders, founded in 1184. The military orders were formed in response to the crusades to care for those wounded in attempts to recover the Holy Land from the Moslems (Kelly & Joel, 1999). The original purpose of the military orders was transporting the wounded from the battlefield to hospitals for care. Thus, the first order of military nurses was known as the Knights Hospitallers (Joel & Kelly, 2002).

Nursing care in early hospitals consisted of basic hygiene, nutrition, and comfort measures. During the Renaissance in the eighteenth century, a process of separation of churches and hospitals began, which vastly improved the physical treatment of the ill and injured.

The Reformation

The Protestant Reformation of the sixteenth century brought about revolt against papal supremacy, which resulted in the formation of multiple protestant churches. Many monasteries and religious orders involved in the care of the sick were closed or dispersed. Protestant leaders then hired nurse deaconesses and elderly women to perform nursing functions, contributing to the almost complete disappearance of male nurses.

Secular nursing was not an attractive option for women. Well-bred women did not work outside their homes, so nursing was neither valued nor accepted. Workhouse inmates provided cheap labor, but often were intoxicated, dishonest, or uncaring; therefore, several nursing orders were revived, providing socially acceptable options for women who desired to perform this work (Joel & Kelly, 2002). The Church Order of Deaconesses, where Florence Nightingale would later receive training, was one such order.

THE DAWN OF MODERNITY: THE INDUSTRIAL REVOLUTION

During England's industrial revolution, important medical breakthroughs kept pace with advancements in mechanization and culture (see Table 2.1). The development of machinery led to the establishment of factories. While upper class women continued the tradition of not working outside the home, factories employed women of lower social status alongside men, and even children. Women caring for the sick were among the lowest status (together with prisoners and prostitutes), and health conditions continued to be abysmal (Kelly & Joel, 1999). As medical and scientific knowledge advanced, so did interest in nurses' training. The stage was set for the founder of modern nursing, Florence Nightingale.

FLORENCE NIGHTINGALE

Called the founder of modern nursing, Florence Nightingale is considered by many to be the most influential person in all the history of illness care

Table 2.1 **Medical and Scientific Advances, 1500–1900 (adapted from Joel & Kelly, 2002)**

Scientist	Dates	Place	Work
William Harvey	1578–1657	England	Described the circulatory system (except capillary system)
Thomas Sydenham	1624–1689	England	Revived Hippocratic reasoning and observation methods
Antonj van Leeuwenhoek	1632–1723	Holland	Improved the microscope to allow visualization of cells and bacteria
William Hunter & John Hunter	1718–1783 1728–1793	Scotland	Founders of pathology
Edward Jenner	1749–1823	England	Smallpox vaccine
Rene Laennec	1781–1826	France	Invented stethoscope
Oliver Wendell Holmes	1809–1894	United States	Developed obstetric practices to improve safety and prevent infection
Louis Pasteur	1822–1895	France	Founder of microbiology, developed pasteurization
Robert Koch	1843–1910	Germany	Founder of bacteriology
Wilhelm Rontgen	1845–1906	Germany	Discovered x-rays

(Joel & Kelly, 2002). In addition to developing a new system of nursing education, she worked to reform social, health care, and military systems. Her nursing model dominated for nearly 100 years, and her influence is still seen today in nurses' notes, nursing research, nursing quality assurance, and nursing care plans (Miracle, 2003).

Florence Nightingale was born May 12, 1820, to an aristocratic English family. Her father taught her Latin, German, Greek, French, and Italian in addition to history, science, art, music and philosophy. She supplemented her education by traveling with friends and family (Joel & Kelly, 2002). She was sensitive, compassionate, and somewhat restless against the constraints of the Victorian age (Keeling, 2001).

While accompanying her mother on visits to the poor, she learned of the appalling health care conditions attendant with this group and determined to contribute "toward lifting the load of suffering from the helpless and miserable" (Bullough & Bullough, 1978, p. 69). When family thwarted her desire for hospital training, she found other creative ways to learn about illness care by studying hospital reports and public health textbooks (Joel & Kelly, 2002).

In 1850, at age 32, Nightingale entered the nurses' training program at Kaiserworth, Germany. This course was more socially acceptable due to its religious focus, and she spent three months there. While there she wrote over 100 pages of detailed notes about her activities and observations. She cared for patients, observed therapies, and assisted in surgery. The most frequently used therapies of the time included poultices, leeches, and fomentations. Poultices consist of hot moist linseed oil, mustard oil, or soap concoctions that are placed between pieces of muslin and applied on the skin for pain, congestion, or swelling. Leeches are bloodsucking aquatic worms used to induce bleeding, which was thought to improve various symptoms. Fomentations are hot wet packs used for pain and swelling.

Nightingale recorded bedside nursing notes every 15 minutes, describing patient's physical, emotional, and spiritual changes. She also took note of the hospital's administrative procedures and details related to outcome measures, delegation of tasks, and motivation of the staff (Dossey, 2000).

During her travels, Nightingale inspected hospitals and made notations on administration, sanitation, and construction as well as the work of physicians. She was negotiating for the position of superintendent of King's College Hospital in London when the Crimean war broke out (Joel & Kelly, 2002).

The British Army was woefully unprepared to manage the thousands of casualties, and the hospital at Scutari (near Constantinople) was "totally lacking in equipment . . . no medical supplies, not even the basic necessities" (Woodham-Smith, 1949, p. 162). Nightingale offered her services and, in a few days, selected 38 nurses and traveled to Scutari. She was never shy about using her influence and wielded control over large financial contributions made by her powerful friends. Despite opposition and resentment from the military, she and her nurses established a kitchen, organized and cleaned the hospital, and made arrangements to control the rats and other vermin. By the end of the war, the mortality rate at Scutari had declined from 60% to 1% (Joel & Kelly, 2002).

Nightingale compiled her experiences into a report entitled, "Notes on Matters Affecting the Health, Efficiency and Hospital Administration of the British Army." It was full of facts and statistical comparisons that argued her case for reform of the British military care system, in addition to gaining her the title of the first nurse researcher (McDonald, 1998).

Following the war, Nightingale founded the first training school for nurses in 1860. She selected 15 students of high character to form the first class. The one-year training program included a nine-hour workday, with bedside teaching and lectures by medical school professors (Joel & Kelly, 2002). Upon completion, students' names were entered into the Register as certified nurses.

Nightingale nurses were in great demand, and Nightingale herself wrote extensively of their education, character, and appropriate work focus. In her most famous publication, "Notes on Nursing: What it is and what it is not" (1859), she articulated for the first time that nursing requires the attainment of a unique body of knowledge (Keeling, 2001). She believed good nursing care facilitated healing, and that nursing was properly concerned with not only disease management, but with environmental manipulation. She was adamant that nursing be the focus: Nurses were NOT to do laundry, cleaning, or errands. She argued for continuing education and equal pay for equal work, stressing nursing observation and communication with the physician, who was not constantly at the bedside as nurses were (Joel & Kelly, 2002).

Nightingale was a truly remarkable woman. In an era when men were dominant and women were poorly educated and seldom active in the public sphere, she managed to reform hospitals, reorganize the medical department of the British army, and establish the nursing profession. Through her research, her many writings, and the establishment of training schools, she greatly affected the development of nursing in the United States and throughout the world.

NURSING IN THE UNITED STATES: THE CIVIL WAR

There were no professional nurses in America when the Civil War broke out. Officials on both sides held the opinion that the war would be very brief and thus were ill-prepared with both medical care and supplies. Immediately after the Battle of Bull Run (July 21, 1861), the appeal for nurses was made, and for the first time, women were asked to leave their homes to serve the wounded. Women on both sides responded, most notable among these were those of the Catholic orders (Wall, 1995).

RESEARCH APPLICATION ARTICLE

McDonald, L. (2001). Florence Nightingale and the early origins of evidence-based nursing. *Evidence-Based Nursing, 4,* 68–69.

McDonald (2001) expounded on Nightingale's influence on the present-day practice of **evidence-based nursing.** Nightingale's philosophy dictated an empirical approach, because she believed natural laws could be discovered through research. Her first work following the Crimean war used this framework. For every soldier in Crimea who died from wounds, seven had died from disease. Nightingale wanted to be sure this never occurred again, so after the war, she worked with an established commission to examine the data and provide recommendations, one of which was the creation of a department to maintain statistics on rates of mortality and morbidity in the British Army. Further, she advocated the collection of similar data in hospitals, which enabled comparisons based on location and other factors. This proposal formed the basis for today's ICD code (Keith, 1988).

A second example of her use of the concepts of evidence-based practice was her landmark study of deaths from puerperal fever. Based upon questionnaires completed by childbirth institutions, she discovered that a number of factors, including maternal age, length of labor, place of delivery, number of pregnancies, and social factors (including socioeconomic status and general health of the mother) affected mortality rates. Then, after examining death rates from puerperal fever among workhouse inmates as compared with mothers giving birth in other venues, Nightingale concluded that delivery location (and availability of trained medical personnel) was more important in preventing death than social factors.

Union Nursing

Dorothea Dix was born April 4, 1802 in Hampden, Maine. She lived on a backwoods farm with her father, an occasional Methodist minister and pamphlet writer; her mother—poor, uneducated and possibly mentally retarded—who was considerably older than her father; and her brothers. Dorothea struggled to fold and stitch pamphlets by the hundreds as well as care for her two younger brothers and do chores her mother was unable to do. A voracious reader, she benefited from occasional trips to Boston to visit her father's parents who were well-to-do. The family moved several times, and at age 12, Dorothea went to live with her

WRITING EXERCISE 2.1

The article discussed above (McDonald, 2001) has presented some of the evidence that Florence Nightingale practiced the concepts of evidence-based nursing. Identify one client from your clinical practice for whom you have applied an evidence-based framework. Write up your assessment of the client and how you specifically tailored your care to include the evidence for best practices, and be prepared to discuss in class.

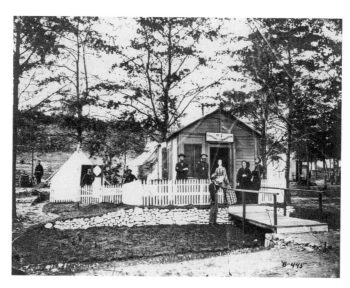

Figure 2.1 **During the Civil War, nurses were key in decreasing the spreading of contagious diseases among wounded soldiers.** Photo courtesy of Corbis-Bettmann.

paternal grandmother in Boston, where she was able to engage in regular study. She was shy and socially awkward, rejecting the social activities of the day as "purposeless" and thus reducing her chances for marriage.

She wrote children's books, edited hymnals and volumes of poetry, and ran an elementary school from her grandmother's home for five years, but was forced to close it due to continued recurrent illness. During a recuperative visit to England, she learned of the deplorable conditions in insane asylums there. Upon her return to Massachusetts, she was mortified to find much the same situation and immediately took up the crusade to improve conditions. In the space of five years she established state hospitals in Massachusetts, Rhode Island, and six other states (Snyder, 1975).

After her work to reform the care of the mentally ill, Dix wanted to organize an Army Nurse Corps in the United States, as Nightingale had in Crimea. After a visit to President Lincoln, she was appointed to help organize army hospitals in Washington, DC. Since there were no nurse training schools at the time, the women trained for one month under physician supervision (Keeling, 2001). The nurses' tasks included supervising and administering the diet ordered by the physician, as well as caring for emotional and physical needs, which included hygiene, dressings, and bed linens; emotional support often took the form of correspondence to loved ones far away (Holder, 2003).

Contrary to the great majority of women at this time, Clara Barton was employed as a copyist in the U.S. Patent Office in Washington when the Civil War began (Holder, 2003). She was adventuresome, independent, and eager to assist in the war effort, but chose not to enlist in the Army Nurse Corps. After the first Battle of Bull Run, Barton and other women could be found working shoulder to shoulder with surgeons and others engaged in hospital duty, and in early August, the women began receiving wages (Oates, 1994). Figure 2.1 illustrates a nursing encampment in the Civil War.

Clara believed that many of the battlefield deaths could have been prevented if care had been available at the site of the injury. She sought and finally obtained permission to deliver supplies to the front lines. Thereafter she was present at many famous

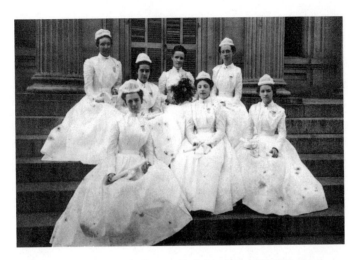

Figure 2.2 **Graduating class of 1900, Touro Infirmary Training School for Nurses.** Photo courtesy of Tuoro Infirmary Archives, New Orleans, LA.

battles, including the Second Battle of Bull Run, Antietam, and Fredericksburg (Holder, 2003). Going from soldier to soldier giving any care and comfort she could earned her the title "Angel of the Battlefield" (Kizilos, 2001). After the war, she went on to found the American Red Cross (Keeling, 2001).

Confederate Nursing

Thousands of Confederate women responded to the call for nurses and worked tirelessly, albeit without benefit of any official government organization or endorsement, as was the case in the north. By 1862 the Confederacy took over the organization of hospitals and care. Several women were appointed superintendents of hospitals, including Sallie Thompkins, the only woman in the Confederacy to hold military rank (Keeling, 2001).

Phoebe Pember was superintendent of Chimborazo hospital in Richmond, Virginia. She wrote of shortages of food, fuel, bandages, and even soap, and of her efforts to enforce cleanliness, discipline, and order (Pember, 1959 cited in Keeling chapter in Chitty, 2001).

The contributions of these and multitudes of lesser-known women during the Civil War advanced professional nursing and changed forever the social perceptions regarding women working outside their homes. Their reform of military hospitals led to great improvements in civil hospitals in many states (Rosenberg, 1987, cited in Keeling chapter in Chitty, 2001).

The contributions of nurses during the Civil War led forward-thinking people to the conclusion that training schools for nurses were needed. In the United States, the first of these was established in 1872 at Bellevue in New York City, as well as at New Haven, Connecticut, and at Massachusetts General Hospital in Boston (Dock, 1907 cited in Keeling chapter in Chitty, 2001). The popular belief of the day held that women were by nature more sensitive and nurturing than men; thus the schools accepted only female applicants for their one-year programs, and the **feminization** of nursing was solidified (Keeling, 2001). As immigration and industrialization increased, so did the number of hospitals. Student nurses provided an inexpensive source of labor to meet care demands, and **nursing education** established an apprenticeship **model** dominated by hospitals and hospital-based care delivery systems (Hood & Leddy, 2003). Figure 2.3 presents nursing graduates of 1900.

SPANISH-AMERICAN WAR

Nursing once again came to the forefront when the United States declared war on Spain in 1898. Originally, only graduates of nurse training schools were eligible to work as army nurses, but as demand increased, others were accepted (Wall, 1995). The Spanish-American War marked the first use of trained nurses in war and was the forerunner of the establishment of a permanent Army Nurse Corps in 1901 (Keeling, 2001).

WORLD WAR I

When the United States entered World War I in 1917, a Committee on Nursing was formed under the Council of National Defense and charged with supplying trained nurses to Army hospitals overseas (Dock & Stewart, 1920). The committee established the Army School of Nursing, recruited nationally, and conducted Red Cross training (Keeling, 2001). As in previous conflicts, World War I demonstrated the effectiveness of using trained professional nurses to deliver care to wounded soldiers. Social changes of the day included the Nineteenth Amendment, granting women the right to vote; the increased utilization of hospitals; and the discovery of penicillin in 1928. At the same time, the Goldmark report was published, advocating that nursing move into the mainstream of higher education with the establishment of collegiate schools of nursing instead of hospital-based diploma programs (Nichols, 2001). The authors of the report believed that university education would advance the profession and provide needed leadership. In 1909 the first baccalaureate nursing program was established at the University of Minnesota and was quickly followed by others (Conley, 1973). Baccalaureate programs were scientifically oriented, in contrast to skill-based diploma programs, and thus began a debate that still rages in many quarters of nursing education.

THE GREAT DEPRESSION

The economic depression following the stock market crash in 1929 affected nursing as surely as all other segments of society. Up to that time, hospitals had been staffed with nursing students, and most professional nurses worked in private homes. Because of economic hardship, many hospitals closed their schools of nursing, and many families could not afford in-home care. Thus, hospitals no longer had access to student labor, and therefore turned to trained nurses, many of whom were unemployed, to fill the empty positions; and the face of hospital staffing was changed forever (Keeling, 2001). Other unemployed nurses found work under government programs providing rural and school health care, improving nutrition, and fighting communicable diseases (Fitzpatrick, 1975).

WORLD WAR II

When the bombing of Pearl Harbor drew the United States into World War II in 1941, nurses were heavily recruited to serve in distant places. This situation resulted in a marked shortage of nurses at home. To remedy this, the Cadet Nurse Corps was founded in 1943. Their goal was to double the recruitment of new nursing students (Petry, 1945). Federal grants provided financial assistance to nursing schools but required that school budgets be separated from those of their affiliated hospitals, further widening the distance from the apprenticeship model of education (Keeling, 2001). The Cadet Nurse Corps was the greatest recruitment of student nurses in history. The Corps was formed in mid 1943, after the United States had been at war for 2 ½ years. It was designed to educate graduate nurses, train

CASE SCENARIO 2.1

You have learned that a program similar to the Cadet Nurse Corps is being considered in an effort to proactively respond to the projected nursing shortage of the next several years. A program representative is scheduled to visit your school.

Case Considerations

1. What questions would you have for the program representative?

2. List and discuss three advantages of a program of this nature from the perspective of the individual, the school of nursing, and the U. S. health care system.

3. List and discuss three disadvantages of a program of this nature from the perspective of the individual, the school of nursing, and the U. S. health care system.

---

nurses' aides, and provide incentives for inactive nurses. In 1941 there were 289,286 RNs in the United States, but only 173,055 were employed in nursing.

Needs were increased both in the military and on the home front. The Red Cross as well as hospitals (both military and civilian) needed nurses, and nursing schools needed teachers. The Nursing Council on National Defense supported government backing for training more nurses in existing schools. The Labor-Federal Security Agency Appropriation Act of 1942 provided funding for refresher courses for inactive nurses, postgraduate education in specialized fields for graduate nurses, and increased enrollment in basic programs.

More than 180,000 young women answered the call. Qualifications included age between 17 and 35 years, at least a high-school education, and good school and health records. Accelerated training was the hallmark of the new programs. To qualify for funds, schools had to reduce the traditional program from 36 to 30 months. During the last 6 months, a Senior Cadet worked in the full time capacity of a graduate nurse. In 1943 the Nurse Training Act was passed, providing grants to finance training for the armed forces, government and civilian hospitals, and health agencies.

Over 100,000 nurses were certified for military service and awarded full commissioned status after the war. In addition, the segregation of African American nurses ended. In 1948 the Brown report again recommended that professional-nursing education be university-based, and that efforts to recruit men and minorities be enhanced (Nichols, 2001)

THE 1950s THROUGH THE 1970s

After World War II, federal funding for medical research, coupled with the rise of medical specialization, led to remarkable advances in care. Sulfa drugs were developed, along with cardiac medications and the defibrillation process (Keeling, 2001). This medical specialization had its negative consequences as well, in the form of increasingly fragmented care. As ground was gained for the belief that health care is a right, government involvement increased, and private health care expanded. From just prior to World War II until the 1960s, the percentage of people covered by private health insurance increased more than threefold, to above 70% (Torrens, 1978). In 1946 the Hill-Burton Act provided funding for hospital construction. In 1953 Congress expanded the Social Security Act by adding Medicare and Medicaid, thus solidifying government responsibility for health care to the poor and aged (Hood & Leddy, 2003).

The increase in the number of hospitals and people covered by medical insurance resulted in an acute nursing shortage. In an effort to cope with the shortage, creating a new model of nursing education: the two-year Associate Degree (AD) (Nichols, 2001). Today, AD graduates are not differentiated from RNs prepared at other educational levels; although both the American Nurses Association (1965) and the National League for Nursing (1982) have for years asserted their positions that the baccalaureate degree be the minimum educational requirement for professional nursing practice.

As the health insurance system expanded, the cost and complexity of the system increased exponentially. By the 1970s it was clear that health care costs were out of control, and as the government began reducing funding, the emphasis shifted to efficiency and cost containment. Initially, the federal government instituted a prospective payment system based upon diagnosis-related groups (DRGs), which paid a prearranged amount for the care of patients covered by Medicare predicated on diagnosis, rather than actual care expenditures (Hood & Leddy, 2003).

This initial change has grown into a massive movement toward health care reform with the goal of cost containment. One response by nursing to the dilemma of cost-plus-access was the development of Nurse Practitioner programs. Nurse Practitioners emerged, in part, to fill gaps brought about by a shortage of primary care physicians (due to the increased specialization discussed earlier) and at the same time meet the public's need for health care services, especially in rural and underserved areas. Today Nurse Practitioners work in multiple specialties, in both primary and tertiary care settings.

As health care costs continued to outstrip inflation in the 1990s, hospital consolidation continued and innovative health care delivery models expanded. Health care providers increased their use of technology, including telehealth care and computer-based monitoring systems, to provide consistent, cost-effective, and accessible care.

THE DAWN OF THE TWENTY-FIRST CENTURY

The major societal processes that will affect nursing into the twenty-first century and beyond include industrialization, technology, and **urbanization.** Through the process of industrialization, the United States economy has shifted to a highly specialized workforce with a service-delivery focus. One example of this is the development of the hospital industry (Schwirian, 1998). As hospitals continue the consolidation processes of the 1990s, nursing-care delivery has changed yet again, with greater numbers of care activities moving into the community. This shift underscores the importance of communication technology to connect remote-care delivery sites. Computers and other telecommunication systems including voice and video capabilities enable nurses, health-team members, and patients to communicate at a distance (Brennan, 1996).

Urbanization is the process of population migration from rural to city dwellings. One result of population shifts is increased diversity. Like the nurses at the dawn of the Industrial Revolution, the nurses of the future must be prepared to provide care to clients from a variety of cultural and social backgrounds in ever-larger urban centers. Ethnic and cultural variations exist in multiple areas and affect spheres of nursing care, including definitions of health, family, the sick role, compliance, and communication patterns. (Schwirian, 1998). The culturally competent nurse must possess an awareness that such variations exist, a willingness to explore them, and the flexibility to adapt care for maximum benefit.

CASE SCENARIO 2.2

Your hospital has appointed you to serve on a committee to make recommendations about how best to prepare the nursing staff to address the health care needs related to the process of urbanization.

Case Considerations

1. How would you begin to research urbanization and its likely impact upon your patient population?

2. What do you think are some effects of urbanization upon patients receiving hospital-based care?

3. What would you recommend the committee do to enhance the ability of nurses employed by your hospital to provide care to those with special needs related to the urbanization process?

CHAPTER SUMMARY

As nursing moves into the twenty-first century, social and scientific changes present ever-more complex challenges. In order to advance our profession and wield our power in service of the greater good, an understanding of the past is critical. The history of nursing is filled with individual and collective examples of bravery, competence, determination, and an uncompromising commitment to serve. May we each resolve to do our part to move our profession forward by improving people's lives as we advance into the future of our own making.

The future is like a corridor into which we can see only by the light coming from behind.

—Edward Weyer, Jr.

REFERENCES

Adler, R. E. (2004). *Medical firsts from Hippocrates to the Human Genome.* New Jersey: John Wiley & Sons.

American Nurses' Association (1965). *Educational preparation for nurse practitioners and assistants to nurses: A position paper.* Kansas City, MO: American Nurses' Association.

Brennan, P. F. (1996). The future of clinical communication in an electronic environment. *Holistic Nursing Practice, 11*(1), 97–104.

Bullough, B., & Bullough, V. (1978) *The care of the sick, the emergence of modern nursing.* New York: Prodist.

Conley, V. (1973). *Curriculum and instruction in nursing.* Boston: Little, Brown.

Dock, L. L., & Stewart, I. M. (1920). *A short history of nursing.* New York: Putnam.

Dossey, B. M. (2000). *Florence Nightingale: Mystic, visionary, healer.* Springhouse, PA: Springhouse Corporation.

Edelstein, E. J., & Edelstein, L. (1975). *Asclepius: A collection and interpretation of the testimonies.* New York: Arno Press.

Fitzpatrick, M. L. (1975). Nursing and the Great Depression. *American Journal Of Nursing. 75*(12), 2188–2190.

Holder, V. L. (2003). From handmaiden to right hand: The birth of nursing in America; *AORN Journal, 78*(4), 618–632.

Hood, L. J., & Leddy, S. K. (2003). *Conceptual bases of professional nursing* (5th ed.). Philadelphia: Lippincott, Williams & Wilkins.

Joel, L. A., & Kelly, L. J. (2002). *The nursing experience: Trends, challenges and transitions* (4th ed.). New York: McGraw-Hill.

Kalisch, B. J., & Kalisch, P. A. (1976). Is history of nursing alive and well? *Nursing Outlook, 24,* 362–366.

Kalisch, B. J., & Kalisch, P. A. (1995). *The advance of American nursing*. Philadelphia: Lippincott.

Keeling, A. W. (2001). Professional nursing comes of age—1859–2000 in Chitty, K. K. *Professional nursing—Concepts and challenges* (3rd ed.). Philadelphia: W. B. Saunders Co.

Keith, J. M. (1988). Florence Nightingale: Statistician and consultant epidemiologist. *International Nursing Review, 35*, 147–150.

Kelly, L. Y., & Joel, L. A. (1999). *Dimensions of professional nursing* (8th ed.). New York: McGraw-Hill.

Kizilos, P. (2001). A Civil War book of the dead, American History, April, p. 36.

McDonald, L. (1998). Florence Nightingale: Passionate statistician. *Journal of Holistic Nursing, 16*, 267–277.

McDonald, L. (2001). Florence Nightingale and the early origins of evidence-based nursing. *Evidence-Based Nursing, 4*, 68–69.

Miracle, V. A. (2003). A closing word—Tidbits about Florence Nightingale. *Dimensions in Critical Care Nursing, 22*(2), 103–104.

Nichols, E. F. (2001). Educational patterns in nursing, in Chitty, K. K. *Professional Nursing-Concepts and challenges* (3rd ed.). pp. 33–63. Philadelphia: W. B. Saunders Co.

National League for Nursing (1982). *Position Statement on nursing roles: Scope and preparation*. New York: National League for Nursing.

Nietzsche, F. (1949). *The use and abuse of history*. Translated in 1874 by Adrian Collins. New York: Liberal Arts Press.

Nightingale, F. (1859; reprinted 1946). *Notes on Nursing: What it is and what it is not*. Philadelphia: J. B. Lippincott.

Nutting, M. A., & Dock, L. L. (1935). *A history of nursing*. New York: G. P. Putnam's Sons.

Oates, S. B. (1994). *A woman of valor: Clara Barton and the Civil War*. New York: Free Press.

Petry, L. (1945). The U. S. Cadet nurse Corps: A summing up. *American Journal of Nursing, 45*(12), 1027–1028.

Schwirian, P. M. (1998). *Professionalization of nursing: Current issues and trends* (3rd ed.). Philadelphia: Lippincott-Raven.

Snyder, C. M. (1975). *The Lady and the president: The letters of Dorothea Dix and Millard Fillmore*. Lexington, KY: The University Press of Kentucky.

Torrens P. R. (1978). *The American health care system: Issues and problems*. St. Louis: C. V. Mosby.

Wall, B. M. (1995). Courage to care: The sisters of the Holy Cross in the Spanish-American War. *Nursing History Review, 3*, 55–77.

Weyer, E. (1959). *Primitive peoples today*. (p. 2.). Garden City, New York: Doubleday.

Withington, E. T. (1894). *Medical history from the earliest times*. London: Scientific Press.

Woodham-Smith, C. (1949). *Florence Nightingale*. London: Constable & Company.

Figure 2.1 (Asclepius) Kalisch, P. A., & Kalisch, B. J. (2004). *American Nursing: A history*. (p. 2). Philadelphia: Lippincott, Williams & Wilkins.

Figure 2.2 (Nightingale) Dossey, B. M. (2000). *Florence Nightingale: Mystic, visionary, healer*. (p. 153). Springhouse, PA: Springhouse Corporation.

CHAPTER 3

Educating the Profession

Angela S. Taylor

Like the moon, light the way for others and they will follow you.
—Hugh Gouldthorpe

LEARNING OBJECTIVES

At the completion of the chapter, the learner should be able to do the following:

1. Discuss how nursing during the Crimean War provided a mechanism for the development of the Nightingale Training School.
2. Explain how nursing leaders at the turn of the century began the process of professionalizing nursing.
3. Analyze how the Flexner and Goldmark Reports transformed nursing education.
4. Discuss the changing experience of black nurses in America.
5. Explain the rise in alternative training programs for nursing.
6. Describe the differences between diploma, associate-degree, and baccalaureate-degree nursing.
7. Discuss the current changes in nursing education and how they will impact nursing practice.
8. Identify the varying needs of the RN to BSN nurse.

KEY TERMS

Associate-degree program

Baccalaureate-degree program

Diploma program

Nursing education

RN to BSN programs

Training school

For over one hundred years, **nursing education** has evolved and continues to evolve. This evolution brought nursing education from work performed primarily by women of questionable backgrounds to a profession replete with the trust and belief afforded to few by society. Nursing is considered to be both a career and a true profession, offering its members autonomy and respect.

EARLY AMERICAN HEALTH CARE

In the mid-1800s nursing was provided primarily by women who were sentenced to care for the sick as part of restitution following arrest for disorderly conduct, public drunkenness, and immoral behavior. A few hospitals were privileged enough to have nuns or deaconesses from religious orders to provide care to the infirm. Lack of education and training in medical concepts did little to facilitate safe or effective nursing care in hospitals. In fact, hospitals were considered to be places where the poor went to die (Kalisch & Kalisch, 2004).

Tension grew between lay trustees of hospitals and physicians during this time as well (Rosenberg, 1987). Trustees retained formal control, while physicians assumed control of procedures and activities to meet the demands of the patients. During the late nineteenth century through the early twentieth century (1880–1910), lay trustees limited their personal involvement and instead, focused their energies and commitment on securing economic responsibilities. Physicians assumed control of medical instruction, patient admission procedures, autopsy policies, staff discipline and performance, and appropriate therapeutics.

As hospitals became medicalized during this time of transition, they evolved into places designed for the middle class to obtain care as opposed to a place primarily intended for the poor and needy (Rosenberg, 1987). As such, the need for nurses to be educated and trained facilitated a move toward training programs that required students to be physically, mentally, emotionally, and morally prepared to undertake the rigorous demands of nursing care.

LADY WITH THE LAMP: THE NIGHTINGALE TRADITION

Florence Nightingale was born in 1820 and became one of the primary contributors to the institution of formal nurses' training, both in Britain and in the United States (Smith, 1951). At age 17 she wrote in one of several private notes that "God spoke to me and called me to His service" (Smith, 1951, p. 12). Eight years after this "call to service," two serious illnesses in her family caused her to realize the necessity of training in nursing.

Nursing Care During the Crimean War

In 1854 when the Crimean War began, Sidney Herbert, Secretary of War for Britain, asked Nightingale to go to Scutari. She was appointed Superintendent of the Female Nursing Establishment of the English General Hospitals in Turkey (Smith, 1951). Nightingale was placed in charge of everything that related to the recruitment, training, and managing of nursing care.

Training Evolution in Britain

In 1859 St. Thomas's Hospital became the focus of a financial battle that would launch the founding of the first Nightingale **Training School** for Nurses (Smith, 1951). A railway line was to be built that would transect the hospital, requiring either the sale or move of the facility. With the mediation services of Nightingale, the facility was moved to Lambeth, and her interest in nursing and nursing reform resurfaced as a priority.

At the same time she was planning for the training school, she wrote *Notes on Nursing,* a book to be used by lay women to provide nursing care for children and family members (Smith, 1951). The five essential points for healthy houses became the beliefs that formed the foundation of nursing (Nightingale, 1969) and included providing the

WRITING EXERCISE 3.1

Essential points for providing a healing environment, according to Nightingale's *Notes on Nursing*, were presented. Select a patient from your clinical practice and discuss how you used these principles in providing care. Write up your discussion and be prepared to discuss it in class.

patient with pure air, pure water, efficient drainage, cleanliness, and light. Other points that facilitaed healing included reducing unnecessary noise; planning patient care to minimize disturbance; providing sensory stimulation through music or visual stimuli; observing and recording patient care and assessment; and the inclusion of vegetables, milk, sugar (for carbon), and gelatin (for nitrogen) in the patient's diet.

Following the publication of *Notes on Nursing,* the Training School for Nurses was opened at St. Thomas's Hospital. While Nightingale's health would not allow her to directly supervise the endeavor, she remained the benefactor and supervisor (Smith, 1951). Mrs. Wardroper, a matron of the hospital, was appointed superintendent of the Nightingale Training School and remained in this position for 27 years. The primary goal of the training school was to prepare highly trained nurses who would elevate the standards of care in the hospital, not to assume positions in private duty. The training school opened in June 1860 with 15 candidates. Only women of "suitable character" were admitted, because Nightingale understood the importance of success in this initial era of reforming the nursing profession.

Every month Wardroper completed a report on each candidate entitled "Personal Character and Acquirements," which included topics on morality and technical ability. In addition, to ensure that the candidates were successful, Nightingale required each to keep a daily diary that was read at the end of each month by both Nightingale and Wardroper. Following one year of coursework and training, the nurses successfully completed an examination and were registered by the hospital as "Certificated Nurses" (Smith, 1951). Even though the training was rigorous and the discipline was painstaking, applications increased as news spread of the success of the training program.

DEVELOPMENT OF U.S. TRAINING SCHOOLS OF NURSING

News of the success of Nightingale's Training School for Nurses quickly spread to the United States. Marie Zakrzewska, a midwife from Berlin, became interested in medicine and attempted to register for medical school. Following the refusal of German medical schools to admit her for training, she emigrated to the United States (Kalisch & Kalisch, 2004). She was introduced to Elizabeth Blackwell, the first woman physician in the United States, in 1854. Blackwell became instrumental in Zakrzewska's admission to Western Reserve University, from which she received her medical degree two years later.

Sensitive to the discrimination of women in medicine, Dr. Zakrzewska founded the New England Hospital for Women and Children in 1862. One of the primary purposes pronounced by the board of directors was the training of nurses under the supervision of the physician (Kalisch & Kalisch, 2004). The first graduate of this program was Susan Dimock. Following her graduation, Dimock traveled to Europe, where she met Florence Nightingale.

Upon her return to the United States, Dimock revised the curriculum for training nurses at the New England Hospital for Women and Children based on guidelines from the Nightingale Training School.

The First U.S. Schools of Nursing

As the first nurse was graduating from Dimock's program (Kalisch & Kalisch, 2004), three schools were preparing to open as the first training schools modeled distinctively after the Nightingale Training School. The first Nightingale school to open was the New York Training School at Bellevue Hospital in New York in 1873. The remaining two included the Connecticut Training School for Nurses at New Haven State Hospital and the Boston Training School for Nurses at Massachusetts General Hospital.

Students desiring to enter one of these early programs were required to meet specific criteria: to be between 25 and 35 years of age, single, and without physical defect. Two character references were required for consideration. Housing consisted of a small room with little lighting and meager furnishings. Meals were served in institutional style. Following dinner, students attended lectures provided by the physicians. Morning began early, with the probationers engaging in simple tasks such as linen maintenance and folding clothes. As time progressed, students were allowed to assume the additional tasks of ironing, folding linen, polishing floors, and cleaning.

Following the second week of work, students passed the probationary period and would become a "junior nurse," with the signing of an agreement providing them with lodging and a stipend in exchange for two years of training service. It was during the next few months that students began to assume patient-care duties and learn nursing skills. As students became a "senior nurse" at the beginning of the second year, they were rewarded with not having to attend evening lectures or take quizzes. They assisted in serving food, administering medications, and were in charge of an entire ward of patients (Kalisch & Kalisch, 2004; Reverby, 1987b).

The National Association of Nursing Superintendents

In 1889 the Johns Hopkins Hospital opened and began recruiting for nursing students. Led by Isabel Hampton, the nursing school opened, training 105 pupils during the first four years (James, 1979). Hampton's goal was to improve society by making nurses' work acceptable and respectable, thereby professionalizing nursing. Forming a Nurses' Journal Club in 1891, Hampton provided opportunities for nurses to engage in discussion on current medical issues both in and out of the hospital.

Hampton (now Hampton-Robb) presented a formal address to the National Conference of Charities and Correction in May 1890, emphasizing nursing's role in medicine, "scientific charity," and the training of women to provide nursing care (James, 1979). Following this, Hampton, along with one of the hospital's administrators, Dr. Billings, presented a paper on "Educational Standards for Nurses" at the International Congress of Charities, Correction and Philanthropy, being held in Chicago in 1893. Figure 3.1 is Isabel Hampton Robb.

As nursing education was being recognized as a means for improving patient care as well as elevating the standing of women in the profession, the conflict between the politics of nursing and the ideals of nursing began to emerge in the minds of several nursing leaders, specifically Isabel Hampton, Lavinia Dock, and Adelaide Nutting. As a means of advancing the profession and addressing these conflicts, the National Association of Nursing Superintendents was begun, with Nutting assuming the leadership of the society upon its inception (James, 1979; Kalisch & Kalisch, 2004). This association was to become the National League for Nursing. Early recommendations from the society included agreement that student nurses should not be sent out to perform private duty nursing, encouragement of training-school alumnae associations, and implementing three-year nursing curricula.

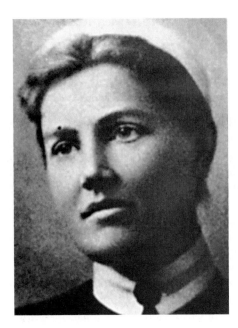

Figure 3.1 Isabel Hampton Robb. Photo courtesy of the American Nurses Association

Shortly after the institution of this society, Hampton founded the Associated Alumnae of the United States and Canada, which would become the American Nurses Association (James, 1979; Kalisch & Kalisch, 2004). This became the professional organization to begin printing the first nursing journal, *The American Journal of Nursing*.

Hospital Training Becomes the Foundation

Between 1890 and 1920 the number of nursing school rose from 35 to 1,775, with the number of trained nurses rising from 16 to 141 per 100,000 population (Reverby, 1987a; Reverby, 1987b). Nursing schools continued to provide hospitals with cheap labor in exchange for training; however, the service needs of the hospital took precedence over the education requirements of the nursing students. If their labor was needed on one ward, it was possible for them graduate without experiences in other areas.

Nursing care responsibilities during hospital training were varied, but controversy existed over the appropriateness of several tasks (Kalisch & Kalisch, 2004; Reverby, 1987b). Whereas it was standard practice for nurses to give baths, dress wounds, give enemas, observe secretions, and gather assessment data, such tasks as catheterization of male patients and massage provoked controversy. Still, even with this controversy, nurses were entrusted with treatments that included leeching and the application of counterirritants, chemicals intended to irritate the skin in an attempt to alleviate disease and promote healing (Kalisch & Kalisch, 2004). Nurses were also the first anesthetists for surgical patients.

Hospital nursing was transformed during the late 1800s and early 1900s by the sanitation movement, the bacteriology revolution, and the advance of technology in patient care (Duffy, 1992; Howell, 1996). With the move from an agrarian to an urban culture, there was a significant influx of people into cities. This rise in urbanization encouraged the growth of the sanitation movement. Towns and cities were able to incorporate new technology into sewer and water systems. Garbage and refuse was systematically collected, and the standard of living improved for the residents, which resulted in improved food, housing, and work conditions (Duffy, 1992). This improvement in living conditions, however, did not necessarily extend to the poor urban areas, with tenement housing and overcrowding being the norm.

While advances were being made in sanitation, another movement was under way. At the turn of the century, laboratories were opening in medical schools. Scientists and physicians were able to isolate and begin to identify bacteria and fungi. In doing so, vaccines and antitoxins were produced, providing mechanisms for preventing and treating some contagious diseases (Duffy, 1992). Through the introduction of antisepsis, surgery became much safer and provided additional options for treatment for those who could afford the procedures and the treatment (Rosenberg, 1987).

By 1925 most communities boasted having a hospital that could provide contemporary services through laboratory and radiologic tests. In essence, technology became the prominent feature of the hospital, with the advantages of improving and individualizing patient care, treating diseases, and improving mortality following surgery (Howell, 1996). It was the implementation of nurse training schools and the use of nurses to provide organized and efficient care that most drastically improved the health outcome of patient care as well as the transformation of the hospital from one that provided indigent care to one that provided care to the middle and upper classes (Rosenberg, 1987).

DEVELOPMENT OF EDUCATIONAL STANDARDS FOR NURSING

As hospitals became more focused on technology, growth, financial security, and expansion, nursing leaders continued to recognize the need for quality nursing education to meet the needs of the changing society. The development of educational standards for nursing was initiated by the work of Hampton, Dock, and Nutting through the implementation of professional nursing associations.

Institution of Regulatory Boards

This work continued into the early twentieth century, with the implementation of the first four licensure laws. These laws were passed in 1903 in New York, New Jersey, North Carolina, and Virginia, providing regulations on educational requirements and the presence of a board of examiners for licensure (Shannon, 1975). The most common problem was that registration was the option of the graduate, not mandatory. New York was the most progressive state, instituting a State Board of Nurse Examiners that mandated minimum requirements for practice and theory to be considered for licensure (Kalisch & Kalisch, 2004). By the 1940s all states had laws to regulate the licensure of nurses, but the transition came slowly and as a result of examinations of both medical and nursing education and the quality of the facilities offering the education.

The Flexner Report

As the hospitals were transformed in providing advanced medical care, the training of physicians remained relatively unchanged at the turn of the century. Investigation of medical education resulted in evaluation and subsequent reformation (Kalisch & Kalich, 2004). With funding from the Carnegie Foundation, Abraham Flexner visited medical schools across the country to evaluate the quality and value of existing programs. Through this investigation, five points were elicited that could be used to judge the programs: entrance requirements, size and training of the faculty, monetary support for the institution, laboratory quality, and the relationship between the school and hospital. The report was published in 1910 and contained serious criticism of the current state of medical education in the United States. As a result, medical education was revitalized, and standards were set to improve the quality of medical education.

THE GOLDMARK REPORT

The Flexner Report and the subsequent transformation in medical education sparked interest in nursing leaders who were passionate about reforming nursing education and implementing standards. The result was a study, taking two and one half years to complete, undertaken by Josephine Goldmark in 1923 to evaluate the quality of education in the 1800 existing nursing schools (Committee for the Study of Nursing Education, 1923). The primary asset of the school's curriculum was the inclusion of symptoms and disease management. Weaknesses included a failure to teach disease prevention and a failure to meet the increased demand for high quality applicants.

Recommendations from the Goldmark Report were to pave the way for the professionalization of nursing education. The committee recommended that the schools which were least able to survive be closed and eliminated. High-school graduation was to be the minimum educational requirement for entrance to a nursing school. Credits for completed courses were to be assigned based on a fixed and standard mechanism. Full-time, qualified instructors were to be used to provide the teaching of theory and practice in their areas of specialty. Equipment and supplies needed to be adequate for learning. In addition, students were to practice skills in a laboratory setting prior to a practice setting in order to ensure standard technique (Committee for the Study of Nursing Education, 1923).

The most provocative recommendations focused on the movement of nursing education from the hospital to the university. The Committee's recommendations relied on the belief that a university setting would unify the education from beginning to end and provide a centralized system for education (Committee for the Study of Nursing Education, 1923). The focus would move from hospital service to liberal education in the arts and sciences (Committee for the Study of Nursing Education, 1923; Kalisch & Kalisch, 2004), with the recommendation that the curriculum span five years and include didactic as well as skills training. The first autonomous university nursing program was opened at Yale University.

ADDING DIVERSITY TO THE PROFESSION

History has often ignored the integration of both black and male nurses into the profession. However, blacks and men have played integral roles in nursing as well as health care in general. In earlier times, their contributions were often limited to times of war. It has only been in recent years that educational and professional opportunities have opened up to these valued members of the profession.

The Development of Black Nursing Programs

Prior to Nightingale and the Nightingale tradition of nursing education, black women served as nurses primarily in two ways: as slaves to the masters of plantations and as servants to clean, wash laundry, and prepare bandages during wartime. Their service was limited, and their abilities were not used to their fullest. No schools of nursing existed for black women until the mid-1870s.

Mary Eliza Mahoney (see Figure 3.2) was born in Boston in 1845 and was admitted to the New England Hospital for Women and Children Training School for nurses, where she graduated in 1879 at age 34 (Bridgewater State College, 2004). After 16 months of training 16 hours a day, seven days a week, Mary Mahoney was the first black woman to graduate from a nursing training school. Not only was she the first black nurse, but out of the 40 students who began the program, she was one of only three persons to complete the 16-month training program. It was not until she graduated that black women who met admission requirements were allowed to attend the school and become trained nurses instead of having to rely on becoming domestic servants. Following her graduation, Mahoney continued to provide nursing care to the black population and was active in the National Association of Colored Graduate Nurses, established in 1908, where she gave the welcoming address at the association's first conference (American Nurses Association, 2006; Hine, 1989).

The first black hospital to be established to meet the needs of the black population was Freedmen's Hospital in Washington, DC. This facility was founded in 1862 to meet the medical needs of slaves who were freed following the Civil War. The Freedmen's Bureau opened this facility, the only federally funded health care facility for blacks in the United States, which initiated the black hospital movement. As such, the Freedmen's Hospital trained both black physicians and nurses at the turn of the century (Duke University Medical Center Library Online, 2005).

Mabel Keaton Staupers was born in 1890 in Barbados, West Indies and emigrated to the United

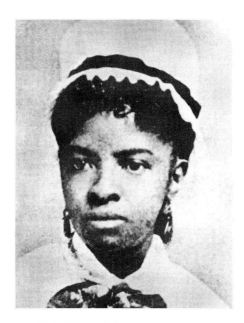

Figure 3.2 Mary Mahoney. Photo courtesy of the American Nurses Association

States with her parents. In 1917 she graduated with honors from the Freedmen's Hospital School of Nursing. Working first as a private duty nurse, as most nurses did following graduation, she later became the executive secretary for the Harlem Tuberculosis Committee, which was a part of the New York Tuberculosis and Health Association. Her duties in that capacity included examining the health needs of blacks in the region. While having an understanding that segregation was inevitable at the time, Staupers worked to create equal rights for black nurses who were being denied membership to the National Association of Nursing Superintendents, which later became the National League for Nursing, and the Associated Alumnae of the United States and Canada, which later became the American Nurses Association (American Nurses Association, 2006; Hine, 1989).

Staupers assisted in the development of the National Association of Colored Graduate Nurses, accepting a position as the first paid executive secretary. It was in that capacity that she helped to break down racial barriers between nursing and nonnursing groups, schools of nursing, and the entry of black nurses into the military. Although Staupers resigned from her position as executive secretary in 1946, she remained active in the organizations, seeing membership into the American Nurses Association opened up to black nurses in 1948 and the dissolution of the National Association of Colored Graduate Nurses in 1949 (Hine, 1989).

The first baccalaureate nursing program in the Commonwealth of Virginia was implemented in 1944 under the supervision of Mary Elizabeth Carnegie, a black woman who was born in Baltimore, Maryland, and attended nursing school while working in a "whites only" cafeteria. She graduated from Lincoln Hospital School for Nurses, earned a sociology degree at West Virginia State College, and later became the assistant director of nursing at Hampton University in Virginia, where she oversaw the development of the baccalaureate nursing program in 1943. Hampton University also holds the distinction of being the state's first nursing program for blacks (American Nurses Association, 2006).

Carnegie not only helped to professionalize the training of black nurses, she was also instrumental in chronicling the history of black nurses through her work in research and as an educator and author. Working to pay tribute to the contributions of black nurses, Carnegie advanced the nursing profession as a whole through her work with the *American Journal of Nursing, Nursing Research,* and as author of *The Path We Tread: Black in Nursing Worldwide, 1854–1994.*

In 1971 the National Black Nurses Association was established in Cleveland, Ohio in an effort to give voice to the concerns of black nurses with regard to health care for black people in the United States. As the official professional organization for black nurses, its vision and mission is directed to the improvement of health care and quality of life for black Americans. This movement was led by such nursing leaders as Mary Harper and Lauranne Sams (National Black Nurses Association, 1999). The outcome has been to more fully recognize the contributions of black nurses and to increase their political involvement as well as opportunities in health care and in nursing education through research, advancement, and achievement of terminal degrees.

The Training of Men in Nursing

There have always been males involved in nursing: in early times, nursing care was almost always provided by men; whether by religious orders or by laymen during times of war, few women were considered qualified for this type of work. With the rise of agrarian societies, however, domestic nursing care shifted from being delivered primarily by men to being provided by women. This shift was necessary as men were needed to work the fields and focus on agricultural development; however, this did not stop some men from pursuing their devotion.

In 1888 two training schools for men were opened, the Mills School for Nursing and St. Vincent's Hospital School for Men (American Assembly for Men in Nursing, 2006). Training men to be nurses proved difficult for many, however, as they were not accepted into the profession readily. In fact, men were excluded from the American Nurses Association until 1930, as female nursing leaders worked to establish equal rights for women through their association in professional nursing organizations.

The Army Nurse Corps was developed in 1901, but men were excluded. They were not allowed to serve as nurses in the military until the Korean War. Male nurses were drafted into military service between 1901 and 1950, but were prohibited from functioning as registered nurses. Nursing schools became sexually integrated after the Korean War and began to admit men to their programs, allowing the numbers of male nurses to increase. Even now, however, the numbers of male nurses is significantly lower than the numbers of female nurses.

NEW EDUCATIONAL MODELS

As nursing became more professionalized, opportunities began to open up for nurses to serve in areas other than hospitals, homes, and the community.

One area where nurses became indispensable was in the military service (Kalisch & Kalisch, 2004). As nurses began to practice in alternate settings, and as the availability of nurses decreased, it was necessary for them to train in new ways to keep up with demand.

Training of Practical Nurses

States sought out ways to train nurses faster in order to meet the rapidly growing needs of their communities (Kalisch & Kalisch, 2004). Some hospitals experimented with decreasing workweek hours, increasing pay, improving work conditions, and employing nursing assistants to fill the void. Others implemented nurseries for the children of nurses. In Seattle, however, legislation was passed to provide for the licensure of practical nurses who had acquired 450 hours of classroom and five months of on-the-job training. Education of this nature, with the preparation of practical nurses to provide some of the hands-on skills in the hospitals, began to bloom across the country. Still the production of new nurses was not able to alter the shortage of nurses to a manageable degree.

ASSOCIATE-DEGREE NURSING EDUCATION

In 1952 Louise McManus undertook a pilot project that was directed at developing nursing education programs at junior and community colleges as a means of further meeting the needs of the nursing shortage (Kalisch & Kalisch, 2004). McManus intended for the nurses who were prepared with a two-year curriculum to provide "beginning general duty" (p. 383). At that time, 90 percent of nursing education was still being conducted in hospital schools of nursing, with the focus on inpatient nursing care. The goal of the **associate-degree program** is to prepare nurses faster, while maintaining a focus on clinical practice in the hospital setting. Less emphasis is placed on general education,

CASE SCENARIO 3.1

You are employed in a facility that is primarily staffed by licensed practical nurses and associate-degree-prepared nurses. The staff that you work with know that you have returned to school to attain a baccalaureate degree in nursing. You are bombarded with comments, including, "I don't know why you want to waste your time going back to school. You won't be doing anything different anyway" and "You must think you are going to be better than us when you get out of school." Tension is increasing each day you work.

Case Considerations

1. What is the primary issue in this scenario? Why is it an issue?

2. What are the differences in preparation and ability for practical nurses, associate degree nurses, and baccalaureate nurses?

3. How will you explain these differences to the staff?

4. Discuss mechanisms you will use to decrease the rising tension on the unit.

making this program distinct from **baccalaureate-degree programs.**

The associate-degree program focuses on technical skills, allowing students to become registered nurses in two years and enter the nursing workforce at a faster pace than with a baccalaureate degree. It is considered to be the entry level for technical nursing practice. The need for nurses during shortages has increased the number of associate-degree nursing programs across the nation; however, many hospitals continue to report a preference for baccalaureate-prepared nurses. Given this preference, the associate degree in nursing is considered to be a point along the educational mobility path for nurses.

UP AND AWAY: TAKING NURSING EDUCATION TO A NEW LEVEL

The impact of the new nursing training models, preparing practical nurses and associate-degree nurses, became evident in the early 1960s. Nursing education was slowly moving away from hospital **diploma programs,** with numbers of associate- and baccalaureate-degree programs steadily increasing (Kalisch & Kalisch, 2004). This change was due in part to the increasing complexity of health care with the institution of critical-care nursing, including intensive care and coronary care.

The shift away from diploma nursing programs can be seen through the changing numbers of existing programs. In the 1970s there were over 800 diploma nursing programs; in 2006, fewer than 100 programs exist across the United States (All Nursing Schools, 2006). The majority of hospital diploma programs continue to exist primarily in the eastern United States, because hospitals have determined that hospital-based nursing programs are not cost-effective for the institutions (Rowett & De Pasquale, 2005), and that these programs educate nurses at a minimally competent level to provide independent nursing care to hospitalized patients (North Carolina Board of Nursing, 2006).

The American Nurses Association First Position Paper

Another cause for the shift in emphasis from diploma to academic education was a result of the publication

RESEARCH APPLICATION ARTICLE

Aiken, L. H., Clarke, S. P., Cheung, R. B., Sloane, D. M., and Silber, J. H. (2003). Educational levels of hospital nurses and surgical patient mortality. *Journal of the American Medical Association*, 290, 1617–1623.

A study in Pennsylvania (Aiken et al., 2003) analyzed the surgical outcomes of 232,342 patients in 168 hospitals. Findings indicated that risk of patient death following surgery was decreased by 5 percent when there was a 10 percent increase in baccalaureate-prepared nurses. Patient mortality was projected to be 19 percent lower in a hospital with 60 percent of the nurses prepared at a baccalaureate level. In addition, years of nursing practice were not found to affect the results of the study. Results of this study indicate that a clear link exists between patient mortality and the level of educational preparation of nurses.

of a position paper on nursing education by the American Nurses Association (ANA) in 1965. It identified three levels of nursing—professional, technical, and assistive—and began a conflict in nursing education that continues to this day. Its primary focus was to identify the baccalaureate degree as the minimum level of preparation for beginning professional nursing practice (Kalisch & Kalisch, 2004; Lynaugh & Brush, 1996). In addition, the ANA identified the associate degree as the minimum level of preparation for beginning technical nursing practice, and vocational training as the minimum level of preparation for assistive nursing practice (American Nurses Association, 2002; Kalisch & Kalisch, 2004).

The New Professional Nurse

As health care needs increase with the aging of Americans and the increasing retirement of nurses, the need for baccalaureate-prepared nurses escalates. More opportunities than ever now exist for accelerated education for baccalaureate education, from **RN to BSN programs** to second-degree programs.

In 2005, 32 states had articulation agreements between associate-degree programs and baccalaureate programs in order to provide hospital diploma and associate degree nurses a seamless transition into a professional nursing education. The baccalaureate programs utilize the basic nursing education provided by the initial training to build a stronger foundation in the sciences and the liberal arts. The focus in the RN to BSN programs is on developing stronger critical-thinking and clinical-analysis skills, and includes coursework in the areas of cultural diversity, economics, policy and politics, and nursing leadership (American Association of Colleges of Nursing, 2005). The added value of the baccalaureate education is seen in Magnet hospitals and academic health centers, where a preference for baccalaureate-prepared nurses is advertised; nurses at these institutions are compensated professionally and monetarily for their advanced education.

Nursing schools have also implemented programs for second-degree students in an effort to provide additional opportunities for individuals to enter the nursing workforce. These accelerated tracks take into consideration that individuals with existing baccalaureate degrees have already completed their general education and liberal arts courses and primarily need to focus on nursing (American Nurses Association, 2002). The courses are intensive and focus on development of nursing skills and critical thinking in health care. Typically, second-degree students are more mature and independent, possessing skills that challenge both themselves and their instructors, making for a rich learning environment.

WRITING EXERCISE 3.2

Nursing education is on the cusp of a new transformation. Discuss why this transformation is necessary at this point in our professional history. What are the issues that affect this change? Describe how this change will affect your practice as a nurse. Write up your discussion and be prepared to discuss it in class.

Specialty Nursing Certification

At this same time, Medicare and Medicaid legislation and the primary health care movement uncovered a disparity between education and practice, indicating that constant retraining was required of hospital nurses (Lynaugh & Brush, 1996). In 1967 the National Advisory Committee on Health Manpower reported that nurses were oversupplied, underprepared, and undercompensated. There was conflict between the responsibility of the nurse and that of the physician.

In an effort to differentiate practice roles, nursing specialty certifications were developed and implemented. The specialty certifications allowed nurses to develop expertise in specific areas of nursing practice based on standards that were nationally recognized (Lynaugh & Brush, 1996). In another attempt to differentiate practice roles and to expand the role of the nurse in primary care was the implementation of nurse practitioner programs, intended to prepare nurses at a graduate level in order to provide cost-effective, high-quality care, specifically in underserved and rural communities (Kalisch & Kalisch, 2004).

GRADUATE NURSING EDUCATION

While the medical community initially opposed the preparation of nurses to provide primary care, the need eventually became evident. Because of that, other specialty nursing roles were developed at universities, with the goal of preparing nurse practitioners in various areas, including family care, pediatric care, women's health care, neonatal nursing, community health, and adult health (Kalisch & Kalisch, 2004; Lynaugh & Brush, 1996). As the needs of society continue to evolve and become more complex, nurses will be required to continue to provide advanced care. As such, nurse practitioners of the future will need to be prepared at a level more appropriate to the care they are to provide. The changes in graduate and advanced nursing education are discussed further in Chapter 20. Table 3.1 describes the historical events that have influenced the evolution of nursing.

CHAPTER SUMMARY

Throughout time, primarily women have delivered nursing care. In the 1800s these women were mentally ill, prostitutes, or the product of the criminal justice system. The Crimean War, which began in 1854, sparked a path for the transformation of nursing education. Through the work of Florence Nightingale, principles were identified that would provide an environment for healing. Using her experience in treating the sick and injured, along with these principles, Nightingale realized a need for standardized nursing education. This standardization was realized as the first Nightingale Training School for Nurses opened in Britain in 1860.

Training schools opened in the United States and followed the tradition set forth by Nightingale.

Table 3.1 Historical Events Influencing the Evolution of Nursing

Date	Event
1923	Studies of nursing education
	Goldmark report
	Founded: Yale University School of Nursing
1926	Burgess report
1929	Stock market crash begins the Great Depression
1933	American Hospital Association endorses Blue Cross
1938	American Medical Association endorses Blue Shield
	Economic Security Program for Nurses
1940	Cost studies of nursing education and service
1943	Founded: Federal Cadet Nurse Corps
1948	Brown report: *Future of Nursing*
1952	*Journal of Nursing Research*
1953	U.S. Public Health Services Studies in Nursing Education
1955	Practical Nursing (Title III) Health Amendment Act
1956	Hughes study: 20,000 Nurses Tell Their Stories
1960s	Created: Medicare and Medicaid
1961	Surgeon General's Consultant Group
1964	Nurse Training Act
1965	ANA position paper on entry into practice
1966	Educational opportunity grants for nurses
1967	First nurse practitioner program, pediatric
1970	Secretary's commission to study extended roles for nurses
1973	Health Maintenance Organization Act
1977	Rural Health Clinic Service Act
	National Commission for Manpower Policy Study
1979	U.S. Surgeon General Report *Healthy People*
1980	Omnibus Budget Reconciliation Act
1982	Budget cut to Health Maintenance Organization Act
	Tax Equity Fiscal Responsibility Act (TEFRA)
1983	Institute of Medicine Committee on Nursing and Nursing Education study
1987	Secretary's Commission on Nursing
1990s	Health care reform

Table 3.1 (*Continued*)

Date	Event
1991	U.S. Department of Health and Human Services *Healthy People 2000*
1997	Agency for Health Care Policy and Research, now known as the Agency for Research and Quality, established 12 evidence-based practice centers
2000	U.S. Department of Health and Human Services *Healthy People 2010*
2002	Nursing shortage clearly identified as a crisis for health care delivery systems

Nursing leaders at the end of the nineteenth century and early part of the twentieth century saw a need to take nursing education one step further. Through the development of professional nursing organizations, leaders such as Hampton, Dock, and Nutting elevated the status of nursing and opened the door to improving the training of nurses.

Following the Goldmark Report in 1923, education facilities revitalized nursing curriculum and began to move nursing education out of the hospitals and into the universities. It was not until the 1950s, however, that the majority of nursing education was being conducted in colleges, universities, and community colleges. The expansion of nursing education into the community college opened a new pathway to licensure as a registered nurse.

In the 1960s the ANA took a stand and proclaimed that baccalaureate nursing education was required as the entry level of professional nursing. This position sparked a conflict that continues into the twenty-first century. While the conflict continues to be discussed in professional and academic settings, nursing education continues to evolve. Graduate nursing education is currently undergoing a revolutionary change, which will elevate the status of the professional nurse to an even higher level. Being led by the American Association of Colleges of Nursing, the new advanced practice nurse will begin her/his career with a doctoral degree instead of a master's degree, leading the nursing profession into the future with a bright path ahead.

> *Only in growth, reform, and change, paradoxically enough, is true security to be found.*
>
> —Anne Morrow Lindbergh

REFERENCES

Aiken, L. H., Clarke, S. P., Cheung, R. B., Sloane, D. M., & Silber, J. H. (2003). Educational levels of hospital nurses and surgical patient mortality. *Journal of the American Medical Association, 290,* 1617–1623.

American Assembly for Men in Nursing. (2006). *The story of men in American nursing.* Retrieved January 8, 2006, from http://www.geocities.com/Athens/ Forum/ 6011/sld001.htm.

American Association of Colleges of Nursing. (2002). *Accelerated programs: The fast track to careers in nursing* [Electronic version]. Retrieved January 8, 2006, from http://www.aacn.nche.edu/Publications/ issues/Aug02.htm.

American Association of Colleges of Nursing. (2005). *Degree completion programs for registered nurses: RN to masters degree and RN to baccalaureate programs* [Electronic version]. Retrieved January 8, 2006, from http://www.aacn.nche.edu/Media/ FactSheets/DegreeCompletionProg.htm.

American Nurses Association. (2006). 1976 Inductee, Mary Eliza Mahoney, 1845–1926. *ANA Hall of Fame,* retrieved January 8, 2006, from http://www. nursingworld.org/hof/mahome.htm.

American Nurses Association. (2006). 1996 Inductee, Mabel Keaton Staupers, 1890–1989. *ANA Hall of*

Fame, retrieved January 8, 2006, from http://www. nursingworld.org/ hof/stauperm.htm.

American Nurses Association. (2006). 2000 Inductee, Mary Elizabeth Carnegie, DPA, RN, FAAN, 1916–Present. *ANA Hall of Fame,* retrieved January 8, 2006, from http://womenshistory.about.com/gi/dynamic/ offsite.htm?zi=1/XJ&sdn=womenshistory&zu=http %3A%2F%2Fwww.nursingworld.org/2Fhof/2Fcarne gie.htm.

Bridgewater State College (2004). *Mary Eliza Mahony, R. N.* Retrieved January 8, 2006, from http://www. bridgew.edu/HOBA/Mahoney.cfm.

Committee for the Study of Nursing Education. (1923). *Nursing and nursing education in the United States.* New York: The Macmillan Company.

Duffy, J. (1992). *The sanitarians: A history of American public health.* Chicago: University of Illinois Press.

Duke University Medical Center Library Online. (2005). *Black history month: A medical perspective.* Retrieved January 8, 2006, from http://www.mclibrary.duke. edu/hmc/exhibits/blkhist/.

Hine, D. C. (1989). *Black Women in White: Racial conflict and cooperation in the nursing profession, 1890–1950.* Bloomington and Indianapolis: Indiana University Press.

Howell, J. D. (1996). *Technology in the hospital: Trans-forming patient care in the early twentieth century.* Baltimore: The Johns Hopkins University Press.

James, J. W. (1979). Isabel Hampton and the profession-alization of nursing in the 1890s. In Vogel & Rosenberg (Eds.), *The therapeutic revolution: Essays in the social history of American medicine* (pp. 201–244), Philadelphia: University of Pennsylvania Press.

Kalisch, P. A. & Kalisch, B. J. (2004). *American nursing: A history* (4th ed.). Philadelphia: Lippincott, Williams & Wilkins.

Lynaugh, J. E. & Brush, B. L. (1996). *American nursing: From hospitals to health systems.* Cambridge, MA: Blackwell Press.

National Black Nurses Association. (1999). *History: National Black Nurses Association.* Retrieved January 8, 2006, from http://womenshistory.about. com/gi/dynamic/offsite.htm?zi=1/XJ&sdn= womenshistory&zu=http%3A%2F%2Fwww.nbna. org%2Fhistory.htm.

Nightingale, F. (1969). *Notes on nursing: What it is and what it is not* (Unabridged republication of the first American edition, as published by D. Appleton and Company, 1860). New York: Dover Publications, Inc.

North Carolina Board of Nursing (2006). Nursing programs leading to diploma in registered nursing. *Nursing programs.* Retrieved January 8, 2006, from http://www.ncbon.com/ Education-nurseprog. asp#DIPLOMA.

Reverby, S. (1987). A caring dilemma: Womanhood and nursing in historical perspective. *Nursing Research, 36*(1), 5–10.

Reverby, S. M. (1987). *Ordered to care: The dilemma of American nursing, 1850–1945.* New York: Cambridge University Press.

Rosenberg, C. E. (1987). *In care of strangers: The rise of America's hospital system.* New York: Basic Books.

Rowett, C. & De Pasquale, S. (2005). Mission accomplished [Electronic version]. *Johns Hopkins Nursing,* Summer.

Shannon, M. L. (1975). Nurses in American history: Our first four licensure laws. *American Journal of Nursing, 75,* 40–42.

Smith, C. W. (1951). *Florence Nightingale, 1829–1910.* Atlanta: McGraw-Hill Company.

CHAPTER 4

Finding and Maintaining Work/Life Harmony

Karin A. Polifko

*Live a balanced life—learn some and think some and draw and
paint and sing and dance and play and work everyday some.*
—Robert Fulghum

LEARNING OBJECTIVES

At the completion of the chapter, the learner should be able to do the following:

1. Verbalize several challenges that one encounters returning to school.
2. Discuss desired outcomes from the professional student.
3. Identify characteristics of the adult learner and how they apply to the returning student.
4. Present an understanding of role, role stress, role conflict, and role overload as they pertain to attending school.
5. Describe significant issues within work/family conflict.
6. Distinguish between work/family spillover and family/work spillover situations.
7. Discuss at least five options or strategies for developing a healthier work/family/life balance.

KEY TERMS

Adult learner	Pedagogy	Social role theory
Andragogy	Role	Spillover
Balance	Role overload	Work/family conflict
Family/work conflict	Role set	
Harmony	Role stress	

RETURNING TO SCHOOL

The decision to return to school for your baccalaureate degree has been made. Maybe the decision was relatively simple: due to life circumstances, whether it was money, family, or other obligations, you could not pursue the BSN degree, and now that the environment has changed, you are afforded this opportunity. For some, the BSN is a requirement for employment or a requirement for promotion. And others may have taken a different path to enrolling in the BSN program by perhaps starting another career that initially was a good fit but somehow changed, resulting in being drawn to the accelerated, second-degree curricular option. Regardless of how you became enrolled in the nursing program, there are several challenges returning students have in common.

Whenever one takes on a new responsibility, there is a need to assess and reprioritize tasks. Given the increasing complexity in everyday lives, being able to prioritize school assignments, work, family obligations, and personal affairs is sometimes difficult and challenging, with many factors competing for a limited amount of time. Time management becomes paramount. Returning to school also brings to light a role transition: new role expectations and sometimes role confusion. If someone is already an RN in a charge nurse role, there may be role confusion, for example, if they complete a leadership clinical rotation on their home unit. Not only is the professional student confused in this situation, so coworkers and staff may be.

Responsibilities of a Professional Student

Returning to school as a professional student holds several responsibilities. Whereas there is a preestablished knowledge base, perhaps in the same content area in a required course, the baccalaureate degree affords the student the ability to synthesize information and experiences while applying these concepts in new ways. Issues may be looked at in manners that expose complexities that may not have been explored previously, necessitating an open mind and curiosity. However challenging going back to school may be, regardless of age, gender, or previous work experiences, it may cause some anxiety and resocialization into the role of student and active learner.

What are some of the expectations and desired outcomes of a student enrolled in nursing studies? First and foremost is the emphasis on communication skills, whether they are written, spoken, or electronically transmitted. If the student is a nurse returning in an RN to BSN program, there may be many years of experiences writing in "nursing shorthand," with abbreviations and incomplete sentences, possibly writing only when there is a positive event to document as in the case of charting-by-exception. In charting-by-exception, much of the documentation is accomplished by check marks on a flow sheet, with the nurse documenting only when there is an event that is out of the ordinary or that does not exist within the parameters set by the institution. Or nurse's notes, as well as other health care provider's notes, are famously written in incomplete sentences.

Further, many of us are familiar with instant messaging, such as using a handheld computer for sending messages. This type of text is often done in an abbreviated fashion such as in incomplete sentences due to space constraints. Both of these scenarios may result in a student having difficulty with writing. The majority of students returning to college struggle with written communication skills and often need refreshers on how to actually write a paper in a logical, cohesive manner complete with full thought development. Writing an outline first is a critical step that is most often missed. Without an outline, a paper often rambles, maybe never even addressing the issues that are required as delineated in the syllabus. Once the outline is completed, a helpful step is to place it next to the requirements found in the syllabus to ensure that the content is addressed. It is not uncommon for a student to miss large components of the written assignment due to simply not checking back once the paper is completed. Another frequent issue in student papers is incorrect grammar and spelling. There are spell-check and grammar-check features in most writing programs; it is advisable to use these frequently when writing and certainly at the completion of a paper before it is submitted.

Most colleges and universities have writing centers, with tutors who can review papers before submission to a professor. Additionally, most nursing schools require that written communications be submitted in a standardized form, which may be an unusual way of documentation that often just requires practice. It is highly recommended that students purchase the publication manual for the chosen format. A common publication format required of nursing students is from the American Psychological Association (APA). A great Web site that offers a quick synopsis of critical APA points may be found at http://www.wooster.edu/psychology/apacrib/apacrib.html After a paper is written, it is often advantageous—and recommended—to have someone else proofread it before turning it in to the professor.

In addition to writing skills, reading skills may take some time to refine. While in school, particularly in the accelerated, second-degree BSN programs, large amounts of reading materials are assigned in a more concentrated fashion than traditional programs. In order to be successful with this skill, the student needs to not only read quickly, but to be able to comprehend and synthesize large quantities of information in several different subjects simultaneously. Many campus writing centers will have useful programs to assist students in reading comprehension.

Likewise, students need to be active listeners and take responsibility for learning. A student's past academic experience may color classroom participation. Questions need to be effectively framed in such a way that the professor can understand the issue and appropriately address the student's concern. Sometimes fear, embarrassment, or simply not understanding the issue may inhibit a student from asking questions. A student needs to realize that professors truly want a student to be successful and to understand the concepts presented; students do not come to class with a full and complete understanding of all topics—if they did, there would be no need for class!

Many college professors lecture to students without seeking and affirming that a student is actually learning and comprehending the material presented. This situation then places the responsibility on the student to inform the professor if there is difficulty with the subject matter, if clarification is needed, or simply whether validation of subject comprehension is needed. It is to be hoped that much of the learning and teaching in the classroom with **adult learners** is more participatory in nature, with the faculty members creating an environment wherein questioning is encouraged, discussions are held, and the student is actively engaged in the discovery of new information (Bevis & Watson, 2000).

Test taking is an area that creates anxiety, from beginning students to doctoral students. A critical factor in successful test taking is being prepared: has all the content to be covered in the exam been read, are there gaps in the student's comprehension of the content, has the student asked the professor about explaining the gaps, has the student attended class, and has the student kept up with any assignments? Like the campus writing center, there are resources that assist a student in test-taking strategies on most, if not all, campuses. Sitting for a multiple-choice test requires different skills and decision trees than does sitting for an essay examination. A significant difference between nursing programs and other collegiate programs is that whereas content mastery is important, many questions are framed as application questions: simple memorization doesn't really assist the student so much as a comprehensive understanding of the concepts. In this case, many students find it valuable to study with other students, especially formulating scenarios wherein there is a need to apply critical-thinking, problem-solving, and decision-making skills.

ADULT LEARNERS: IT'S DIFFERENT THIS TIME AROUND!

Most RNs return to school due to employer demands, as a means of achieving career goals, or simply personal satisfaction and the love of a challenge. Students enrolled in the accelerated, second-degree programs may have already held successful positions in a career (or two) and have come to the conclusion that current needs are not being met, and they desire a career change. Both categories of returning student pose challenges and opportunities for both the faculty member and the student, as previous learning becomes integrated into the present learning environment.

Reed and Beaudin (1993, p. 1) state that the age cohort of those students 35 years and older is "expected to increase dramatically and become the largest growing category of students at the postbaccalaureate level." The U.S. Department of Education surmised that almost 75 percent of students enrolled in undergraduate studies are defined as "untraditional," encouraging educators at the postsecondary levels to reframe how

they teach (National Postsecondary Student Aid Study, 2001). For many educators, including nursing educators, with students beginning their careers later than the majority—traditionally 18 to 22 years of age—of students, there is a need for awareness of adult-learner characteristics and expectations.

Generally speaking, the adult learner is more mature, more self-assured, and certainly more experienced in life and career choices than the traditional-age student. They are more likely to be returning to school for intrinsic goal attainment rather than pure employment need (Richardson & King, 1998). Adults are more likely to bring life experiences into the classroom, using work, family, and social examples to explain certain phenomenon, rather than just relying on a textbook or profession for explanations.

Adult learners have had to juggle multiple responsibilities, including work, family, social and personal obligations, and now, educational responsibilities. They are used to setting priorities, making choices, streamlining their lives, and may even expect their teachers to understand when choices are prioritized that may not place school at the top. Given the multiple priorities and decisions to be made, time management is often an issue, with competing issues and concerns (Richardson & King, 1998; Knowles, 1968).

WRITING EXERCISE 4.1

As mentioned in the above narratives, there are numerous reasons for returning to school to earn the BSN; and probably just as many reasons not to return to school. In a brief one-page paper, answer the following questions: (1) What are your prime motivating factors for returning to school? (2) Identify any issues that may have held you back in your decision to return to school; (3) Other than attaining the degree, what other goals do you have for the program, both personally and professionally? These goals can be identified as learning opportunities or outcomes that you will achieve once you have graduated.

THE UNIQUENESS OF THE ADULT LEARNER

Compared with the traditional-age student, adult students have numerous, unique qualities that bear discussion. Adult students, or nontraditional students, have busy lives that are filled with multiple responsibilities, including work, the nuclear family as well as extended family, house maintenance, and now school. With the majority of nurses being women, there is a strong possibility that they may be the primary caretaker for the family, resulting in additional stresses and responsibilities. With the fullness of everyday life, adult students have also learned to prioritize, multitask, and manage their time, albeit maybe not always effectively.

O'Brien and Renner (2000) found that adult learners are more intrinsically than extrinsically motivated. Whereas the employer may value the RN returning to school, often it is intrinsic factors such as self-esteem, self-worth, recognition, and both public and personal acknowledgment of achievement that drive the adult's decisions.

A hallmark of the adult learner—and perhaps different from the younger student—is the need to immediately apply newly learned information. Because of the vast experiences they bring into the classroom, these students want the subject matter to be logical and applicable to past life and career experiences, with the ability to build on current expertise. Knowles (1968, 1980) wrote about these traits, further commenting that adults are more active learners than their younger counterparts and desire independence and self-directed learning; perhaps this is why many adults dislike group projects! What is important to glean from this information is that many nursing programs have been rather traditional in the ways in which they teach the curriculum; most adults are working, and having several days (or evenings) tied up with a class can wreak havoc on most schedules. Shane (1983) even wrote about the "returning to school syndrome" wherein

the returning RN starts a baccalaureate program with enthusiasm and excitement, only to become conflicted with life's responsibilities and demands.

In order to have a win-win scenario between the returning student and school, both parties need to understand that adult students have different experiences, socializations, and expectations than younger students, and that maybe there needs to be increased flexibility and understanding of these concerns at the beginning of the journey.

A BRIEF OVERVIEW OF ADULT LEARNING CONCEPTS

Merriam and Cafferella (1991) group the adult-learning theories into three primary categories: "those anchored in adult learners' characteristics, those based on an adult's life situation, and those that focus on changes in consciousness" (p. 249). One of the most widely discussed theories of adult learners is developed from Knowles (1980, p. 43), who defined the notion **andragogy** as the "art and science of helping adults learn." Knowles contrasted the term andragogy with that of the accepted term **pedagogy,** which is simply the art and science of helping children learn. In pedagogy, the teacher is the one with authoritative focus, planning, directing, and evaluating of learning experiences. In contrast, teachers with an andragogical focus believe that learning is mutually collaborative, with the students actively participating in the planning, design, and evaluation processes in conjunction with others. Self-directed learning (when the student takes responsibility) is conceptualized in addition to Knowles by Houle (1980) and Tough (1979). Jarvis, McHale, Holford, and Griffin (2003) developed the Model of Learning Process for the adult learner wherein students actively reflect and assess the gaps between their current knowledge and the desired knowledge, again further emphasizing the need for professors to allow adult students the opportunities for self-evaluation. Chapter 14,

Teacher/Learner, will go into much more depth regarding adult education and the mutual expectations between the two constituencies.

ROLE, ROLE STRESS, AND ROLE OVERLOAD

Roy's Adaptation Model (Roy & Andrews, 1999) explains that a **role** is what society defines as set expectations that others have toward one another. A **role set** consists of those multiple roles that someone holds simultaneously, such as father, husband, student, professional. Common among adult learners is the concept identified as **role stress,** which is the pressure or strain resulting from the variety of expectations that the multiple roles require, and may be exhibited as physical and psychosomatic symptoms, such as headaches, anxiety, stomachaches, or shortness of breath.

Everyone has a certain role that they carry out, whether it be student, mother, husband, caretaker or wage earner; adults usually have multiple roles they perform, sometimes not equally as well. Roles and social positions often define who and what we are, what our place is in society, and are viewed within context of one another. Some societies are hierarchical, with a certain gender or caste having more privileges than another, whereas other societies allow more equality between peoples. Roles identify patterns of behavior that correspond to expected reactions by others. Regardless, **role overload,** particularly in women, is found to be detrimental and is caused by "multiple and conflicting expectations from others" (Nelson & Burke, 2002, p. 5). Role overload occurs when there are multiple expectations without fulfillment in any one of the roles or their corresponding expectations. Historically, women have had a higher workload, with the primary responsibility of dependent care, housework, plus vocational career work. According to Frankenhaeuser (1991), women averaged 78 hours a week of workload as compared with 68 hours for men.

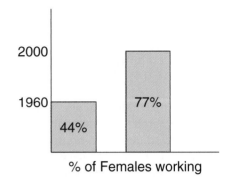

Figure 4.1 **Female employment in the US 1960 and 2000**

Inasmuch as men may be increasing their contribution to the running of the household and time spent with children, Bond, Galinsky, and Swanberg (1998) found that over a 20-year study the gaps are still insignificant and only slightly improving.

LABORING IN AMERICA

According to the U.S. Census Bureau 2004–2005 report, women continue to increase in the workforce, whether it is as a full-time or a part-time participants. The number of working women has more than doubled over the last two decades, with almost 60 percent of able women employed, as compared with 44 percent four decades ago, with the largest increase in married women: 41 percent in 1970 as compared with 62 percent in 2003 (U.S. Census Bureau, 2005, p. 377). Figure 4.1 illustrates female employment in the U.S. (1960 and 2000). One of the largest female professions in the United States is that of registered nurse; of the almost 2.5 million holding licenses, over 92 percent are women, followed by the teaching profession of elementary and middle school teachers who are 82 percent female (U.S. Census Bureau, 2005, p. 386).

One area of great increase in the labor statistics is that of working women with children and very young children (under 6). When many of the baby boomers

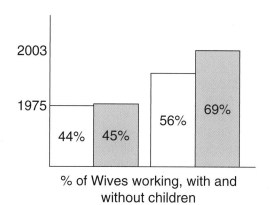

Figure 4.2 **Percentage of wives working in the US, with and without children 1975 to 2003**

were growing up, it was more of an exception than the norm to have a mother who worked outside the home; instead, the conventional picture was that of the father who worked all day and the mother who stayed home to raise the children, keep the house, and await the return of her husband. According to the U.S. Census Bureau, in the twenty-first century, the more typical scenario is that of a dual-earner family. The percentage of working wives without children has grown from 44 percent in 1975 to almost 56 percent in 2003, whereas the percentage of working wives with children has increased from 45 percent in 1975 to more than 69 percent in 2003 (see Figure 4.2). The largest increase in working wives has been in the category of those with children 14 to 17 years of age, growing from 54 percent to 81 percent from 1975 to 2003; however, almost 60 percent of those wives with children under 6 are working (U.S. Census Bureau, 2005, p. 377). For single mothers, the numbers increase to 77 percent who work, and over 82 percent of single fathers work (U.S. Census Bureau, 2005, p. 378). In putting all these numbers together, one can conclude that families will continue to have both wage earners working, placing further demands, stressors, and expectations not only on the couple, but on the children as well. Barnett (2004) discusses the need to understand that whereas many may believe that motherhood and marriage are "natural" roles for most women, and

that employment can be a huge source of discontent, there is a need to further explore the implications of multiple roles and whether one can handle them all simultaneously—and successfully. It is often with the overlapping and multiplicity of roles that one engages in that leads to conflict, whether intrapersonal or interpersonal conflicts. Much of the literature has illustrated the negative consequences for working parents, yet there are as many positives as there are challenges.

SOCIAL ROLE THEORY

According to the tenets of **Social Role Theory,** men historically have been the primary workers outside the home, responsible for earning the paycheck, and women have been the primary caretakers of the home and children. Because of these imbedded roles in American society, many still look to women to be associated with parenting and men to be associated with outside employment (Eagly, Wood, & Diekman, 2000). With the most common situation in the United States being a dual-earner family, wherein both the mother and father work to provide financial support for the family, there are numerous opportunities for continual role conflicts. Part of the conflict occurs when roles are either reversed or compounded, sometimes resulting in negative reactions by members of society, or internal conflicts within the person who carries a nonaccepted societal role. In particular, men who are stay-at-home dads may have a hard time earning acceptance among other fathers who work. Mothers who work, either by choice or necessity, may also have a difficult time gaining approval from stay-at-home moms; in fact, much has been written in the literature about this topic in particular (Marks & Houston, 2002).

There are some that hold the belief that it is the social responsibility of the female to focus on her children rather than career development, and that regardless of situation, all females should want to become mothers, and that the primary identity of a woman is that of mother. Similarly, there is a notion that one must accept that a career is "sacrificed" for the good of the children, and that a mother will always be available for her family, regardless of the situation. Russo (1976) labels this the "motherhood mandate."

Likewise, part of social-role theory speaks to the feminine and masculine characteristics that are expected by women and men in the United States. Our social roles dictate that women are soft, agreeable, caring, and consensus building, skills that are consistent with being a caretaker. Women who work are sometimes seen as less nurturing and less committed to their families than women who stay home with their children (LeMaster, Marcus-Newhall, Casad, & Silverman, 2004). Men, on the other hand, are expected to be assertive, competitive, and outgoing, skills that assist in working in the outside world. Again, much of the role conflict occurs when there is a misperception of expectations that others have and the attendant labeling. People mostly expect women to have feminine characteristics and men to be masculine. Women who are assertive and forthright or employed in male-dominated fields are often labeled pushy, difficult, and less feminine. Men who are in alternate social roles or who work in predominantly female professions are mislabeled as feminine, less ambitious, and less competent, leading to numerous societal misperceptions.

BACKGROUND OF WORK/FAMILY BALANCE

Historically, men and women have always worked while they had families, regardless of the decade in which they lived. What may have changed over time is the amount of work, the type of work, and whether it was paid or unpaid. Only as more mothers moved into the workplace and, increasingly, as single parents headed families, did the literature begin to reflect the notions of work/family balance. Other events that initiated this focus include the women's movement in the 1970s; the issue of quality of life; and, with the advent of technology and computerization, telecommuting. Much of the research and literature in the area of work/family balance began in the late 1970s and continues today (Burke, 2004). As hours at work increase, time available to spend at home, in leisure activities or simply with family members, correspondingly decreases. The notion of work/family balance encompasses several topical areas, including time at work, time at home, childcare, sick care, marital issues, leisure time, and both work and life satisfaction.

Women are becoming just as important to the family's finances as men in the dual-earner families; or they are becoming (either by choice or situation) the single wage earner in the family. According to Townsend (2005), over 85 percent of women work outside of their home, adding even more stressors in the form of commuting, childcare, sick care, and life obligations. Additionally, many women are challenged by not only being a mother to their children, but also by being caught in the "sandwich" generation wherein they are the primary caregivers for aging parents who may not be able to care for themselves. Even though parents may not be so infirm as to need total care, assisted-living expenses are often beyond the means of the normal family finances; and with elders living longer, these situations require long-term thinking, not only about health issues, but finance issues as well.

The traditional man-as-primary-wage-earner scenario is slowly disappearing as job security decreases while living expenses increase, thus necessitating two incomes in most families. By the same token, more men are becoming involved with family life and household responsibilities, which is very different from the days when only women were the accepted homemakers. Men, while perhaps still not the primary caretaker of the home and children in a dual-earner family, are contributing more time to these responsibilities than even a decade ago, often assisting with additional housekeeping chores including meal preparation, cleaning, and childcare.

WORK/FAMILY BALANCE— OR IS IT?

Family at-home time and work have been considered separate entities until the last few decades. While having a second income, usually from the wife, was considered "play" money, in today's economy, two incomes are almost a necessity. Correspondingly, more and more unmarried men and women are becoming parents, many by choice (Burke, 2004). Work influences home life, and home life invariably influences the work situation, with both scenarios having a direct effect on personal well-being.

When one thinks of balancing work and family, it conjures up the image of a scale, wherein one side tips downward as the other tips upward. When one area is in conflict, then the balance is askew, resulting in an imbalance between the two domains. There is oftentimes an imbalance between work and family life, with an experience of dissatisfaction in both areas, which is colored by the individual's perception of satisfaction and their ability to meet the demands of both domains.

Early on, the review of literature on work/family interactions began with a discussion of how the two areas developed into conflict; hence much of the literature even today focuses on that conflict (Lewis, 2002). After the conflict was identified, the research focused more on work/family balance: how to achieve and master it . A third movement in this arena has appeared, which is researching work and life integration, rather than focusing on the concept of pure balance (Rapaport, Tailyn, Fletcher, & Pruitt, 2002).

Rapaport and fellow researchers refer to work/family integration rather than balance, because they feel that balance connotes the total, with work, for example, taking 60 percent and leaving 40 percent for family, or vice versa. They believe that the term *integration* implies that individuals can sometimes participate as fully and entirely equally in both domains, it just depends on what level of satisfaction they wish to achieve. The term *work/family integration* can be as equally applied to singles as it can to those who are married.

Like Rapaport and colleagues (2002), this author believes that work and family issues cannot be easily compartmentalized, with overflow from one domain encroaching on the other domain. Instead of integration, the term *harmony* is introduced within the context of work/family/life. **Harmony** is defined as "congruity of parts with one another and with the whole" (www.hyperdictionary.com). Harmony illustrates the concept of being in synchrony, being in accordance, and being in agreement with all facets of work/family/life. How many times does one give up something in one domain to fit the demands and requirements of other domains? For example, whose turn is it to stay home with a sick child? Is it the spouse with the less hectic meeting schedule? Is it always the mom? Or the dad? Or is it the one with the most flexible or generous sick leave?

Harmony also connotes satisfaction with one's life situation, without pitting one domain against another. Unlike **balance**, which can be perceived as give and take, in a harmonious situation, everything can coexist without struggle, and with acceptance. Like integration, harmony speaks to achieving inner peace, having resilience, and going about life with grace, humor, and enthusiasm. Harmony is working together, rather than competing against; having reached a comforting equilibrium.

WORK/FAMILY CONFLICT

Much of the literature's research has focused on two predominant areas: the work domain and the family domain. There are, however, additional domains that need to be considered when discussing **work/family conflict,** and they are the life domain and the social domain. Not everything occurs at work, nor are issues found distinctly within the family domain; there are personal life issues such as need and self variables, and there are variables that address the social domain that may include the person's place in the community or society at large and their contributions.

As defined in the literature, work/family conflict occurs when there are pressures in one role due to interference from another role. Greenhaus and Beutell (1985) define work/family conflict as "a form of interrole conflict in which the role pressures from the work and family domains are incompatible in some respect" (p. 77). Oftentimes it is the overlapping of the roles and the "juggling" that creates the stress and conflict, which at times can be almost overwhelming. To go further, there are situations where work interferes with family (WIF) and situations where family interferes with work (FIW). To offer two examples, work can interfere with family when there is a specific time needed to be at work, and childcare is unavailable at that time (perhaps an 11pm to 7am shift). Family can interfere with work when a frail elderly parent needs their child to transport them to the physician's office during a time that an out-of-town business trip is planned. Both can be equally as problematic because they can create conflict.

Likewise, there is some evidence in the research that is contradictory; some may find that when there is a need to balance two or more roles, there are rewarding situations that lead to life satisfaction and a sense of accomplishment (LeMaster et al., 2004). Whether it is WIF or FIW conflict, employers especially are interested because these types of conflicts can have negative consequences, including undesirable work outcomes (absenteeism, turnover, incomplete work) or undesirable family outcomes.

THE CONCEPT OF IMBALANCE

For the past few decades the concept of imbalance has prevailed in the literature as the primary consequence of work/family and **family/work conflicts.** Hall and Callery (2003) define imbalance occurring when "goals were in jeopardy and

processes were unacceptable over the longer term" (p. 409). **Imbalance** occurs when one domain takes precedence over the other; one becomes subordinate and one dominant, either consciously or subconsciously. Compromise is no longer an option, or it may be totally exhausted, or setting of priorities is no longer an easy task. One of the major disruptions that creates an imbalance is childcare for an acutely ill child: who stays home? On the other hand, with the increasing longevity of people's lives, many are caught in the sandwich generation, which can easily cause a stressful situation in a work environment.

What are the symptoms of imbalance? Because of the necessity for setting priorities, there is guilt over the one area taking time from the other; there is also disappointment along with anger, isolation, weariness, or mental as well as physical exhaustion. Depression and feelings of helplessness or lack of control may also be present. When work is involved, there may be a corresponding decrease in productivity, an increase in mistakes, and resentment that one cannot be as equally as devoted to work obligations as to family responsibilities. Real issues of financial concern may also be present when there is a significant and longer-term imbalance between work and family. And lastly, when someone on a career trajectory needs to temporarily move off the path for family reasons, there may be issues of personal failure, career viability, and professional aspirations.

People progress on paths, or trajectories, that lead to the achievement of goals and desires, both in their family life and professional careers. Trajectories are often determined by values and goals and may change depending upon circumstances. As long as goals are being met, either personally or professionally, the situations are viewed as being in balance and become unbalanced when current goals are not achieved (Hall & Callery, 2003). When one works toward predetermined objectives and is successful in achieving those objectives, there is a feeling of accomplishment, success, and personal fulfillment. We need to feel that there is positive, forward movement toward meeting our goals and objectives as opposed to regressive or no movement. It is when our

CASE SCENARIO 4.1

Multitasking several different obligations at the same time is one of the more difficult things to do. Very few people can honestly say, "I am bored and have nothing to do, and I am all caught up with everything." Part of the challenge of going back to school is adding another obligation into an already full life. In light of this situation, answer the following questions:

Case Considerations

1. Right at this moment, do you feel you are in total control of your life?

2. How many roles are you taking on right now? Is this more or less than in the past?

Is there role overload? Role stress? Role ambiguity?

3. How do you prioritize obligations? How far ahead can you plan? Or do you?

4. Do you feel there is an issue with work/family balance? What seems to be more in imbalance, work or family? Is one area proving to be a more challenging area than the other? Is there conflict?

5. Who can you count on when there are conflicting situations? What are the most common conflicting situations that you find yourself in? How do you solve the issues? Can they be avoided?

---

personal and professional goals appear to be in conflict with one another that we experience imbalance and struggle to rectify those conflicting situations or expectations by eliminating the causative factor or trying to accomplish too much. A disruption in one or more trajectories can cause a reevaluation of priorities, negotiation, compromise, and a reassessment of goals. Different goals may become reemphasized or deemphasized, depending on the desired effects and who and what they impinge upon.

SPILLOVER

Most of us are looking for that perfect fit between work and family life, hoping that there are qualities in both domains that energize, fulfill, and satisfy us. Yet reality is such that many times there is a tug between the differing obligations and commitments that we not only personally have, but that we in turn maintain for our family

members and outside organizations. Unfortunately, there is probably a higher incidence of negative issues that occur as a result of these conflicts than there are of peaceful coexistence and harmony. Nevertheless, there is recent documentation of positive outcomes from work/family or family/work influences (Moen & Yu, 1999). Many career women could not imagine staying home full time if they have children, and there are probably a few career men who don't at least daydream about working from home; then there are those in both categories of workers who become stronger and more actualized if they are part of the workforce in some manner.

Spillover is another term mentioned in the literature that describes the extent to which family life interferes with work, or vice versa. When there is spillover, "carryover stress" (Greenhaus & Parasuraman, 1987) occurs, which becomes significant when one area, such as work, interferes and places demands onto another area, such as family life. These negative stressors have potential for emotionally, physically, and socially affecting an individual, resulting in a variety of outcomes and consequences. For example, if a spouse becomes ill, is out of work, and is unable to contribute to the running of the household and assist with the children, the other spouse may very well have spillover into the work domain. The consequences of the family/work spillover may include bad decision making due to lack of sleep, poor quality of work, decreased productivity, inferior people-management skills, missed deadlines, and fewer hours spent on the job. By the same token, stress from spillover could result in anxiety and short tempers at home, poor sleep patterns, longer hours at the office, and house maintenance responsibilities possibly placed on hold. Carryover stress can equally upset and negatively affect the individual and family and, depending on the situation, the employee's organization as well.

As families members age, work demands also grow and expand. For example, it is noted that while every age of child rearing has its challenges, those who work full time while taking care of preschoolers are under additional pressures and challenges that other workers who may have more scheduling flexibility are not. And, as discussed previously, as workers enter midlife with growing job duties, there may be demands to take care of aging parents in addition to their own children. Women are probably affected more than men by this phenomenon known as being in the "sandwich generation," because they are usually the primary caretakers for both their children and their parents. Within the context of spillover, it may be assumed then that conflictive and negative spillover increase through a worker's midlife due to simultaneous strains and anxieties.

WORK QUALITY AND FAMILY INTERFERENCE

Like home, work environments have diverse variables that influence people and their stress. A small body of research looks at these influential variables, including the age and presence of children, the professional status of spouses, marital status, racial and cultural markers, work roles, and family responsibilities, including dependent relationships outside of children. Numerous results occur when family variables mix with work variables, and a potentially large number of conflict-oriented situations can arise as a result of these interferences. For example, work/family conflict can manifest in the presence of issues of job satisfaction, life satisfaction, family satisfaction, role overload, and role ambiguity. An inadequate work environment can result in tremendous anxiety and stress, both mental and physical, eroding confidence, resulting in self-doubt, feelings of powerlessness, poor self-esteem, not to mention decreased productivity, higher levels of mistakes, and inferior quality of work.

What are some of the work stressors that may not be so obvious? Job monotony, nonautonomous decision making, and unpleasant environments can lead to innocuous stress that is not as easily defined. Sometimes it is the little annoyances that are more stressful, such as being closely monitored daily for time at work in a salaried position; being evaluated for quality of results can lead to a conflict-based scenario easier than ensuring that the supervisor discussing his or her thought processes during a problem-solving session. Likewise, Frye and Breaugh (2004) found that a supportive supervisor could greatly decrease stress and resulting conflict, particularly among parents of preschoolers. Parents who found their supervisors to be supportive, sympathetic, and flexible when there was a family emergency were less likely to feel work/family or family/work conflicts.

One of the more negative results of work/family interference is that of job turnover; when there is gross dissatisfaction with work, an employee has the tendency to withdraw. Part of the dissatisfaction with work and the resulting conflicts is the serious consideration of turnover or thoughts of quitting. Resignation is a permanent way of eliminating the conflict between work and family, better meeting the needs of the family (Boyar, Maertz, Pearson, & Keough, 2003).

RESEARCH APPLICATION ARTICLE

Grzywacz, J. G., Almeida, D. M. & McDonald, D. A. (2002). Work-family spillover and family stress in the adult labor force. *Family Relations*, 51, pp. 28–36.

People do not work twenty-four hours a day, seven days a week. We all have outside lives and obligations, with increasing numbers of workers, including women, who also have family commitments to maintain. Although there has been a fair amount written in the literature in the past several decades about work and family interactions and subsequent challenges, little has been explored in terms of research studies that address the issue of work/family spillover and its effects on both the employee and the employee's family.

Grzywacz and colleagues (2002) examined the National Study of Daily Experiences, which is a component of the National Survey of Midlife Development in the United States, to ascertain the level and extent of work/family spillover in adults who work. These two samples were part of a grant to examine those predictors of aging in the areas of physical and psychological health as well as social responsibility. More than 3,000 adults aged 25 to 72 were randomly chosen to be interviewed via telephone, and later completed two written surveys. The average age for both samples was 42.31; females comprised 54 percent of the sample; nearly 70 percent were married; the average number of hours worked per week was 43; and only 12 percent were childless. Income averaged $46,000 per year. There were four dependent variables: positive work/family spillover, positive family/work spillover, negative work/family spillover, and negative family/work spillover. Statistics used to examine the effects of independent variables (age, gender, race, number of children, marital status, hours worked per week, annual salary, and livelihood) on the dependent variables included both bivariate and multivariate analyses. Some of the results were that women stated more negative spillover effects than men and that negative spillover increases as one ages through young and early years and declines in later midlife. Predictably, those with children under 6 had a higher level of negative family/work spillover. Alternately, those employed in managerial and professional roles experienced a higher level of negative work/family spillover stress than those in service careers. This study provided several interesting insights into the issues of spillover, family life, and work-related stressors.

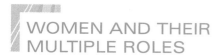

WOMEN AND THEIR MULTIPLE ROLES

Women have always worked. The change that has occurred in the last 50 years or so is where the work is done; in earlier decades, women worked in the home, taking care of the house, the bills, and the children. Today, although approximately 16 percent of the female workforce remains childless, the vast majority of women hold employment outside the home while simultaneously taking care of children. In fact, 63 percent of women with infants are

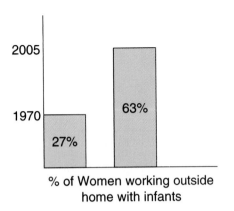

Figure 4.3 Percentage of women working outside the home with infants

working outside of the home (Newsweek, May 4, 2005), as compared with 1970 when the rate was only 27 percent, illustrated by Figure 4.3. Marks and Houston (2002) note that the longer a woman works before having a child, the more likely she will be to return to work, either part or full time, after the child is born. The years between 25 and 35 are important for establishing a career basis, and with women waiting longer to have their families, one area of critical concern is timing: even though a career may be more developed, an older mother experiences different stressors that may affect career choices than a younger mother.

Further, increasingly women are earning higher-education degrees, illustrating their dedication to building a career. The professional schools of medicine, law, and veterinary science are seeing more women apply, in some cases more than males (vet school), and in business schools almost a third of the enrollees are women. On college campuses, more than half of the students are women, with more females earning their degrees than their male counterparts. Barnett (2004) notes that for females, the probability of getting married increases with the number of years of education. With college and graduate school attendance going up for females, it appears that many plan on having multiple roles that include marriage, work, and more than likely,

children, further adding to the likelihood of life stressors.

LIFE SATISFACTION

As previously discussed, there are numerous variables that contribute to work, family, social, and life satisfaction. Gender, age, educational attainment, marital status, having children (particularly preschool-age children), and occupation are probably the most common issues that affect satisfaction levels in the different domains. Satisfaction occurs when one is content with one's decisions or if gratification is present. When viewed in light of work or life satisfaction, another consideration is how closely the results concur with the values to which one is emotionally tied.

Hochschild (1997) writes that there are several issues that may make work seem like a refuge from the stressors at home, most particularly experiencing a divorce, having preschool children (especially if the wife is working full time), and a higher-level career position. Another key satisfaction aspect is that of financial stability; the more financially secure a family is, the fewer work/family stressors arise from financial concerns. However, it is curious and perhaps an econmic sign of the times that in many cases, family incomes are rising due to dual-income earnings, rather than one spouse earning a significantly higher income.

Another major satisfaction variable is the number of hours worked versus being at home. It can be assumed that many professionals and managers work longer than the typical 40 hours per week, sometimes bringing work home and working weekends, but would probably work fewer hours if given the opportunity. Similarly, many lower-paid workers would probably work more hours and earn more money than currently. It is not uncommon that in higher- and dual-income families, one of the spouses—and not necessarily the wife—may decrease the hours worked or choose to stay home as a way to ease family, social, and life stressors. Work can also become less rewarding and less satisfying, resulting in resentment and a

WRITING EXERCISE 4.2

Part of being an adult is having some sense of where you are going in life. Can you easily identify your life's goal(s) in any detail? Other than the obvious, such as happiness, contentment, a family, what are the mapped out goals that you have for yourself? Many times, you need to lay a path and follow it, as most achievements don't just happen and require thoughtful preplanning and goal direction. How can you best accomplish your life goals, and what measurable steps can you take to begin successfully working toward them?

desire to shift priorities to home. Part of the difficulty, at least with some of the predominantly female professions such as staff nursing, librarianship, social work, elementary-school teaching, and restaurant workers is that they are lower paying, have less autonomy, and additionally may have nontraditional or restrictive schedules that often conflict with childcare options. Coupled with less opportunity for advancement, some of these variables inextricably add to spillover stress between work and home life and may also decrease satisfaction significantly.

COPING STRATEGIES TO DEVELOP HARMONY BETWEEN WORK/FAMILY/LIFE

When one is faced with a multiplicity of roles, with often competing objectives and desired outcomes, stress is sure to follow. For example, when your child is too sick for daycare or school, what are your choices when you have a critical meeting or a presentation to make at work? However, for as many men, women, and families that struggle with the daily balancing act, there are those who are successful in establishing and maintaining harmony within the factions in their lives.

Are there effective coping strategies to employ in decreasing the spillover stress from either the work or family domain—or maybe even both? Numerous articles have been published, as have many books, on the subject of balancing work and family issues, but again, this thread needs to go further into creating harmony between the domains. Some of the suggestions are as follows:

1. Promote an equal (or as equal as one can) division of household family work, such as laundry, grocery shopping, cleaning, and childcare tasks.

2. Encourage nontraditional roles for the wife and husband; perhaps it makes good sense that the father stays home with the young children if daycare services are not optimal and the mother can be the primary breadwinner.

3. Promote the authenticity of being childless and single by choice.

4. Acknowledge that perfection is not the goal, especially when it comes to household tasks and childrearing.

5. Acknowledge that parenting is difficult and challenging as well as being tremendously rewarding and fulfilling.

6. Understand that when one spouse is having a particularly arduous time at work, the other spouse can take on extra home chores, such as meal preparation, taking children to and from activities, and other cooperative tasks.

7. Is part-time rather than full-time work a temporary possibility?

8. Employers can offer flexible scheduling and alternative work schedules.

9. Employers can also offer on-site child care that is affordable and, in the case of workers with unusual scheduling, offer expanded hours. One type of daycare that can be both a recruitment and retention tool is to offer sick-day care for children of employees too sick to go back to school, but not necessarily sick enough to be at home by themselves.

10. Managers and supervisors need to be supportive, understanding, and flexible with employees with sick children, especially those with preschool children and without close family support mechanisms.

11. Employing organizations can actively encourage the values of work/family balance by developing and implementing family-friendly policies. In some organizations, there may need to be a major attitude shift as well as behavioral changes implemented.

12. Better time management goes without saying: do you really need to go to the grocery store every night after work, or can you prepare several meals in advance and freeze them so that you won't be as stressed-out coming home from work.

13. Realize that having a family should not be a career liability for women, the logistics just need to be figured out.

14. Priority setting becomes paramount. Reassess often and regularly your priorities at work, at home, and in your social circles. What are the obligations that are truly necessary and which are the ones that can be eliminated?

15. Regarding priorities, who comes first, your children? Your spouse? Your work? You?

16. Realize that life is not perfect, and a certain amount of chaos and imperfections are normal and to be expected.

17. Understand that one cannot be in two places at the same time, and give yourself enough time to go from point A to point B.

18. You can not meet anyone else's needs successfully if your needs are not met first.

19. If possible, choose to live in an area that is geographically close to work, children's school, home, and basic shopping needs. With the average commute to work continuing to increase, the less time in the car, the better for everyone. Is living near extended family a possibility?

20. Can someone else be hired to do the housework? The gardening? Repair minor household problems? The more things that can be delegated, the more time one has to do those things that are more pleasurable.

21. Is there some way to carve out some personal time? As crazy as it may be to do, a little down time can make the world of difference in destressing and becoming refocused.

What is the ultimate goal in life? For most of us, it is the ability to be self-fulfilled with a sense of contentment with choices made, regardless of whether they are career, family, or life choices.

CHAPTER SUMMARY

Adult learners have different learning styles as compared with traditional students. Adult students can add to the classroom experience by bringing in life examples rather than looking to the book or professor for further explanations. A key point about adult learners is that while enrolled in school, they are coordinating multiple responsibilities, including work, family, and community obligations along with meeting class deadlines. Due to their numerous responsibilities, above all, adult learners don't like to waste time! For many, going to back to school presents numerous opportunities as well as challenges. Time management, priority setting, decision making, and simply juggling schedules

CASE SCENARIO 4.2

As the manager of an extremely busy and at times stressful Emergency Department, you work with a variety of nurses, but interestingly most are single. Lately, however, there is one staff nurse, Marissa, who has been coming in late, calling in sick more frequently, appears distracted at work, and is increasingly unhappy and just plain negative. She has two children, both under 5, and is recently separated from her husband. Fortunately, she has a supportive mother, but her father's health is in rapid decline, requiring Marissa's care when she is not at work. Several staff members have come to you requesting that you "do something about Marissa."

Case Considerations

1. As the manager, what are your professional obligations as far as offering your assistance to Marissa? What are your personal boundaries?

2. What do you see as some of the issues in the above-mentioned scenario? Which one has priority and why? Which one can be placed lower on the priority listing and why?

3. How would you assist Marissa in identifying support mechanisms, and what are they?

4. Likewise, what are some coping strategies that you may suggest to Marissa to help her? Which ones are personal, which ones are professional, and should you be involved in both domains as her manager?

5. How would you respond to the staff when they want you to "do something about Marissa?" How far should you go in assisting her? What could be some of her options and how could she implement them?

become even more difficult and more complicated as lives become busier.

With more two-income families than ever in history, the established scenario of the husband going to work and the wife staying at home with the children is fast fading, as almost 75 percent of all traditional families have both the mother and father working. Family becomes intertwined with work, work becomes part of family life, and the two, oftentimes under stress, result in conflict and imbalance. Regardless of the domain where the conflict originates, conflict is a driving force behind the proliferation of books and articles on achieving balance. It appears that in spite of the marital status, parental status and age, Americans are experiencing more stressful lives than previous generations. Luckily, there are quite a few beneficial coping strategies that one can take advantage of in an effort to find, establish, and maintain harmony in both one's work life and in one's family life, and fortunately, the two can peacefully coexist.

Everyone should carefully observe which way his heart draws him, and then choose that way with all his strength.

—Chinese Proverb

REFERENCES

Barnett, R. C. (2004). Women and multiple roles: Myths and reality. *Harvard Review of Psychiatry, 12*(3), 158–164.

Bevis, E. O. & Watson, J. (2000). *Toward a caring curriculum: A new pedagogy for nursing.* Sudbury, MA: Jones and Bartlett and the National League for Nursing.

Bond, J. T., Galinsky, E., & Swanberg, J. E. (1998). *The 1997 national study of the changing workforce.* New York: Families and Work Institute.

Boyar, S. L., Maertz, C. P., Pearson, A. W., & Keough, S. (2003) Work-family conflict: A model of linkages between work and family domain variables and turnover intentions. *Journal of Managerial Issues, 15*(2), 175–190.

Burke, R. J. (2004). Work and personal life integration. *International Journal of Stress Management, 11*(4), 299–304.

Eagly, A. H., Wood, W., & Diekman, A. (2000). Social role theory of sex differences and similarities. In T. Eckes & H. M. Trautner (Eds.). *The developmental social psychology of gender* (pp. 123–174). Mahway, NJ: Erlbaum.

Frankenhaueser, M. (1991). The psychology of workload, stress and health: Comparisons between the sexes. *Annals of Behavioral Medicine, 13,* 197–204.

Frye, N. K. & Breaugh, J. A. (2004). Family-friendly policies, supervisor support, work-family conflict, family-work conflict, and satisfaction: A test of a conceptual model. *Journal of Business and Psychology, 19*(2), 197–220.

Greenhaus, J. H. & Parasuraman, S. (1987). A work-nonwork interactive perspective of stress and its consequences. *Journal of Health and Social Behavior, 24,* 300–312.

Greenhaus, J. H. & Beutell, N. J. (1985). Sources of conflict between work and family roles. *Academy of Management Review, 10*(1), 76–88.

Grzywacz, J. G., Almeida, D. M., & McDonald, D. A. (2002). Work-family spillover and family stress in the adult labor force. *Family Relations, 51,* 28–36.

Hall, W. A. & Callery, P. (2003). Balancing personal and family trajectories: An international study of dual-earner couples with pre-school children. *International Journal of Nursing Studies, 40,* 401–412.

Hochschild, A. R. (1997). *The time bind: When work becomes home and home becomes work.* New York: Metropolitan Press.

Houle, C. O. (1980). *The inquiring mind*, 2nd ed. Madison: University of Wisconsin Press.

Jarvis, P., McHale, J. V., Holford, J., & Griffin, C. (2003). *The theory of practice and learning.* U.K.: Routledge.

Knowles, M. (1980). *The modern practice of adult education: From pedagogy to andragogy.* New York: Cambridge Books.

Knowles, M. (1968). Andragogy, not pedagogy! *Adult Leadership, 16,* 350–352.

LeMaster, J., Marcus-Newhall, A., Casad, B. J., & Silverman, N. (2004). Life experiences of working and stay-at-home mothers. In J. L. Chin (ed.), *The psychology of prejudice and discrimination.* Westport, CT: Praeger.

Lewis, S. (2002). Work and family issues: Old and new. In R. J. Burke & D. L. Nelson (eds.), *Advancing women's careers* (pp. 67–82). Oxford: Blackwell Publishing.

Marks, G. & Houston, D. M. (2002). Attitudes toward work and motherhood held by working and non-working mothers. *Work, Employment and Society, 16*(3), 523–536.

Merriam, S. B. & Cafferella, R. (1991). *Learning in adulthood.* San Francisco: Jossey-Bass.

Moen, P. & Yu, Y. (1999). Having it all: Overall work/life success in two-earner families. *Research in the Sociology of Work, 7,* 109–139.

National Postsecondary Student Aid Study. Retrieved March 28, 2005, from http://nces.ed.gov/programs/coe/2002/analysese/nontradtional/index.asp

Nelson, D. L. & Burke, R. J. (2002). *Gender, work stress and health.* Washington, DC: American Psychological Association.

O'Brien, B. & Renner, A. (2000). Nurses on-line: Career mobility for registered nurses. *Journal of Professional Nursing, 16,* 13–20.

Reed, N. & Beaudin, B. (1993). Adult students and technology in higher education. *Collegiate Microcomputer, 11*(1), 1–4.

Richardson, J. & King, E. (1998). Adult students in higher education: Burden or boom? *Journal of Higher Education, 69*(1), 69–83.

Roy, C. & Andrews, H. A. (1999). *The Roy adaptation model,* (2nd ed.). Stamford, CT: Appleton & Lange.

Russo, N. F. (1976). The motherhood mandate. *Journal of Social Issues, 5,* 143–153.

Shane, D. (1983). *Returning to school: A guide for nurses.* Englewood Cliffs, NJ: Prentice Hall.

Tough, A. (1979). *The adult's learning projects: A fresh approach to theory and practice in adult learning.* (2nd ed.) Toronto: Institute of Studies in Education.

Townsend, L. (2005). Top work/family challenges and solutions. Retrieved April 14, 2005, from http://www.bluesuit,om.com/career/balance/challenges.html

U.S. Census Bureau, Statistical Abstract of the United States, 2004–2005, p. 372. Retrieved April 13, 2005, from http://www.census.gov/prod/2004pubs/04statab/labor.pdf

CHAPTER 5

Seeking and Managing Information

Pamela J. Sherwill-Navarro

*Knowledge is of two kinds. We know a subject ourselves, or
we know where we can find information upon it.*
—Samuel Jackson

LEARNING OBJECTIVES

At the completion of the chapter, the learner should be able to do the following:

1. Describe the difference between professional publications (journals) and popular press (magazines).
2. Discuss the concept of peer reviewed or refereed publications.
3. Compare and contrast the types of information available via libraries and their electronic resources and Web sites.
4. Analyze the differences between databases and Internet search engines, and describe when to use each.
5. List at least five sites that can be useful to locate literature-based resources for health care.
6. Define what a writing style is, and list two that are commonly used in nursing publications.
7. Identify several methods to facilitate lifelong learning and staying current with developments in your profession.

KEY TERMS

Databases	Peer reviewed	Search engines
Evidence-based resources	Referred	

Two fields that are changing very rapidly are health care and information. This chapter deals with the integration of both fields. They are intimately related because identifying, locating, managing, and disseminating information is necessary to maintain nursing skills and knowledge, improve patient care, increase efficiency and facilitate lifelong learning. Changes in the field of information have increased the options and the amount of information available to nurses. An important part of your nursing education is to develop skills that will be needed now, as a student, and later as a health care professional. These skills are known as information literacy, and they are a competency that American Association of Colleges of Nursing expects both new and experienced nurses to possess.

Approximately 5000 biomedical journal articles are published each day. If you count only the number of randomized control research studies, there are about 50 each day (Glasziou, DelMar, Salisbury, & NetLibrary, 2003). Those numbers make the task of keeping up with the current literature daunting. Because it is impossible to read and retain everything in a field, developing the skills to locate what is needed quickly and efficiently is critical. It is estimated that 50 percent of what residents learn during their residency will become obsolete by the time they have completed it (Bush, 2001). Predicting which 50 percent that will be is impossible. A similar prediction can be made for nursing education, so it is necessary that nurses have the skills to efficiently and effectively locate the information that they need when they need it.

SIGNIFICANT TRENDS IN HEALTH CARE INFORMATION

Bibliographic databases index journal articles, and the content of individual journals, and most are now accessible via the Internet. More and more nursing journals are available online but most require a subscription (individual or institutional) or charge for one-time access. A number of professional organizations, government agencies, and universities have sites that are freely available and contain useful information, especially in the area of evidence-based practice, a trend that continues to fuel the need for skills to locate and evaluate relevant literature.

LITERATURE TYPES

The preferred source of current information is the journal article. Books are often considered out of date by the time they have been published due to the time required for the publication process. Books are not without value, however, because they are excellent sources for established information. They answer questions such as "What is the normal range of values for a particular laboratory test?" or "What are the symptoms exhibited by a patient with cystic fibrosis?" These are known as background questions, about general methods or knowledge of a disorder. To answer foreground questions, which deal with specific knowledge relevant to a patient (e.g., determining the most effective therapy for hypertension), research journal articles are the preferred source. There are multiple types of research studies. Certain study designs are better suited to answer particular research questions. Generally randomized control trials are the preferred study type for questions about therapy. In your research courses you will learn about this in greater detail.

Journals differ from popular press or magazines in several ways. They are usually published or sponsored by a professional organization. Articles tend to be longer, use technical language or jargon, contain references, and are peer reviewed or refereed. The authors of journal articles are considered experts in the field, and their credentials are provided. The format of journal articles tends to be more uniform or structured, containing an abstract, a review of the literature, a discussion, results, a conclusion, and references or a bibliography. Illustrations are included to support the text and are usually graphs, tables, charts, or relevant photos.

Articles in magazines or the popular press tend to be shorter and do not follow a specific format. The author is usually a staff writer or journalist who is not an expert on the subject and does not have credentials. When an expert opinion or information is needed, an expert is interviewed or quoted.

These articles are written in everyday language and avoid the use of professional jargon. Illustrations tend to be glossy photos that are used more for getting attention than to support the text. These articles lack footnotes and rarely have a formal bibliography.

Peer-Reviewed or Refereed Publications

Professionals who are writing about research they have conducted or programs they have implemented wish to disseminate this information to their colleagues. They are usually the authors of professional journal articles. Prior to publication, experts review these articles blindly (the author[s] names and institution are removed) and make recommendations that an article be published as written, after revisions are made, or that it be declined from publication with that particular journal. This review process is known as peer review. A publication that utilizes this procedure is known as a refereed publication. It is important to note that not all professional publications utilize this process. Publications that have undergone this rigorous procedure are considered to be more significant than those that have not.

There are several methods of determining if a journal is peer reviewed or refereed. If you conduct a literature search in the following databases, there is the option to limit the search retrieval to only articles that have undergone this process: CINAHL, Expanded Academic ASAP, EBSCO Academic Search Premier, Social Sciences Index, ProQuest, Health and Wellness Resource Center, and ABI/Inform. The following journal full-text databases index only peer-reviewed journals: ACS Web journals of the American Chemical Society, JSTOR Retrospective Journals, Kluwer Academic Press Journals, Project MUSE Journals, Elsevier Science Direct, and Wiley Interscience Journals. The most authoritative source is Ulrich's International Periodical Directory. This resource is available in both print and electronic formats. The journals that are peer reviewed or refereed will have an icon of a referee's

striped shirt in front of the title. Journal Citation Reports, one of the ISI Web of Science databases, is another source of determining if a journal is refereed. If these sources are not available to you, there are a few alternatives. The first is to examine an issue of the journal and check the page that contains the editor's name and subscription information. This page is often located in the beginning of the journal, but if it is not, check the back of the journal and look for the words "peer reviewed" or "refereed." There are several other print publications to assist you that may be available at your library. The Medical and Health Care Books and Serials in Print: an Index to Literature in the Health Sciences and The Serials Directory contain entries that will inform you if the journal is refereed. If your library does not have any of these tools, contact one of the librarians to determine what they have available.

Professional literature is fact based rather than opinion based; therefore, statements must be credited to their source and background information must be documented. Footnotes direct the reader to the original source of the information while bibliographies provide a detailed account of the sources used for the review of the literature and historic information provided.

LOCATING INFORMATION

Now that you know there is a plethora of information available, how do you efficiently locate what you want when you need it? One option is to physically enter the library, pull journals off the shelves, and review the tables of contents to try to locate articles on your topic. Since this method can be very time consuming and inefficient, it is not recommended. Another option is to use an Internet search engine. However, anyone who has done this knows the amount of information retrieved can be overwhelming and sometimes of questionable quality. Searching the Internet for the answer to a question can be like finding the proverbial needle in a haystack. There is another option, however—bibliographic databases. These specialized databases index journal articles that can be searched to locate the desired information.

Search Engines versus Databases

It can be confusing to comprehend the difference between Internet search engines and searching databases, especially since most databases are accessed via the Internet. Databases are collections of records with multiple searchable fields. Depending upon the purpose and intended audience for the database, the records may be specific to a topic, such as cancer in the Cancer Lit database or Clinical Practice Guidelines in the National Guidelines Clearinghouse database. Other databases are much broader such as PubMed (the "900-pound gorilla" biomedical database that covers the history of medicine, dentistry, space life sciences, cancer, bioethics, toxicology, aids, complementary medicine, and nursing) and CINAHL (Cumulative Index to Nursing and Allied Health Literature), which indexes the literature of nursing and the various allied health disciplines.

Databases may also index a particular type of material. For example, Dissertation Abstracts is a database that indexes PhD candidates' dissertations. The Internet Movie Database (http://www.imdb.com) is a database of movies that includes a description of the plot, a listing of the characters (with links to the credited actors' biographies), the genre, and ratings/opinions of viewers about the film. A search using an Internet search engine also produces a database of material, but this database is the set of records containing the search keywords. As for the type of material, they are all Web pages. Some will be commercial Web sites designed to sell a product or service that is reputable or not, a government agency Web site created to disseminate information, university/college sites, sites developed by organizations to provide information to members and prospective members, and finally, sites created by individuals.

The Internet is a larger and less organized collection that numerous people have contributed to with little cooperation, organization, or quality

control. It's your responsibility to determine if the information is reliable and current. When searching the Internet, you use a search engine that employs several different methods of locating information (such as bots or spiders that search known pages and then follow the links found on them). That means that if a page is not indexed, it can be impossible to find. This information is used to create an index. When the spiders or bots identify a new page, it is added to the index. This information may not be added to the index immediately, and it is not available to a searcher until it has been added. Each search engine has different criteria about how and what it indexes, which is why the results from two different engines will be somewhat different.

Google is a search engine that is considered more complete in its indexing than some of the others (Sullivan, 2002). The portion of the Web that is accessible by search engines is known as the invisible Web. It is estimated that only about one-third of the Web is visible. It uses keyword searching to identify a match in locating the keywords that you entered. Each search engine utilizes a ranking method to determine the order in which the information retrieved is listed. It is important to note that sometimes the ranking is based upon compensation paid to the search engine company or the skill of the Web site designer (and not the actual relevance to your topic).

Web sites are created for a variety of purposes by a variety of people. There is no quality control or guarantee about the quality of the information retrieved. Whereas it is possible to locate relevant and reliable information from the Internet, this is usually not the most efficient method for identifying research articles. Locating peer-reviewed research literature using an Internet search engine is not recommended. The number of "hits" retrieved from a search engine can often number in the tens or hundreds of thousands. Sifting through these can be the modern equivalent of sitting on the floor in the library and flipping through a large number of journals trying to locate the needed information. Although surfing the Internet is not the most efficient method of researching the professional literature, it can be very useful in obtaining information and publications from professional organizations such as practice standards, clinical guidelines, licensure information, continuing education, and employment opportunities, to name a few.

TIPS FOR INTERNET SEARCHING

There are a few things that can be done to reduce the amount of retrieval and to increase the relevance of the retrieval when using an Internet search engine. The following hints are generic, so checking the help section of your favorite search engine is recommended.

1. Use capital letters only for proper nouns. Never type the entire query in capitals.

2. Use quotations on a phrase so it is searched as a phrase instead of individual words.

3. Find your favorite search engine and become familiar with its search rules and capabilities.

4. Use Boolean operators "and" "or" and "not" correctly. Boolean operators allow you to combine multiple terms in a search by connecting the terms with "AND"; allow you to search for synonyms simultaneously by connecting the terms with "OR"; and to exclude terms, for example, aspirin NOT Tylenol.

5. Use synonyms when the initial search terms do not retrieve the desired information.

6. Use truncation to retrieve multiple endings—**nur*** will retrieve "nurse," "nurses" or "nursing"; **nur*** will also retrieve "nurture," "Nuremberg" or "nurseryman." Figure 5.1 illustrates Boolean logic.

Figure 5.1 illustrates Boolean logic.

EVALUATING WEB SITES

Anyone can create a Web site and publish anything that they wish. There is no peer review or evaluation of material published on the Internet. Therefore, it is a case of "buyer beware," so the user should use some basic criteria to evaluate Web sites. Figure 5.2 offers several suggestions for evaluating Web sites.

RECOMMENDED WEB SITES

Web sites produced by professional nursing organizations can be an excellent source for position statements, credentialing information, professional news, employment listings, grant-funding information, and publications. Access to some sections, however, might be limited to members. Government

Boolean Operator	Example	
AND	Rum **AND** Coke	A drink containing both rum and coke
OR	Rum **OR** Coke	A drink that may be only rum, may be only coke, or may contain both rum and coke
Not	Coke **Not** Rum	A drink that is only coke
	Rum **Not** Coke	A drink that is only rum

Figure 5.1 Boolean Logic.

Web Page Characteristics	Check List
Accuracy	Is the information reliable and error free? Does the site contain contact information?
Authority	Is there an author listed? Is he qualified or an authority?
Objectivity	Is the purpose clearly stated? Why was the page created? Who is the intended audience?
Content	Is the information accurate? Do links go to authoritative sites? What is covered? What is the level of coverage?
Currency	Is there a date on the page? When was the last update? Do the links work or are they dead?

Figure 5.2 **Web page evaluation.**

Web sites such as the CDC, FDA, and the various institutes of health are useful to access government publications (usually accessible to all on the Internet). The state board of nursing for each state can be an excellent source for licensure requirements. Some universities and colleges may have research centers that can also be useful.

The last section of a URL (uniform resource locator) or Web address often provides some information about the type of page. Government sites usually end in .gov. The extensive state of Florida Web site, developed to make state information easily accessible to its citizens, ends in .com (myFlorida.com), so be aware that this is a guide and not a guaranteed rule. Educational institutions commonly end in .edu. The most common endings are .com, .gov, .mil., .edu, and .net. A site that ends in .com or .biz (or .co if it is a U.K. site) is usually a commercial site. Foreign Web sites may end with two letter endings such as .de for Germany, .ch for Switzerland or .za from South Africa. Checking the ending of a URL may give you some indication of the type of page it is.

Here are the URLs of some professional Web sites:

American Nurses Association:
    http://www.nurisngworld.org

Sigma Theta Tau International:
    http://www.nursingsociety.org

American Association of Critical Care Nurses:
    http://www.aacn.org/

AORN Online: The Association of Perioperative Registered Nurses:
    http://www.aorn.org

Oncology Nursing Society (ONS):
    http://www.ons.org

Keywords versus Subject Headings

Internet searching is only keyword or free-text searching. Many databases allow keyword searching but can also be searched by subject headings. Subject headings are a more powerful way of searching because it allows you to search with more precision and efficiency. Imagine you are doing a search to locate all of the information in a database about nonsteroidal anti-inflammatory drugs or NSAIDs. If you choose to search by keywords, imagine all of the words you must enter to make the search comprehensive! Some of the terms that should be entered would be Motrin, Advil, Tylenol, Bextra, Celebrex, Aspirin, Ibuprofen, Salsalate, Diflunisal, Diclofenac, misoprostol, Etodolac, Arthrotec, Lodine, Dolobid, Voltaren, Fenoprofen, Dalfon, Flurbiprofen, Ansaid, Indomethacin, Indocin, Ketoprofen, Orudis, Orvuail, Ketorolac, Torodol, Naproxen and so forth to make the search comprehensive. Obviously, this is not a very efficient way to conduct a search.

Using subject headings instead of keywords is a more efficient and effective method of searching. Subject headings are terms assigned to records by indexers in databases that use a controlled vocabulary. When searching for all records about nonsteroidal anti-inflammatory drugs in such a database, the only term that needs to be entered would be the subject heading that the database assigned to convey the concept of nonsteroidal anti-inflammatory drugs or NSAIDs. There is no need to enter all of the other related terms that would be necessary in a keyword search.

Different databases have different terms for subject headings. Sometimes they call it controlled vocabulary, thesaurus, MeSh (in PubMed) and CINAHL Headings in CINAHL. When using a new database, try to locate this feature. In most databases the controlled vocabulary is a database that can be searched to locate the best term to use. Many databases use a feature known as mapping, which attempts to take the entered term and locate related subject headings. When mapping is not able to identify relevant subject headings, it may be necessary to try synonyms. Another benefit of using subject headings in databases like CINAHL and PubMed is that an option is provided for using subheadings that allows the search to be focused on a particular aspect of that subject, such as psychosocial factors, drug therapy, etiology, adverse effects, or other options.

RECOGNIZING INFORMATION NEEDS AND DEVELOPING SEARCH STATEMENTS

When you have an assignment or a question in the clinical area that requires finding facts, research, or information, you have an information need. The first step is to convert the need into a search statement. Next, you must determine what the main concepts are, then decide if there are there any particular aspects of the question that are important. Finally, you must think about the type of information needed.

Imagine you have been given an assignment to write a paper about high blood pressure or hypertension. The assignment also states that you must use a minimum of 8 references. At least 6 of the references must be research articles from peer-reviewed journals published within the last 5 years. An initial database search reveals that there are thousands of articles about hypertension, so you revise your topic to focus on the treatment of the disorder. Now let's take the information need and turn it into a search statement.

What are the main concepts?
- Hypertension

What are the particular aspects?
- Treatment

What types of information?
- Peer reviewed
- Research articles
- Recent—published in the last 5 years

What is the search statement?

I am looking for articles about the treatment of hypertension from journals that are peer reviewed and report research that were published in the last 5 years.

Suppose the information you need is the type that would be found in research articles but factual information, such as what the range is for a complete blood count or standard dosing of erythromycin. How would you go about locating that type of information? When looking for established knowledge such as laboratory values, symptoms of congestive heart failure, or standard dosing of a sertraline, a textbook in print or electronic format is the place to look.

Developing a Search Statement

What are the main concepts?

- Compete blood test

What are the particular aspects?

- Normal laboratory values

What types of information?

- Established facts

What is the search statement?

What are the normal expected ranges from a complete blood test?

What are the main concepts?

- High cholesterol or hypercholesterolemia
- Alternative or complementary products

What are the particular aspects?

- Therapy
- Effective
- Safe

What type of information?

Research articles

What is the search statement?

I am looking for recent research articles about safe and effective alternative or complementary therapies for hypercholesterolemia.

INFORMATION RETRIEVAL

After clarifying your search statement and determining what type of information is needed, the next step is to locate and retrieve the desired information. Next, you must determine what database or databases would be best for conducting the search. After completing the database search and reviewing the results, there are usually some articles that the searcher wants to read entirely (not just the abstract). Depending upon the database and provider purchased by the library, the database may contain some of the articles in full text. If more full-text articles are needed, check with the library staff to determine if there are other options for obtaining full texts. Occasionally, articles can be located free of charge online. These articles may be in a sample issue of the journal available online, or it may be a continuing education article. Sometimes you can find an article online by typing the article title in quotations and searching for it on Google. If these

CASE SCENARIO 5.1

You have a patient assigned to you in your clinical rotation who has been diagnosed with high cholesterol, and his or her physician has prescribed Zocor, a statin to lower the cholesterol levels. The patient does not want to take the medication and wonders if there is any research about alternative or complementary therapies that would be as effective and safe.

Case Considerations

Take this information need and create a search statement.

methods are not successful, contact the library staff to see if the library owns the journal in print or electronic format. When a medical library does not have print or electronic access to an article that you need, they can order it via an efficient interlibrary loan service managed by the National Library of Medicine. If you are using PubMed, your library might allow you to register as a user of Loansome Doc if they offer this service. Loansome Doc allows you to enter interlibrary loan orders directly through the PubMed database. Libraries may offer this service to their users for a fee. Check with the library at your school or hospital to obtain more information about interlibrary loan policies and charges. Many online journals allow users to purchase access to individual articles but the cost may be high.

USEFUL DATABASES

The primary nursing database is CINAHL or Cumulated Index to Nursing and Allied Health Literature. Another very useful database is MEDLINE or PubMed, which is a biomedical database that also indexes nursing literature. Nursing is a very diverse and multidisciplinary field. Depending upon your area of specialization, PsychLit, which provides access to the psychological literature, might be a useful database. ERIC indexes the educational literature. Sociology Abstracts covers the sociology literature. Sometimes the business literature will need to be accessed, and there are a number of databases that could be useful. Your librarian can assist you in determining which specialized databases are available and would best serve your needs.

CINAHL

CINAHL is a database that covers material from 1982 to the present and indexes journal articles, books, dissertations, videos, computer files, pamphlets and other formats related to nursing and allied health. The format of the subject headings are based upon the basic structure and content of those in MEDLINE; however CINAHL is much more specific and detailed with regard to areas of interest in nursing and allied health. If this database is available to you, it should be your first choice when looking for information about the nursing process, nursing history, and issues related to the specific education level of nurses, nursing theory, or other nursing subjects.

CINAHL uses a controlled vocabulary. There are a number of different vendors that produce the database, so it is difficult to be specific about the mechanics of the database because it varies. If your institution provides access to the EBSCO Host version of the database, there is an interactive tutorial available that might be helpful. http://www.library. health.ufl.edu/help/'CINAHL/index.htm

PsycInfo

PsycInfo indexes the psychological literature. CINAHL and MEDLINE index some of the psychological literature, but to be comprehensive in this area it might be necessary to search all three. This database uses subject headings, but the level of detail is not as great as it is in either CINAHL or MEDLINE. PsycInfo is unique because it indexes back to the 1800s. This database is available only by subscription, so check with your institution to see if you have access.

MEDLINE (PubMed)

The scope of MEDLINE is much broader than either CINAHL or PubMed, and is seen in Figure 5.3. This is a biomedical database that covers the literature of medicine, dentistry, veterinary medicine, preclinical sciences, health care administration, and nursing, to name the major areas of coverage. There are over 12 million citations in 70 languages from almost 5000 journal titles dating back to the mid 1960s. It is possible to search only the nursing literature, and although there is some duplication of the journals indexed in CINAHL and MEDLINE, the list is not identical.

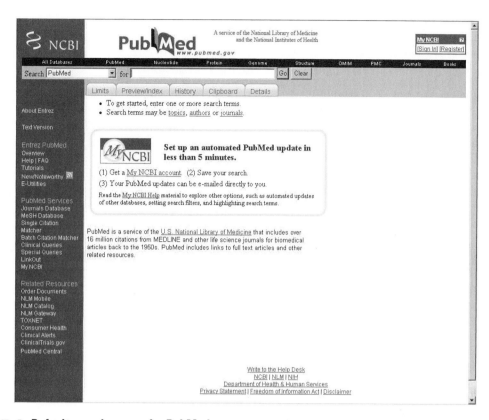

Figure 5.3 Default search screen for PubMed. © NLM National Library of Medicine. Reprinted with permission.

The National Library of Medicine produces the MEDLINE database. The information is available from a number of commercial database producers or in the PubMed format, which is available without charge to anyone with an Internet connection. PubMed is an example of a database that does an excellent job of mapping keywords to subject headings. The immense number of records in this database makes it prudent to utilize the power of the controlled vocabulary and other features to restrict the search to exactly what is desired. For example, a search of PubMed with the keywords "high blood pressure" retrieves over 158,000 records, and a search of "hypertension" as a keyword produces more than 240,000 records. Suppose you are only interested in the nursing care of patients with hypertension. If the search is changed to the keyword search "hypertension and nursing," the number of results is reduced to over 1480. If the search is "high blood pressure and nursing," the results are over 900. When this search is done using the subject headings or MeSH and the subheading "nursing," the results are over 300. The use of subject headings reduces what librarians refer to as false hits. False hits are results that contain the terms entered but are not actually about them. For example, a keyword search for citations about Florence Nightingale would contain some citations that contain the words Florence Nightingale but are not about her. In London there is a nursing school named the Florence Nightingale School of Nursing and Midwifery. Doing that keyword search will retrieve material that is not about Florence but is written

WRITING EXERCISE 5.1

The assignment for class is to prepare a presentation about the complications of using Vancomycin, a very powerful antibiotic. The research must be recent (last five years), in English, published in nursing journals, consist of randomized control trials, and be limited to middle-aged adults. The only database you have access to is PubMed (www.pubmed/gov).

1. Take your information need and write a search statement:

   I need research about the complications of using vancomycin on middle-aged adults. The research articles need to be written in English, published in nursing journals, published in the last five years, and be randomized control trials.

2. What are the main concept(s)

   Vancomycin and complications

3. What type of information do you need?

Randomized control research articles in English that are recent

4. What type of subjects?

   Middle-aged adults

Now go to the MeSH browser in PubMed.

What subject heading are you going to search to locate?

   Vancomycin

Are there any appropriate subheadings?

   Adverse effects

Now run the search and then use the "Limit" function to limit the search.

Language: English

Publication type: Randomized control trial

Age: Middle age, 45–64

Subset: Nursing Journals

Publication date: The year that will limit the results to the last five years

---

by faculty from that institution. MEDLINE also includes a feature called "Limits," which serves as another tool for focusing in on the desired information. Limits allows citations restricted to English, a particular date range, sex of subjects, age groups, type of publication (editorials, meta-analysis or randomized control trials, to name a few), or subject areas such as nursing literature.

To locate this database go to http://www.pubmed.gov. The National Library of Medicine has created a helpful tutorial available from a link on the left side of the screen in the blue side bar. Using this database for general information can be deceivingly easy, but obtaining focused relevant results take some skill and practice.

HAS THE INTERNET MADE LIBRARIES OBSOLETE?

With the proliferation of electronic journals, electronic books, and databases, is there still a need for libraries? Contrary to commonly held belief, many of these resources are not available for free. Often the library at your college, university, or hospital provides access to many of these resources either on-site or remotely. Libraries also provide access to print books and journals; not every book and journal is available in electronic format. When a library does not own the book or the particular issue of a journal you need, they can usually borrow it from another library through interlibrary loan. This service is provided for free or at a cost usually less than what you would pay for electronic access on the Web. Librarians can assist you in locating material full text, suggesting the best databases for what you are looking for, and identifying the best subject headings. Medical librarians are health information specialists. You are the expert in knowing what information you need. Together, imagine how successful the search will be.

EVIDENCE-BASED PRACTICE RESOURCES

The concept of evidence-based practice is becoming an important movement in nursing. If you are not yet aware of this area, you soon will be. The most commonly used definition of evidence-based practice is the integration of the best research evidence with clinical expertise and patient values (Sackett, Straus, Richardson, Rosenberg, & Haynes, 2000). Basically, what evidence-based practice does is to utilize synthesized research literature and use it to make clinical decisions. Clinical practice should be based upon what research has proven is effective. There is a variety of quality resources both free and through subscription on the Internet. The following is a list of some of those resources:

- AHRQ—Agency for Healthcare Research and Quality
  http://ahcpr.gov/clinic/epcix.htm
- United States Preventive Services Task Force
  http://www.ahrq.gov/clinic/uspstfix.htm
- Bandolier
  http://www.jr2.oix.ac.uk/bandolier/index.html
- The Joanna Briggs Institute
  http://www.joannabriggs.edu.au/
- McMaster University Evidence-Based Health Care Resources

  http://www.cochrane.mcmaster.ca/evidence-based.htm
- National Guideline Clearinghouse
  http://www.guidelines.gov
- Sarah Cole Hirsh Institute
  http://www.hirshinstitute.com/default.htm
- University of York Centre for Evidence-Based Nursing (EBN)
  http://www.york.ac.uk/depts/hstd/centers/evidence/ev-intro.htm
- University of Rochester Center for Nursing
  http://www.urmc.rochester.edu/son/research/crebp.html
- Cochrane Collaboration
  http://www.cochrane.org
- EBN Online
  http://ebn.bmjjournals.com

WRITING RESOURCES

Each profession uses writing as an essential tool of communication between members of the profession. Nursing is no exception to this tradition. Nurses write for a variety of purposes: to complete a writing assignment for a class, to communicate the results of research, to document innovative programs or practice techniques, and to express opinions that are either personal or professional. Professional writing tends to be written in the active voice and in the third person. Each profession tends to use one predominant style for citations and references. Nursing uses APA or the American Psychological Association style. Periodically, this style is updated as new items (such as how to cite a Web page or e-mail in a bibliography) are added to stay current. It is important to always use the latest version when writing. It is strongly suggested that if this is the style your school requires for written assignments, you purchase the APA manual. It is available in most bookstores and at Internet bookselling sites. Here are some Web sites that might be helpful.

- The APA site
  http://www.apastyle.org/elecref.html
- OWL Online Writing Lab Purdue University
  http://owl.english.purdue.edu/handouts/research/r_apa.html
- Bedford Martin Online: Using Principles of APA Style to Cite and Document Sources
  http://www.bedfordstmartins.com/online/cite6.html
- Dr Mary Ellen Guffey APA Style Formats Electronic
  http://www.westwords.com/guffey/apa.html

LIFELONG LEARNING AND STAYING UP TO DATE

Keeping up with the literature can seem overwhelming because so much is written every year; but there are some services that can be helpful. Once you begin practicing, you will develop an area of expertise, and this will somewhat narrow the type of research that interests you. Labor and delivery nurses have little need or interest in congestive heart failure or Alzheimer's disease unless family members have these conditions. Many databases such as CINAHL and PubMed allow you to save search strategies, and they will rerun the search periodically and e-mail the results to you. Another tool is receiving the table of contents of select journals electronically. The increasing number of electronic journals makes more available. To have the table of contents e-mailed to you, simply do a Web search for a journal Web site and look for e-mail or electronic table of contents. This service is usually available without requiring a subscription. Other electronic services include listservs where members post questions, answers, and information that other listserv members may find useful.

Another service is Nurse Linx. You can register for this service at (www.nurselinx.com) and receive an e-mail each weekday of selected journal citations and abstracts from a variety of current journals that are predominantly nursing but occasionally medical when the topic is relevant. The majority of the specialties are medical, but there is a general nursing and a nurse practitioner option.

CHAPTER SUMMARY

In this chapter, some of the differences between professional publications and popular press articles are discussed. The concept of peer-reviewed or refereed publications is introduced and its value in maintaining the quality of professional literature is discussed.

The type of information located with a search of the Internet with a search engine and a bibliographic database is presented. The type of material available in libraries is also presented. CINAHL, PubMed, and PsychInfo are the main databases for searching the nursing literature. Using the controlled vocabulary and other database features can focus the results of a search and limit the retrieval to citations that are closer to the topic being searched. Several Web resources for nursing information are presented. Web sites that offer tips about the use of APA format are included. To facilitate lifelong learning, several options are listed.

> *Technological progress has merely provided us with more efficient means for going backwards.*
>
> —Aldous Huxley

REFERENCES

Bush, J. (2001). Is it time to re-examine family practice? *Family Practice Management, 8*(8), 43–48.

Glasziou, P., Del Mar, D., Salisbury, J., & NetLibrary, I. (2003). *Evidence-based medicine workbook*. London: Bmj. from http://www.netLibrary.com/urlapi.asp?action=summary&v=1&bookid=103832

Sackett, D. L., Straus, S. E., Richardson, W. S., Rosenberg, W., & Haynes, R. B. (2000). *Evidence-based medicine: How to practice and teach EBM* (2nd ed.). Edinburgh: Churchhill, Livingstone.

Sullivan, D. (2002). *How search engines work.* Retrieved July 22, 2005, from http://searchenginewatch.com/webmasters/article.php/2168031

ADDITIONAL RESOURCES

Evaluating web sites: Criteria and tool (2004). Retrieved July 22, 2005, from http://www.library.cornell.edu/olinuris/ref/research/webeval.html

Beck, S. E. (2005). *The good, the bad and the ugly: Or why it's a good idea to evaluate web pages*. Retrieved July 22, 2005, from http://lib.nmsu.edu/instruction/eval.html

Fitzpatrick, J. J. & Montgomery, K. S. (2003). *Internet resources for nurses* (2nd ed.). New York: Springer Pub. Co.

Thede, L. Q. (2003). *Informatics and nursing: Opportunities and challenges* (2nd ed.). Philadelphia: Lippincott, Williams & Wilkins.

CHAPTER 6

Theoretical Basis for the Practice of Nursing

Vicky P. Kent

Words are a form of action, capable of influencing change.
—Herman Melville

LEARNING OBJECTIVES

At the completion of the chapter, the learner should be able to do the following:

1. Define theory.
2. Define nursing theory.
3. Describe the historical evolution of the development of nursing theories.
4. Identify domain concepts relevant to nursing.
5. Compare and contrast the definitions of the domain concepts of selected nurse theorists.
6. Describe the relationship of theory to nursing practice.
7. Identify controversial issues regarding the use of nursing theories.

KEY TERMS

Domain concepts: Person, Nursing, Health, Environment

Grand theory

Metaparadigm

Middle range theory

Nursing theory

Practice theory

The vocabulary of nursing theory

Theory

This chapter emphasizes the importance of clear and precise language as a means to define nursing and nursing theory. It provides the reader with a historical overview of the development and use of theories in nursing practice. It is not meant to be an exhaustive summary of all theories developed or used by nurses, nor a critical evaluation of existing theories. On the other hand, it is meant to give the reader a broad sense of how theories inform practice, research, and subsequent knowledge development in the discipline.

NURSING AS A PROFESSION

Dictionaries such as the Oxford English Dictionary (1971) tell us that the term *nurse* has existed in English from at least as far back as the fourteenth century from an older word meaning to nourish. The nurse suckled or practiced a form of childcare. From that meaning, a nurse came to mean a person, usually a woman, who tended to the sick.

These days, the practice of nursing encompasses the domain of four concepts: **person, health, nursing,** and **environment**. By person, we refer to the human being interacting with the nurse for health reasons. Nursing includes an analysis of the patient's situation, a diagnosis, devising a plan for healthcare, putting that plan into action, and a postaction analysis of the healthcare provided. This is what we refer to as the nursing process. Health is not only a state of not being ill, it includes an evaluation of how people interact with their environment. The environment is the place, time, and situation in which the patient and nurse exist.

Nurse scholars have developed numerous frameworks, models, and theories that incorporate the four concepts indicated above. The theories this chapter will examine claim that the relationship connecting the four concepts is unique to nursing. One characteristic of a profession is that it has a unique body of knowledge; the development of nursing theories and their application to the care of society is one way in which nursing distinguishes itself as a profession.

DERIVATION AND DEFINTION OF THE WORD *THEORY*

A **theory** is a fundamental set of propositions about how the world works. Its meaning is derived from the Greek word *theoria,* "contemplation, speculation, a looking at, things looked at," from *theorein* "to consider, speculate, look at," from *theoros* "spectator," from thea "a view" + horan "to see." *Theater* comes from Greek *theatron* "theater," literally "place for viewing," from *theasthai* "to behold" (Online Etymology Dictionary, 2005).

Senge (2005) suggests that theories are invented for the same reasons as theater, to bring forth ideas to help us better understand our world. Theories also provide a discipline with a foundation for examining truths.

A theory is a way of analyzing facts and finding the relationships that the latter have to one another. It is a hypothesis or an educated guess. A theory is a system by which we link a set of principles to a particular perspective, as well as being the idea behind our actions. Practice, or praxis, is the series of actions that the nurse performs. These actions are supported by existing theory and in some cases form the basis of new theory in nursing.

Nursing theory uses its own terminology to link the work nurses do to the core principles of the profession of nursing. Nursing theory is not the explanation of the career; it is the tools with which to understand the correlation among concepts central to the practice and to those actions that define and describe the work of the profession. Theories consist of concepts, propositions, and laws, which can be communicated; it is invented, rather than found (Dickoff & James, 1968). Meleis (1997) states that nursing theories are "reservoirs for answers to significant nursing phenomena" (p. 13). Thus, in developing, describing, and using theory, nursing theorists create a way to communicate the essence of nursing values and practices to each other and to practitioners of other disciplines.

HISTORICAL OVERVIEW OF THEORY DEVELOPMENT IN NURSING

Florence Nightingale's work marks the beginning of theoretical development in nursing. Her observations, actions, and evaluation of those actions establish the basis for nursing practice as we know it. It is from her writings in *Notes on Nursing* (1946) that the **metaparadigm** concepts of person, nursing, health, and environment emerge as essential conditions for the discipline of nursing. Nightingale clearly delineates a set of guidelines and propositions about how nurses are to proceed in caring for their patients. It is her view that knowledge is essential for any profession, and that nursing knowledge is different from medical knowledge (Nightingale, 1946). Furthermore, the practice of nursing as both an art and a science requires that nurses continue to learn and grow as professionals.

For the remainder of the nineteenth century and well into the twentieth century, nurses derived their knowledge from the biological and social sciences and were dependent on physicians' orders to provide guidance for practice. The medical model of disease and pathology is the focus of nursing interventions. According to Chinn and Kramer (2004), administrators of hospital-based schools of nursing believe that knowledge of theory is unnecessary and would, in fact, be detrimental to the nurse.

Spurred by the movement of nursing education from hospital-based training schools to universities and the desire to demonstrate that nursing has its own scientific body of knowledge, nurses begin to explore and test theories that would distinguish nursing from medicine (Joel, 2003). It would take one hundred years from Nightingale's initial writings, however, before any work was published related to theory in nursing. The first published theory and text,

Interpersonal Relations in Nursing, which describes the interpersonal relationship between the nurse and the client is that of Hildegard Peplau in 1952. Peplau's theory stimulates considerable debate among nursing scholars about the use of and need for theories that are uniquely nursing.

Interest in the development of nursing theories abounded during the decades of the fifties and sixties. Predominant nurse theorists and scholars of the time focused their efforts on establishing nursing as a scientific discipline. To this end, nurse scholars began to debate the use of borrowed theories and their relevance to nursing practice versus the development and creation of theories specific to an applied practice discipline. Donnelly (2001) writes, "by the end of the 1960s, the nursing community began to identify the writings of many scholars as theories even though the writers themselves did not necessarily claim their work as theories" (p. 332). During this period there was also considerable discussion in the literature about the importance of the philosophy of science and its impact on the development of nursing theories and knowledge development.

All of these discussions continued well into the twentieth century. During the 1970s and 1980s nurse scholars and researchers continued to refine their ideas. Building on the work of Nightingale, Fawcett (1984) writes about the core concepts that are central to the domain of nursing practice: nursing, person, health, and the environment. These metaparadigm concepts originally articulated by Nightingale (1946) and formalized by Fawcett in 1984 became the underlying framework from which scholars developed theories and models.

The next step in the formalization and validation of nursing theory took place in 1985. The creation through legislation of the Center for Nursing Research (NCNR), later known as the National Institute for Nursing Research (NINR) and housed within the National Institutes of Health (NIH), is a defining moment in the recognition of the contributions nurses make to creating and maintaining a healthy society (Joel, 2003). With the establishment of the NCNR, monies became available for nursing research. As funding became increasingly available for research, nurse scholars began to examine and evaluate the extent to which existing nursing theories and models were useful and relevant for practice. It was also during the 1980s that nurse scholars developed extensive criteria by which professionals could determine the reliability, validity and applicability of existing theories (Fawcett, 1980; Meleis, 1997).

Much of the work of the late twentieth century and into the twenty-first century focused on the development of middle-range theories and practice theories. Middle-range theories and practice theories are, according to Fawcett (2000) and Meleis (1997), less abstract than grand theories. The midrange theories have articulated more clearly the relationships among the concepts, are applicable to practice situations, and are more appropriate for empirical research than grand theories (Liehr & Smith, 1999; Young, Taylor, & Renpenning, 2001). Liehr and Smith suggest that refinement of existing middle-range theories is essential to continued theory and knowledge development as the discipline moves into the twenty-first century.

LEVELS AND TYPES OF NURSING THEORIES

Nursing theory incorporates the four concepts of person, health, nursing, and environment, which represent the metaparadigm or worldview of the discipline. A metaparadigm, according to Fawcett (1984), is the broad perspective that describes and explains the phenomenon of interest in the discipline and helps explain how the discipline deals with that phenomenon. Throughout the history of nursing, theorists have returned to these principles as the basis from which to develop ideas about and recommendations for nursing practice.

Fitzpatrick and Whall (1996) describe three levels of theory as relevant and important to the development of nursing knowledge. These nursing theories are **grand, middle-range,** and **practice theories.** Grand theories are the most abstract in

nature, providing us with broad definitions of the domain concepts, their relationship to practice, and the fundamental actions of nurses (Jacox, 1974). Middle-range theories are less abstract, contain fewer concepts, and provide us with definitions and expectations of the nurse/client interaction that are more precise. Middle-range theories, according to Joel (2003), are the most testable and have the greatest relevance for practice. According to Chinn & Kramer (1995), however, middle-range theories do not cover the complete range of phenomenon of interest in the profession, but do cover a broad enough scope of issues that are of concern to the discipline. Practice theories are the least abstract and delineate specific actions for practice (Higgins & Moore, 2000).

Scholars such as Dickoff and James (1968) characterize nursing theories not according to their level of abstraction, but according to their ability to describe, explain, predict, or prescribe phenomena of interest in the discipline. These types of theories are factor isolating (descriptive), factor relating (explanatory), situation relating (predictive), and situation producing (prescriptive). According to Dickoff and James, the ultimate goal of theory development is to move beyond merely describing and explaining the phenomena of the discipline. Nursing theories need to be able to predict and be useful to prescribe the phenomena of concern.

In this chapter, we describe the work of four celebrated theorists: Florence Nightingale, Hildegard Peplau, Martha Rogers, and Sister Callista Roy, whose theories are characterized as grand theories or models by some nurse analysts (Whall, 1996; Roy & Andrews, 1999), but lend themselves to the development of middle-range theories. Peplau's Theory of Interpersonal Relationships, however, has also been called a middle-range theory (Fawcett, 2000). These theories have also been categorized according to the underlying philosophy or worldview of the writer and in some instances according to the emphasis each theorist places on one of the four metaparadigm concepts (Meleis, 1997).

Regardless of how one categorizes the work of each of these theorists, all of these and many others

---

BOX 6.1   Common Elements of Nursing Theories

If the nurse understands theory as thought and reasoning based on fact, what are the facts of nursing? Some commonly accepted certainties are

- People (individuals, families, and communities) are the recipients of nursing care. (Person)
- All people have varying states of health. (Health)

- Nurses assist clients in coping with their health needs. (Nursing)
- Some variables that affect health are environment, genetics, and economic circumstances. In addition, the client or client caretaker makes choices daily about the client's health. (Environment).

---

have contributed to the body of knowledge that is nursing and have laid the foundation for the development of practice theory, or how people function in their everyday lives (Stevenson, 2005). These theories offer a pragmatic approach to the actions deemed useful and necessary to function in the discipline. Each theory incorporates the metaparadigm concepts of person, health, nursing, and environment, which are essential concepts relevant to the practice of nursing. Figure and Box 6.1 describe the common elements of nursing theories.

OVERVIEW OF SELECTED NURSE THEORISTS

Florence Nightingale, Hildegard Peplau, Martha Rogers, and Sister Callista Roy are some of the more notable theorists in the profession of nursing. Their work contributed tremendously to the development of nursing knowledge. Each of their theories identifies and defines what it is that nurses do which is particular to the discipline of nursing and different from the discipline of medicine.

Although Florence Nightingale did not explicitly state that nurses need a theoretical basis for practice, she recognized that nursing knowledge is distinct from medical knowledge and that a profession needs

to have a distinct body of knowledge (Nightingale, 1946). The others, Peplau (1952), Rogers (1970) and Roy (1970), stated in their early works that there is a need for a theoretical basis for nursing practice.

During their respective lifetimes, Nightingale, Peplau, and Rogers left three distinct legacies that still have a major impact on current developments in nursing theory. As of this writing, Roy continues her work as a professor and nurse theorist at Boston College.

Florence Nightingale

Florence life's accomplishments were extraordinary. Women of her time were not expected to have any interest outside family and social obligations. She had a keen desire to improve the welfare of others and expressed endless frustration about her inability to fulfill what she believed to be her responsibility to use her social position to right societal injustices (Nightingale, 1946). At the age of 31 she was finally able to extricate herself from her family and realize her dream of becoming a nurse. Her remarkable accomplishments include improving the British military health care system, thus influencing military nursing, improving sanitation conditions in hospitals in England, and developing nursing schools.

It was Nightingale's vision to train nurses to be hypervigilant in the war against unsanitary conditions and impurities in the environment. Her goal for the

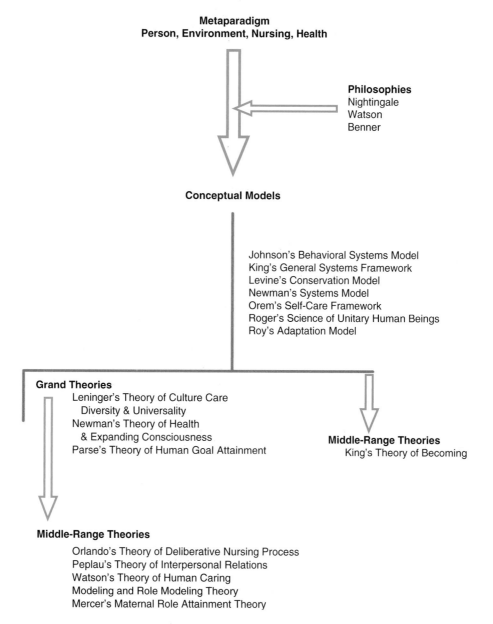

Figure 6.1 Structural hierarchy of contemporary nursing knowledge components.

SOURCE: Based on information from Meleis, A. I. (1997). *Theoretical nursing: Development and progress* (3rd ed.). Philadelphia: Lippincott.

patient was to raise the nurse from the level of merely a servant/companion who doles out medicine and makes no real decisions to that of a keen observer of the environment and the main decision maker for the least obstacles to health for the patient.

Nightingale emphasized that the focus of nursing care is the patient, not the illness. Nursing activities encompass health promotion, disease prevention, recovery from illness, and environmental control issues. Nurses can bring about change in the patient's condition by using "fresh air, light, warmth, cleanliness, quiet, and the administration of a [proper] diet" (Nightingale, 1946, p. 5). In Nightingale's model, the nurse must take charge of the surroundings to provide the most positive impact on the patient. The control of noise and light are important factors in the patient's recovery.

Hildegard Peplau

Hildegard Peplau was a first generation American born in 1901 to Polish immigrants. Like Nightingale, she also had a vision for nurses and nursing. She was a psychiatric nurse whose ideas developed as a result of her experience and understanding of interpersonal relationships. Peplau believed that "the principles which underlie interpersonal relations would transform nursing situations into learning experiences and these experiences could be a reference source of hypothesis that could have relevance for all nursing situations" (1952, pg. xi.). In Peplau's Interpersonal Relations Theory, nursing is psychodynamic. It is characterized by its wholeness.

As did Nightingale, Peplau envisioned the work of nursing as the elevation of the patient to the highest degree of wellness possible: the resolution of illness. According to Peplau's theory, the nurse and patient build a relationship that allows both to gain knowledge from the experience. The nurse acts in many different capacities and takes on many roles while assisting the patient to achieve independence.

Peplau identified four phases as integral to the therapeutic relationship. These include orientation, identification, exploitation, and resolution. Identifying problems and factors that motivate the client to seek help is the fundamental goal of the orientation phase. Clarification of the problem is ongoing in the identification phase; the client assesses the nurse's ability to help and begins identifying with the nurse based on the client's belief that the nurse is capable of helping. During the exploitation phase, the client begins to make use of all available resources. The resolution phase of the relationship is marked by the emergence of new issues, once the original issue has been resolved.

Although the potential for professional growth is a hallmark of Interpersonal Relations Theory, the key to a successful therapeutic relationship is for the nurse to understand that the client's needs are the focus of the relationship. The nurse must heed and use the following self concepts when engaging in a safe interpersonal relationship with the client: anxiety, pattern interactions, self, and modes of experiencing (Peplau, 1989). Understanding and applying these concepts decreases the potential for conflict and confusion that may occur when the nurse's needs instead of the client's become the focus of the relationship. It is the shared relationship, the interpersonal process, characterized by the four distinct, yet overlapping phases that enables the nurse to assist the patient to move forward (Peplau, 1952, 1997) from a point of dependence on health care providers to self-reliance.

According to Peplau, the nurse/client relationship begins as two strangers who interact. The key is building trust through open and honest communication. To Peplau, nursing is a process of assisting the client to move from a state of dependence to independence and self-reliance. It is the nurse's responsibility to help the client identify constructive resources. In a modern setting, Peplau would help the client work on psychological and sociological problems, all the while working to resolve the client's physical problems. For example, Peplau might refer the client with alcohol problems to Alcoholics Anonymous. She might further refer the client's family to Al-Anon or Alateen groups. The nurse educates the client to deal with new or tangential psychological or sociological issues that develop simultaneously or as a result of the client's physical problem. The nurse provides the tools to help clients help themselves. As the client's condition improves, both the nurse and the client develop a positive relationship that ultimately improves the confidence and competence of the nurse. It is important that the nurse's professional growth not occur at the expense of the client.

Martha Rogers

As did Nightingale and Peplau before her, Martha Rogers believed that nursing is uniquely different from medicine. It was her desire to demonstrate the unique and distinct body of nursing knowledge that prompted her to develop the theory of Unitary Human Beings (Rogers, 1970), which later became known as the Science of Unitary Human Beings (SUHB) (Rogers, 1983). Rogers' theory emphasizes the importance of viewing the person as a unified whole in constant interaction with the environment. The SUHB theory examines nurses and clients within the context of an evolutionary multi-dimensional energy system.

The theory draws on principles of quantum physics, offers that at the particle level all matter is energy. This energy, organized as a field, is a fundamental unit of man and his environment. The human energy field that is referred to as unitary man is irreducible. There is constant interaction between man and the environment. This relationship is described as a multidimensional or pandimensional energy field. It is a shared process characterized by openness, pattern and organization, four-dimensionality (pan dimensionality), and mutual energy fields. Embedded in the SUHB theory, which Rogers revised in 1970, 1980, 1983, and 1989 are the principles of integrality, resonancy, helicy, and integrality. These principles suggest that there is an ongoing exchange of energy between the persons and the environment (integrality). Life processes have high and low frequency wave patterns that are rhythmical in nature (resonancy), and that these patterns are nonrepetitive, with increased diversity (helicy).

The goal of nursing is to assist humans to achieve the highest level of health possible by promoting symphonic interaction between the person and the environment. Nurses achieve this goal by directing and redirecting patterns of interaction (Rogers, 1983). Nurses are also human energy fields. They are an integral part of the patient's environment, and a mutual interaction of energy exchange occurs during the nurse/client relationship.

As did Nightingale, Rogers emphasized the importance of the environment. For Rogers, the environment extends beyond the course of an episode of health or illness and includes health care professionals, family, home, and community. The client is more than just a person with a disease. He is part of everyone and everything in the universe and, as such, is affected by a constant exchange of energy. The focus of nursing care should be the positive interaction between the client and his environment. People are continually in the process of "becoming." Both wellness and illness are part of the continuum of a client's ongoing life. Imagine a nurse in a modern day who has just come on to the unit in a hospital. Does this nurse seek a positive interaction with each patient? Does the nurse resist coming to work hungover or otherwise impaired so that she is at her best and most functional when taking care of sick people? Mood and energy level have a direct impact on the well-being of the patient. For Rogers, the nurse's self-awareness helps patients to be aware of how best to meet their own needs. Nurses who subscribe to the SUHB theory view clients as inseparable from their environment. Nursing interventions ensure that the client understands this relationship of health, illness and environment. Nurses work collaboratively with their clients to direct or redirect energy to promote harmony and ultimately positive interaction between the client and the environment.

Sister Callista Roy

Roy (1978) acknowledges that events in her personal, as well as her professional life, influence the development of her model. The second child of a large family, she joined a religious order when she graduated from high school. She completed her undergraduate education as a Sister of Saint Joseph at Mount St. Mary's College in California. She developed the Roy Adaptation Model (RAM) in 1964 while she was a graduate student at the University of California.

The Roy Adaptation Model, first published in 1970 was derived from principles of Helson's adaptation theory. Helson's premise was that one's ability to respond positively to a changing environment is dependent upon the degree of change and the person's ability to cope with change and is essentially a pooled effect of multiple influences (Roy, 1976, 1997). Roy's observation of children's adaptive responses to illness serves as the foundation for the development of her adaptation model for nursing. Some present-day scholars believe that Roy's own neurological illness in 1966 may have served as the impetus for the refinement of her theory and for subsequent publication of the theory and use as a conceptual model for nursing education and practice (Boston College. com, 2003).

The core concept of the RAM model is adaptation, which is "the process and outcome whereby thinking and feeling persons, as individuals or in groups, use conscious awareness and choice to create human and environmental integration" (Roy & Andrews, 1999, p. 30). Humans are whole, open, and adaptive systems capable of responding to stimuli in their environment using special coping mechanisms, the latter of which allow for successful adaptation to a dynamic environment. Adaptation is considered a positive response to change.

According to this model, persons are adaptive systems who experience multiple stimuli (inputs), develop methods for handling the stimuli (coping processes), and generate responses (outputs). Stimuli may arise from internal or external sources and are classified as focal, contextual, or residual. Two subsystems, the regulator and the cognator, control adaptive or ineffective responses. The client uses these innate or acquired mechanisms to deal with a changing environment (Roy & Andrews, 1999). The regulator works through the autonomic nervous system, while the cognator deals with information processing. These control mechanisms function to maintain the integrity of the client in one of four adaptive modes: physiologic needs, self-concept, role function, and interdependence. Responses to stimuli manifest through the adaptive modes, thus revealing the adaptation level of the client.

Nursing is "a profession that focuses on human life processes and patterns and emphasizes promotion of health for individuals, groups and society as a whole" (Roy & Andrews, 1999, p. 4). The goal of nurses using the RAM theory is to assist adaptation in each of the four modes in health and illness. This is accomplished using a six-step nursing process: assessing behaviors and stimuli that affect the adaptive modes, identifying appropriate nursing diagnoses, developing and implementing interventions to enhance the adaptive functions, and evaluating the interventions.

Roy's premise is that patients are dependant and must adapt to whatever is going on in their lives. Every person has an innate ability to adapt. It is the nurse's responsibility to identify and to bring forward that ability. Imagine an amputee who must safely transfer from a bed to a chair. Imagine another patient who has lost a job and needs agency resources and support. Imagine a third patient who has recently given birth, but whose postpartum depression is an obstacle to her successfully functioning as a mother. In each case, imagine that Roy's intervention would be to help the patient adapt for survival. Assess the problem, determine the basic need, and help the client develop the innate ability to adapt. Whether it is physically helping a patient transfer from one location to another, providing information about useful community resources, or helping find needed counseling, the nurse who uses Roy's model reasons that if health care professionals cannot remove the obstacle to survival, the only answer is to help the patient survive through adaptation to the new situation.

There are similarities and a subtle difference in the way each theory incorporates the terminology used to describe nursing, nursing activities, the patient, and the environment. These differences can be attributed to the historical time period in which the theorists develop their ideas, as well as their philosophical way of viewing the world. A very common theme, however, that is clearly evident in each of the theories cited is that nurses as professionals are responsible for actions conducted for the benefit of improving, maintaining and sustaining health. Table 6.1 provides a succinct description and comparison of each of the described theories. It includes basic assumptions underlying the theories and a description of the metaparadigm concepts of person, health nursing, and environment.

Table 6.1 Table of Theorists

Theorist	Metaparadigm Concepts	Assumptions
Nightingale	Person: biopsychosocial, physical, intellectual, spiritual being who is suffering; has the potential to change.	People are unique. Disease is a reparative process.
	Nursing: an art and a science; activities are directed toward changing the patient's environment.	Good observational and interpersonal relationship skills are essential.
	Health: not the opposite of illness; affected by the environment.	It is the imbalance between the patient and the environment that causes illness.
	Environment: the external conditions that contribute to illness or well-being.	
Peplau	Person: an organism who lives in an unstable environment.	The kind of person each nurse becomes makes a difference in what the patient will learn as care is given.
	Nursing: an interpersonal therapeutic process; actions promote forward movement of the patient to constructive living.	Good interpersonal relationships are essential to life.
	Health: word symbol; implies forward movement of personality and other ongoing processes.	The nurse has a legal responsibility for actions and consequences of those actions.
	Environment: external forces that exist within the context of culture.	
Rogers	Person: an organized energy field; irreducible; characterized by pandimensionality; constant interaction with the environment; a unified whole.	Life is a shared process characterized by openness in pattern and organization, pandimensionality and mutual energy fields.
	Nursing: learned profession; a science and an art; studies man's development in relationship to constant interaction with the environment.	Energy fields are open, dynamic, unique.
	Health: patterns that denote behaviors of high or low value.	Wave patterns change continuously and become increasingly complex.
	Environment: irreducible, pandimensional energy field, an infinite, open system, change continues and is mutual with the human energy field.	
Roy	Person: bio-psycho-social being in constant interaction with the environment who has capacity for self-determination.	Individuals adapt to coping with stimuli from the environment.

(*continues*)

Table 6.1 *(Continued)*

Theorist	Metaparadigm Concepts	Assumptions
	Nursing: science and practice of promoting adaptation in situations involving health and illness.	Adaptation is a dynamic process.
	Health: state and process of becoming whole; adaptive response to stimuli.	Stimuli (input) are controlled two subsystems of coping mechanisms: regulator and cognator.
	Environment: contains input to person; includes internal and external stimuli.	Stimuli are focal, contextual, and residual.
		Persons have the creativity, capacity, and ability to cope with stimuli.
		Adaptation is the positive response to the stimuli.

SOURCES: Nightingale (1946), Peplau (1952), Rogers, (1970, 1989) Roy (1970), Roy & Andrews (1999).

WRITING EXERCISE 6.1

This chapter describes four nursing theories: Nightingale's Environmental Theory, Peplau's Interpersonal Relations Theory, Rogers Science of Unitary Human Beings, and Roy's Adaptation Model. (1) Develop a brief paper comparing and contrasting the common elements of each theory. (2) Describe the client's environment and health in your own words. (3) Discuss the way your definitions of environment and health may be similar to or different from the perspectives and conceptual frameworks of the theorists presented in his chapter.

As you read the following case studies, use these guide questions to apply a theorist's model to the case in question.

1. What are the most important elements of this theorist's model?

2. What definition does this theorist use for person, nursing health, and environment?

3. What are the facts to consider in this case scenario?

4. Looking at the case scenario through the eyes of the perspective of the theorist you have chosen,

   ▪ What person or people are the principle players in the story?

   ▪ What is the role of the nurse in this case?

   ▪ How does health become an integral element of this case scenario?

   ▪ What is the environment of this case?

CASE SCENARIO 6.1

A male client, 58-years-old, requires an angioplasty for treatment of a myocardial infarction. His wife of 30 years and their daughters, ages 16 and 25, accompany him to the hospital on the morning of the procedure. The nurse directs the family members to the waiting room and takes the client into the preoperating holding suite.

While the nurse prepares the client for surgery, the latter expresses anxiety about the surgery. "My physician explained the procedure, and it sounds like a fairly routine operation. I'm just a bit nervous, though; I've never had major surgery." The nurse responds with gentle reassurance and encourages the client to express his feelings. The nurse finishes the preoperative routine and wheels the client into the operating suite.

The nurse transfers the client to the operating table, covering him with a warm blanket after he is secured on the table. She stays in the room with the client until the surgeon begins the procedure. The nurse notifies family members that the procedure is underway.

Periodically, the nurse assesses the status of the patient during the procedure. The surgery proceeds without complication. The surgical outcome at this stage is successful. The nurse takes the client to the postanesthesia care unit (PACU). After he awakens, the nurse takes family members to see him. The client complains of pain and is teary eyed. His wife and 25-year-old daughter remain composed, but his 16-year-old daughter begins to cry, which in turn, causes the client to cry. The PACU nurse observes the interaction. She approaches the bedside, assesses the patient, and determines that he is recovering without problems. She reassures the patient and family members, instructs the family about postoperative expectations, and encourages them to return to the waiting room. The nurse inquires about additional support systems and determines that the rabbi and a member of the synagogue are present.

Case Considerations

1. How do you define client? Given your definition, who is the client in this situation?

2. Can you apply one theory to this situation better than another? Which one?

3. How does the data support your choice? According to the perspective of the theory you have chosen for this case scenario,
   - Who is the client?
   - What is the environment?
   - What is health?
   - What is the role of the nurse?

4. What additional data would help you decide which theory is applicable in this situation?

THEORY AND PRACTICE

Two essential questions arise when one considers the theory/practice connection. How does nursing theory relate to the practice of nursing?

What can the use of theory do to improve the quality of nursing? Figure 6.2 illustrates the relationships between theory, practice, and research. Nurses all work within a structural framework of acceptable and recommended practice. The advantage of work related to theory is that clinicians observe, decide, and act according to their education. Theory guides practice and is refined

CASE SCENARIO 6.2

A community-health nurse makes a home visit to a young family with a new baby. The nurse first met this family when he went to eat at their restaurant. It happens that he has been assigned by his agency to evaluate the family's response to the now 9-month-old baby. The nurse assesses the family members. He finds that the infant is achieving all developmental milestones, and that the mother's work and health are fine. She expresses concern about her husband, 33-years-old with a history of depression, who recently stopped taking his antidepressants, although this prescribed medication kept his depression under control.

The husband seems to have achieved great success. His marriage is stable, he adores his wife and baby, and he is a talented chef and owner of a renowned restaurant. He confides to the community-health nurse that he experiences episodes of sleeplessness and gastric distress. He reports, "I've lost about 15 pounds without even trying."

The wife tells the nurse that the client is always unhappy. She states, "It is difficult for me to see him suffer. We have decided to sell the business. That is the only thing that will make him happy, I'm sure of it."

Case considerations

1. According to Peplau's theory of Interpersonal Relations, how should the nurse proceed in this case? What are the key questions that the nurse should ask the client about medication? About sleep routine? About gastric distress?

2. What role does the wife play in helping the nurse help the client? What are the responsibilities of the nurse to educate the wife of the client?

3. What conflict of interest might be a factor for the nurse as a restaurant customer? According to Peplau, whose needs must be considered the most important in nurse/client interaction?

4. What advice should the nurse give the client? Is it necessary to involve the prescribing physician in the question of noncompliancy in taking prescribed medications?

5. Who is the most vulnerable person in this family? Why? What steps can the nurse take to protect the entire family?

through testing and research. The usefulness of theory is made obvious by its practical application. Florence Nightingale insisted that nurses learn from their observations. "Observations are for the sake of saving life and increasing health and comfort" (Nightingale, 1946, p. 70). Her work exemplifies the theory/practice connection.

Nightingale's observations and subsequent writings about those observations, the patient's reactions to the environment, interactions with others, and responses to nursing actions are the basis for how and why nurses practice nursing. Nightingale does not call her ideas a theory of or for nursing;

it is evident, however, that her observations prompted the development of strategies to improve the health of her patient. Meleis (1997) suggests that the ultimate benefit of theory application is improvement in nursing care.

"Through theory nurses can systematically derive and develop nursing interventions that can be tested, evaluated and linked to measurable outcomes" (MacPhee as cited in Sessanna, 2004, p. 225). The essence of nursing is demonstrated through successful resolution of client problems identified as nursing specific. Research using nursing theory as the basis for nursing interventions

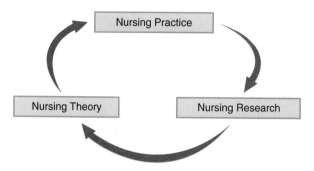

Figure 6.2 **Process and interdependence of knowledge development: nursing practice, theory and research.**

provides the discipline with scientific knowledge about the usefulness of the theory. Theories cannot be proved or disproved:` the data collected either support or fail to support the theory. It is only through continual application of theory in multiple settings with multiple clients and populations that we can determine the extent to which any of the theories developed by nurse theorists are actually useful in guiding nursing practice. A sample of current research, which uses one of the four theories described in the chapter, is found in Box 6.2.

BOX 6.2

Connecting Research, Practice, Theory (Selected Examples from the Literature)

Nightingale

Sessanna, L. (2004). Incorporating Florence Nightingale's theory of nursing into teaching a group of pre-adolescent children about negative peer pressure. *Journal of Pediatric Nursing: Nursing Care of Children & Families,* 19(3), 225–31.

Whall, A., Shin, Y., & Colling, K. B. (1999). A Nightingale-based model for dementia care and its relevance for Korean nursing. *Nursing Science Quarterly,* 12(4), 319–323.

Peplau

Douglass, J. L., Sowell, R. L., & Phillips, K. D. (2002). Using Peplau's theory to examine the psychosocial facts associated with HIV-infected women's difficulty in taking their medications. *The Journal of Theory Construction & Testing,* 7 (1), 10–17.

Schafer, P. & Middleton, J. (2001). Examining Peplau's pattern integrations in long-term care. *Rehabilitation Nursing,* 26(5), 192–197.

Rogers

Lewandowski, W. A. (2004). Patterning of pain and power with guided imagery. *Nursing Science Quarterly,* 17(30), 223–41.

Davidson, A.W. (2001). Person-environment mutual process: Studying and facilitating healthy environments from a nursing science perspective. *Nursing Science Quarterly, 14*(2), 101–108.

Roy

Dobratz, M.C. (2004). Life-closing spirituality and the philosophic assumptions of the Roy Adaptation Model. *Nursing Science Quarterly,* 17(4), 335–338.

Cunningham, D. A. (2002). Application of Roy's adaptation model when caring for a group of women coping with menopause. *Journal of Community Health Nursing,* 19(1), 49–60.

RESEARCH APPLICATION ARTICLE

Cunningham, D. A. (2002). Application of Roy's adaptation model when caring for a group of women coping with menopause. *Journal of Community Health Nursing*, 19(1), 49–60. Women in the throes of menopause experience myriad symptoms that affect their daily functions. In this study, Cunningham (2002), the researcher uses the Roy Adaptation Model (RAM) to examine women's responses to stimuli (focal, contextual, and residual) associated with menopause and to develop a program that would enhance adaptation (positive response) within the four adaptive modes (physiological, self-concept, role function, and interdependence). Data collection, nursing diagnosis, and subsequent interventions and evaluations are based on a six-step process. These steps include assessing behavior, assessing stimuli, developing nursing diagnosis, setting goals, intervening, and evaluating.

Data reveal that participants experience ineffective adaptation in the self-concept and interdependence modes. Nursing diagnoses include a disturbance in body image related to menopause and social isolation related to the inability to discuss menopause with immediate family and friends (Cunningham, 2002, p. 54). A facilitated group process and educational intervention approach to address the participant's responses to menopausal changes is implemented. Results of the study indicate that participants successfully achieve the goals of voicing enhanced confidence in body image and identifying at least one person with whom the participant can speak freely about menopause (Cunningham, 2002, p. 58).

Cunningham concludes that the Roy Adaptation Model, which emphasizes a holistic approach to assessing, analyzing, and developing treatment strategies to enhance adaptation (Roy & Andrews, 1999) provides the theoretical approach that enables the researcher to assist clients in achieving adaptation. The study sample is small (N=3); therefore, the results cannot be generalized. The researcher suggests that facilitating small groups using the Roy model may provide women with the support they need to adapt to menopause.

WRITING EXERCISE 6.2

1. Select one of the theories presented in the text.

2. Develop a set of questions that the theorist might ask a client.

3. Write a short dialogue between you and a client. Have each person (nurse and client) express what matters to him or her in basic nursing care. Consider the fact that a client may be an individual, family, or community.

4. Comment on clues you look for in the client's attitude, appearance, and ways of answering your questions that will help you understand the client's needs.

5. Formulate a plan of care for your client based on the theoretical model you have chosen.

6. Write a brief paper and be prepared to discuss your application of theory in class. Justify your choices.

CURRENT CONTROVERSY: ARE NURSING THEORIES NEEDED?

In essence, scholars ask what is the present state of the discipline? This chapter serves as an introduction to the many theories of nursing. Borrowed theory, theory specifically for nursing, and grand, middle, and practice theory constitute the substance of the debate among scholars. In the ongoing discussion of the profession of nursing, scholars revisit the advantages and limitations of each theory's perspective and parameters. Donnelly (2001) suggests that nursing theories are not scientific theories. For a theory to be considered scientific, it typically requires a "real" analysis based on data about the state and condition of a specific population. Logical steps of empirical analysis build the foundation for each particular scientific theory's premise. According to Donnelly "nursing theories are merely descriptions of the way nurses want things to exist instead of actual states of affairs" (p. 339).

Nursing theories as they are currently depicted provide insufficient evidence to support nursing as a scientific discipline (Cash, 2001). Theories serve the purpose of encouraging dialogue, but serve no value to advance the profession unless they can be tied to action. Cash (2001) and Donnelly (2001) believe that nurse theorists have failed to demonstrate the usefulness of their theories to nursing practice. However, the literature is replete with examples of how nurses apply existing nursing theories to practice situations and how nurses use theories to improve the quality of nursing care.

There are scholars that validate the correlation between nursing theory and practice (Pearson, 2002; Fawcett, 2000). At best, critics consider nursing theory as an integral element of the profession and a necessary foundation from which to further the discipline. Parker and Cody, theoretical scholars, in conversation with Fawcett (2003a & 2003b) propose that nursing theory does guide practice. The study and advancement of theory depends upon the follow-through of research and practice.

Clear connections between theories, research, and practice constitute the foundation of nursing as a discipline from which new ideas and changes will stem. "Nursing theory, regardless of its level of abstractness, is connected to practice; nursing theories reflect nursing and are used by nurses to frame their thinking, action and being in the world" (Parker as cited in Fawcett 2003a, p. 131). Theorizing requires ongoing dialogue among members of the discipline.

CHAPTER SUMMARY

The continual development, refinement, and application of nursing theories contribute to the body of knowledge that is uniquely nursing. The professional nurses' awareness and understanding of the historical context and ongoing development of theories is essential for their professional growth. "The maturity of a discipline as well as a profession is, according to Joel (2003), dependent on the direction its theory building will take" (p. 205). Furthermore, scholars such as Liehr and Smith (1999) suggest that the challenge of the twenty-first century is to move the discipline forward by developing, then conducting, research to evaluate middle-range theories.

Continuous dialogue and examination of the usefulness and relevance of nursing theories provides stimulus for intellectual development. Knowledge development is one way in which a discipline demonstrates the unique contributions it has to offer society. In this chapter, nursing theory validates itself as a support to actions that enhance the quality of care. Theory is the cornerstone on which nurses base research and practice.

All observers are not led by the same physical evidence to the same picture of the universe, unless their . . . backgrounds are similar, or can in some way be calibrated.

—Benjamin Whorf

REFERENCES

Boston College (2003). *Office of the nurse theorist.* Retrieved April 29, 2005, from http://www2.bc.edu/~royca/.

Cash, K. (2001). Editorial: Theory as resistance. *Nursing Philosophy, 2*, 1–3.

Chinn, P. L., & Kramer, M. K. (1995). *Theory and nursing: A systematic approach.* (4th ed.). St. Louis: Mosby.

Chinn, P. L., & Kramer. M. K. (2004). *Integrated knowledge development in nursing.* (5th ed.). St. Louis: Mosby.

Cunningham, D. A. (2002). Application of Roy's adaptation model when caring for a group of women coping with menopause. *Journal of Community Health Nursing, 19*(1), 49–60.

Davidson, A.W. (2001). Person-environment mutual process: Studying and facilitating healthy environments from a nursing science perspective. *Nursing Science Quarterly, 14*(2), 101–108.

Dickoff, J., & James, P. (1968). A theory of theories: A position paper. *American Journal of Nursing, May-* June *17*(3), 197–203.

Dobratz, M. C. (2004). Life-closing spirituality and the philosophic assumptions of the Roy Adaptation Model. *Nursing Science Quarterly, 17*(4), 335–338.

Donnelly, E. (2001). An assessment of nursing theories as guides to scientific inquiry. In Chaska, N. (Ed.) *The nursing profession: Tomorrow and beyond.* Sage Publications.

Douglass, J. L., Sowell, R. L., & Phillips, K. D. (2002). Using Peplau's theory to examine the psychosocial facts associated with HIV-infected women's difficulty in taking their medications. *The Journal of Theory Construction & Testing, 7*(1), 10–17.

Fawcett, J. (1980). A framework for analysis and evaluation of conceptual models of nursing. *Nurse Educator, 5*(6), 10–14.

Fawcett, J. (1984). The metaparadigm of nursing: Current status and future requirements. Image: *The Journal of Nursing Scholarship, 16*, p. 84–87.

Fawcett, J. (2000). *Analysis and evaluation of contemporary nursing knowledge: Nursing models and Theories.* Philadelphia: F. A. Davis Co.

Fawcett, J. (2003a). Theory and practice: A conversation with Marilyn Parker. *Nursing Science Quarterly, 16*(2), 131–136.

Fawcett, J. (2003b). Theory and practice: A discussion by William Cody. *Nursing Science Quarterly, 16*(3), 225–231.

Fitzpatrick, J., & Whall, A. (1996). *Conceptual models of nursing: Analysis and application* (3rd Ed.). Stamford, Connecticut: Appleton & Lange.

Jacox, A. (1974). Theory construction in nursing. *American Journal of Nursing, 23*(1), 4–13.

Joel, L. (2003). *Kelly's dimensions of professional nursing.* (9th ed.). McGraw-Hill.

Higgins, P. A., & Moore, S. M. (2000). Levels of theoretical thinking in nursing. *Nursing Outlook, 48*, 179–183.

Lewandowski, W. A. (2004). Patterning of pain and power with guided imagery. *Nursing Science Quarterly, 17*(30), 223–41.

Meleis, A. I. (1997). *Theoretical nursing: Development and progress.* (3rd ed.). Philadelphia: Lippincott.

Nightingale, F. (1946). *Notes on nursing: What it is and what it is not.* Philadelphia; J. B. Lippincott Co.

Online Etymology Dictionary (2005). Retrieved June 4, 2005 from http://www.etymonline.com/

Pearson, A. (2002). Nursing in theory and practice. *International Journal of Nursing Practice, 8*, 117.

Peplau, H. (1952). *Interpersonal relations in nursing.* New York: G. P. Putnam's Sons.

Peplau, H. (1988). The art and science of nursing: Similarities, differences and relations. *Health Science Quarterly, 1*(1), 8–15.

Peplau, H. E., (1989). Anxiety, self & hallucinations. In A.W. O'Toole and S.R. Weld (Eds.), *Interpersonal theory in nursing practice: Selected works of Hildegard E. Peplau* (pp. 287–295). NY: Springer Publish. Co.

Peplau, H. (1997). Peplau's theory of interpersonal relations. *Nursing Science Quarterly, 10*(4), 162–167.

Porter, S. (2001). Nightingale's realist philosophy of science. *Nursing Philosophy, 2*, 14–25.

Rogers. M. (1970). An *introduction to the theoretical basis of nursing.* Philadelphia: F. A. Davis.

Rogers, M. (1983). Science of unitary human beings: A paradigm for nursing. In I. W. Clements & F. B. Roberts (Eds.), *Family Health: A theoretical approach to nursing care.* New York: John Wiley & Sons.

Rogers, M. (1989). Nursing: A science of unitary human beings. In J. Riehl-Sisca (Ed.), *Conceptual models for nursing practice* (3rd ed.). Norwalk. Ct.: Appleton & Lange.

Roy, C. (1970). Adaptation: A conceptual framework for nursing. *Nursing Outlook, 18*, 42–45.

Roy, C. (1971). Adaptation: A basis for nursing practice. *Nursing Outlook, 18*, 254–257.

Roy, S. C. (1974). *Introduction to nursing: An adaptation model.* Englewood Cuffs, N. J.: Prentice Hall, Inc.

Roy, S. C. (1997). Future of Roy Model: Challenge to redefine adaptation. *Nursing Science Quaterly, 16*, 42–48.

Roy, C. & Andrews, H. A. (1999). *The Roy Adaptation Model.* (2nd ed.). Appleton & Lange: Stamford, Connecticut.

Schafer, P. & Middleton, J. (2001). Examining Peplau's pattern integrations in long-term care. *Rehabilitation Nursing, 26*(5), 192–197.

Senge, P. (2005). *Society for organizational learning. Developing capacity for inspired results.* Retrieved May 29, 2005, from http://www.solonline.org/organizational_overview/lexicon/

Sessanna, L. (2004). Incorporating Florence Nightingale's theory of nursing into teaching a group of pre-adolescent children about negative peer pressure. *Journal of Pediatric Nursing: Nursing Care of Children & Families, 19*(3), 225–31.

Stevenson, C. (2005). Practical inquiry/theory in nursing. *Journal of Advanced Nursing, 50*(2), 196–203.

The Compact Edition of the Oxford English Dictionary. (1971). Oxford University Press.

Whall, A. (1996). The structure of nursing knowledge: Analysis and evaluation of practice, middle range, and grand theory. In J. Fitzpatrick, A. Whall (Eds.) *Conceptual models of nursing: Analysis and application.* (3rd ed.). Stanford, CT: Appleton & Lange.

Whall, A., Shin, Y., & Colling, K. B. (1999). A Nightingale-based model for dementia care and its relevance for Korean nursing. *Nursing Science Quarterly, 12*(4), 319–323.

Woodham-Smith, C. (1951). *Florence Nightingale.* New York: McGraw-Hill.

Young A., Taylor, S. G., & Renpenning, K. (2001). *Connections: Nursing research, theory and practice.* St Louis: Mosby.

CHAPTER 7

Evidence-based Practice

Sheila Cox Sullivan

Facts are stubborn things; and whatever may be our wishes, our inclinations, or the dictates of our passions, they cannot alter the state of facts and evidence.
—John Adams

LEARNING OBJECTIVES

At the completion of the chapter, the learner should be able to do the following:

1. Trace the historical development of evidence-based practice.
2. Discuss a framework for determining the quality of evidence.
3. Discuss the importance of evidence-based practice to constituents of health care.
4. Describe how the use of clinical practice guidelines are utilized to improve nursing care.

KEY TERMS

Clinical practice guideline
Evidence-based practice

Randomized clinical trial

Research utilization

Imagine taking your ailing parent or child to a physicians's office to receive treatment for an acute bacterial upper respiratory infection. Following the collection of a history and physical, the health care provider confirms your suspicions. The prescribed treatment is a hot mustard plaster and peppermint tea at bedtime. Feeling distressed at the chosen therapy, you voice your concern. The health care provider benevolently smiles and replies, "This is how we did

it fifty years ago when I was in school." No doubt, you would take your loved one to another health care provider immediately and caution your friends against the first one.

Historically, many health care practices evolved from traditions or superstitions. However, as scientific knowledge advanced, it became clear that practioners must rely on the evidence provided by diligent research to deliver the best health care. The purpose of this chapter is to trace the roots of the evidence-based practice movement, to review criteria for accepting or rejecting evidence, and explicate one current model for implementation of evidence-based practice (EBP).

DEFINING EVIDENCE-BASED PRACTICE

Dr. David Sackett, one of the moving forces behind EBP, defines it as the merging of personal clinical expertise with the best available research results according to patient preferences and values (Sackett, Rosenberg, Muir-Gray, Haynes, & Richardson, 1996). Experienced health care personnel must keep up with the ever-changing landscape of treatment options in order to offer their patients the best choices for care. However, with new information emerging on a nearly daily basis, keeping abreast of the literature is a daunting and overwhelming task. One acquires the ability to review the literature effectively through education and practice (Tod, Harrison, Morris-Docker, Black, & Wolstenholme, 2003).

EBP occurs when a health care worker, or more commonly a group of health care workers, searches the available evidence to formulate a plan of care consistent with the client's wishes. Searching the evidence requires a synthesis of extant literature because many studies are likely available for review. From this synthesis, the workers generate a **clinical practice guideline** or treatment protocol to suggest actions to others who will face similar treatment issues. To ensure achievement of the desired outcome, an evaluation process follows implementation.

A clinical practice guideline (CPG) provides an algorithm for making clinical decisions about patient care. Specifically, the Institute of Medicine of the National Academy of Sciences (1990) defined CPG as "systematically developed statements to assist practitioners and patient decisions about appropriate health care for specific clinical circumstances." Multidisciplinary teams working on a particular

disease process, such as congestive heart failure, is a common way to develop clinical practice guidelines. McPheeters and Lohr (1999) defined four essential components of a CPG: (1) It should be developed in a systematic manner; (2) The CPG must be usable by both providers and patients for informing and collaborating in treatment/care decisions; (3) The treatment must be pertinent to the patient's condition; and (4) The CPG must clearly address well defined "clinical concepts" (p. 100).

Some nursing literature uses the terms **research utilization** and **evidence-based practice** interchangeably. Although there are clear similarities between the concepts, the terms are not fully synonymous. Polit and Beck (2004) define research utilization as "the use of findings from a disciplined study or set of studies in a practical application that is unrelated to the original research." Whereas research utilization begins with a concept and seeks how to best implement the concept into client care, EBP begins with a practical problem and seeks to determine how to solve that problem based upon the evidence provided by disciplined research. (Muir-Gray, 1997).

Consider the following example: The nurses on a surgical floor are experiencing difficulty with unplanned nasogastric tube (NGT) extubations or stabilization of NGTs. They decide to review extant literature addressing these concepts. Their search does not yield information on NGT stabilization; however, a substantial body of literature exists on stabilization of endotracheal (ET) tubes. The nurses extrapolate information from the ET studies and apply it to NGT practices on their unit. These nurses have used research.

However, following success in decreasing unplanned NGT extubations, the nurses share the literature they found on ET tube stabilization with their colleagues in the critical-care area. After reviewing all the studies and summarizing the findings, the critical-care nurses completely revise their ET stabilization policy to reflect currently published knowledge. The new clinical-practice guidelines offer alternatives shown to be effective that allow patients and nurses to choose which is most comfortable

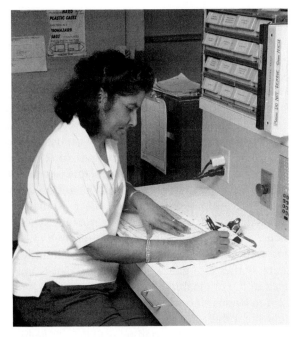

Figure 7.1 **A registered nurse reviews a patient's progress on his critical pathway.**

while maintaining ET tube security. The critical-care nurses in this case exemplify evidence-based practice.

Another example can be drawn from developing education policy and procedures for a rural clinic in an underserved, largely ethnic population. Rather than using standard educational interventions, the staff reviewed literature on learning styles and preferences in that unique population. Clinic nurses developed procedures unique to the clinic and population and enhanced the efficacy of nursing education in the clinic.

Outcomes of EBP

Having defined the concept of EBP, one must consider the outcomes and sequelae of implementing this process. The first desirable outcome is generally accepted as improved health or disease management. However, each intervention designed to achieve these states creates a cost, many of which may be substantial. EBP has the potential to increase the cost

of health care overall in the following ways: "Treating conditions that were previously untreatable, treating people who would previously have been untreated, providing more expensive types of treatment, and more intensive clinical practice" (Muir-Grey, 1997, p. 26.) In the current climate of health care that values cost control, health care managers are responsible for carefully weighing the ratio of cost to benefit. Further, personnel education regarding new procedures, the purchase and maintenance of new equipment, and monitoring outcomes all require capital. Identification of a funding source for these activities may create a barrier to implementation of evidence-based practice. Even though public policy initiatives may address the capital outlay, they do not consistently cover the long-term issues of education and maintenance. Ironically, many advocates of EBP cite cost containment as an advantage of this approach to health care. Because health care providers are more informed regarding the efficacy of tests and treatments, they do not waste health care dollars on activities not needed for particular conditions. Figure 7.1 illustrates the test review.

HISTORICAL PERSPECTIVE

The purpose of this section is to establish a foundation for evidence-based practice based upon historical context and current health care trends. Sociopolitical antecedents of the evidence-based practice movement from a global perspective will be addressed.

Economics

Prior to the 1970s a technology explosion in health care greatly increased the types of treatments available for disease. Among these advances were heart-lung bypass machines in the 1950s, paving the way for coronary artery bypass grafting; external cardiac defibrillation in the 1960s; and mechanical ventilation (which was motivated by the polio epidemic in the 1950s). As with any advance in technology, the accompanying increase in health care costs spiraled ever upward from 5 percent of the U.S. Gross Domestic Product (GDP) in 1960 to over 14 percent in 2002 (Jones, 2005). However, this phenomenon was not isolated to the United States; other industrialized countries experienced similar changes in health care spending.

The global oil crisis precipitated by the 1973 Arab-Israeli War abruptly ended America's supply of inexpensive petroleum. The increase in daily costs of living generated by this crisis caused health care leaders to become more aware of expenditures and to attempt to improve the efficiency of the health care dollar. In essence, Muir-Gray describes health care in the 1970s as "delivered for the shortest time, in the least expensive place, by the least expensive professional, using the cheapest possible drugs or equipment to ensure effectiveness and safety" (Muir-Gray, 1997, p. 18).

In the 1980s, however, quality improvement became the new emphasis. Far more informed than their predecessors were, maturing baby boomers demanded easily accessed, safe, and effective health care (Muir-Gray, 1997). Therefore, health care providers began to acknowledge that cost control was only one variable in cost effectiveness; instead, consumers should receive the best treatment at the best price.

Health Care

In 1972 rather ahead of his time, Archie Cochrane published *Effectiveness and Efficiency: Random Reflections on Health Services* in the U.K. This text deplored the lack of a scientific basis to justify health care practices. Specifically, Cochrane believed that in a world of finite resources, decisions for using these resources in the most effective way for the most people required scientific evidence. He identified **randomized clinical trials** (RCTs) as a highly reliable way to gain the desired evidence. Cochrane's views led to the development of the Cochrane Collaboration, a database of RCTs categorized by specialties. This international collaboration facilitates retrieval of evidence in a variety of medical specialties, facilitating understanding, and provision

of the best-known interventions for patients (The Cochrane Collection).

Cochrane's work corresponded with a 1978 report from the U. S. Congressional Office of Technology Assessment suggesting that technologies and tests in use during that period had evidence-based validity less than 20 percent of the time. This finding energized the health care community as well as health care constituents. Economics and medicine aligned, and the quest for consistent evidence-based practice in health care began in earnest. Polit and Hungler (2004) consider EBP "a major paradigm shift for health care education and practice" (p. 678).

One of the most ringing endorsements for EBP came from the Institute of Medicine's report, *Crossing the Quality Chasm: A New Health System for the 21st Century* (IOM, 2001). In this document, the IOM promotes embracing EBP as a way to improve patient safety and decrease the potential for risk. The text goes on to recommend six aims for the health care system: safe, effective, patient-centered, timely, efficient, and equitable. EBP effectively addresses each of these goals.

Nursing

Nurses have also been incorporating research findings into practice. Conducted by the Western Interstate Commission for Higher Education Research (WICHE), the first federally funded nursing research utilization study took place in the 1970s. This series provides a strong example of basing nursing practice on evidence. The seminal publication from this effort considered the needs of grieving spouses (Dracup & Breu, 1978). Other utilization projects, such as Conduct and Utilization of Research in Nursing (CURN), considered very pragmatic issues such as reducing diarrhea from enteral feedings (Horsley & Crane, 1981) and pain management (Horsley & Crane, 1982).

Nursing began to shift from educational issues to clinical concerns in the mid-1980s. In 1986 the development of the National Institute for Nursing Research (NINR) allowed nursing research to expand greatly due to improved funding opportunities.

Numerous new journals joined the effort to disseminate these new findings. Sigma Theta Tau International cites the development and dissemination of research as one of the organization's major goals.

British nurses took the lead in developing evidence-based nursing (EBN). Centers for EBN exist in numerous countries, including the United States, Germany, Australia, and Canada (Ciliska, DiCenso, & Cullum, 1999). Similar to the Cochrane Collaboration, these centers conduct literature reviews designed to facilitate development of evidence-based policies and procedures in nursing. They also conduct workshops to facilitate EBN in other locations and disseminate results from their initiatives via Web sites, presentations, and journals.

> *Quality care should not exist on a patchwork basis across the United States. Patients have a right to expect that we afford them the best care that science presently offers.*
> Grif Alspach

Concerns Regarding EBP

While EBP seems logical, some practitioners have been critical of this philosophy of health care. One criticism suggested that EBP addressed the concerns of health care managers rather than patients (Grahame-Smith, 1995). A major concern of this faction deals with quality of life issues; these practitioners are concerned that following the CPG may deprive some clients of their choice of treatments (McPheeters & Lohr, 1999). Some physicians feared that the prescriptive nature of following clinical-practice guidelines restricted their freedom to practice (Colyer & Kamath, 1999). These groups are concerned with "cookbook" medicine approaches that limit the collaboration between the practitioner and the patient. Other critics feel that RCT populations are not consistent with the general population and,

further, feel that services in practice areas are not comparable to those available in medical centers where RCTs usually occur (McPheeters & Lohr, 1999). Conversely, French (2002) suggests that the very concept of evidence-based practice is so blended with the meaning of nursing as to be indistinguishable. Nevertheless, nurses continue to emphasize the role of research in daily judgments about patient care.

SYNTHESIS OF THE LITERATURE

To determine the best-known information given a certain topic, there are two major barriers to overcome. First, one must conduct an exhaustive review of the literature and second, decide whether the studies are useful. While many studies are published in the literature, not all of them are worthy of consideration; some study results disagree with others, and different definitions of outcomes make synthesis of the literature challenging.

Finding the Evidence

The most effective way to locate evidence is a search via an online database. The most common database used in nursing is the Cumulative Index of Nursing and Allied Health Literature (CINAHL). MedLine and PubMed are also helpful for locating health care related studies. Most colleges have access to these databases online, but it takes time and training to become proficient in searching. A reference librarian at a Health Sciences library is an invaluable resource in guiding one through a literature search. However, online databases are not always complete because search terms chosen by authors and editors determine the categorization of the studies. Therefore, additional sources of information may require exploration. Another source of information is the reference lists of articles found to be valuable for further coverage of the topic.

WRITING EXERCISE 7.1

Using online databases, search for a nursing topic of interest to you. How many different articles on the subject could you find? Limit your search to research articles. How much difference did this limitation make in the number of articles available? Does the National Guideline Clearinghouse offer an evidence-based protocol or clinical-practice guideline in this area?

Evidence-based practice centers, such as the Cochrane Collaboration or one of the multiple centers in the United States, have resources to assist with literature searches and information on literature synthesis. Some journals, such as *Evidence-Based Nursing*, choose to publish only those articles that meet specific criteria of rigor and summarize that information (DiCenso, Ciliska, Marks, et. al., 2004). These journals, some of which are online, are excellent resources for finding evidence regarding a topic. The National Guideline Clearinghouse also readily offers a number of established medical protocols or clinical practice guidelines at http://www.guideline.gov.

Research Designs

Determining the quality of the published evidence requires knowledge of research methodology beyond the purposes of this chapter. However, research methodology in nursing may be broadly divided into two types: qualitative and quantitative. While qualitative research attempts to determine the meaning of events, quantitative research proposes to determine cause and effect relationships (Fain, 1999). From the perspective of evidence-based medicine, quantitative design is preferred due to larger sample sizes and the ability to provide information in large samples of participants regarding the efficacy of particular interventions.

Many researchers consider the randomized clinical trial the gold standard of clinical research (Murdaugh, 1999). For considering a study an RCT, Polit and Beck (2004) suggest the study have the following characteristics:

- A purpose of determining whether a clinical intervention is more effective than current practice
- A large heterogeneous sample, which prevents results from being affected by race or gender
- Multiple research sites, which limit the probability that the effect is due to location
- That participants undergo random assignment to either the experimental or control group

The major reason that RCTs are so valued is because the randomization of participants to differing control groups minimizes the effect of unknown or confounding variables on the outcome. The minimization of these extraneous effects occurs because these variables are assumed to be equally distributed between the control and experimental groups (DiCenso, Cullum, & Ciliska, 1998). This assumption is a limitation of any RCT.

An example of an RCT is the Antihypertensive and Lipid-Lowering Treatment to Prevent Heart Attack Trial (ALLHAT). This study enrolled over 24,000 participants at 625 centers in the United States and Canada (Davis, 2000). This trial randomly assigned participants to receive either doxazosin or chlorthalidone, and only the researchers knew which drug a participant took. Known as double blinding, this technique prevents participants from responding in what they may consider the desired way and further prevents observers responsible for collecting the data from being influenced by knowing which treatment a participant is receiving (Polit & Beck, 2004). The ALLHAT study exerted a profound impact on the treatment of these major risk factors for cardiac disease.

A meta-analysis is a common strategy employed to summarize multiple RCTs investigating similar interventions and outcomes. This statistical technique considers each study as a unique data point, combining these results to cause a more reliable outcome. A larger "sample size" created by combining the studies results in a more accurate estimation of treatment efficacy than can be obtained from individual studies alone (Polit & Beck, 2004). This complex process is common in the research literature, but EBP consortiums may employ the technique during the synthesis process. An excellent resource for further information regarding meta-analysis is available from http://www.edres.org/meta/.

It is important to note that nurses must remain aware that other types of evidence exist. The qualitative perspective capably captures elusive concepts such as personal beliefs, experiences, and feelings (DiCenso, Cullum, & Clilska, 1998). These authors further stated "good evidence does involve more than RCTs and systematic overviews . . . the key is ensuring that the right research design is used to answer the question posed" (p. 39). Although synthesis models for qualitative methods exist (Noblit & Hare, 1988), their use is infrequent.

Finally, nurses have other ways of learning and understanding concepts or ideas that help them give the best possible care to each patient. Whereas research is clearly a major component of a nurse's knowledge, clinical experience, patient experience, and contextual knowledge also play a role in determining the best intervention for a given situation (Rycroft-Malone, Seers, Titchen, et. al., 2004). Even though EBP acknowledges the importance of clinical experience, it is very important that patient knowledge and the information gleaned from the setting are not eliminated from the equation of making health care decisions.

Evaluating Research

Instructions on trying to decide what research studies are appropriate for inclusion are beyond the scope of this text. However, the Agency for Healthcare Research and Quality (AHRQ) has reviewed existing systems for assessing the strength of evidence (2002). This summary of extant guidelines found over 100 systems for evidentiary review, which naturally yielded conflicting results when applied to studies. However, in their report (available at http://www.ahrq.gov/clinic/epcsums/strengthsum.pdf), critical concepts to be reviewed are given for varying types of research designs. Additionally, any research text will offer guidance in the critique of research articles.

Read the articles under consideration with a research textbook or other evaluation rubric open to the chapter on analyzing research studies. Excellent frameworks for research evaluation are Rosswurm and Larrabee's (1999) or a research evaluation checklist found in the American Journal of Critical Care, Sept. 2002 issue. Look for the critical elements that the rubric suggests. Not having a clearly stated statistical hypothesis may be an editorial deletion; however, failing to define adequately the operational concepts may cast serious doubt on the validity of the study. Be very aware of the ability of the study to apply a concept known as generalization to the exact setting in which the researcher's interest lies. For example, consider a student researching nursing interventions aimed at preventing pneumonia in postoperative patients. Although numerous publications address prevention of ventilator-associated pneumonia in critical-care units, much of this data will not apply to a routine patient following gallbladder removal. The causative mechanisms are not similar, and therefore, the results are not generalizable to the different population.

The U.S. Preventive Services Task Force (USPSTF) developed a system for rating guideline recommendations noted in Table 7.1. The five possible ratings (A, B, C, D, and I) are assigned according to the strength of the evidence and the degree of the overall benefit to harm ratio as noted in Table 7.2.

Table 7.1 The U. S. Preventive Services Task Force (USPSTF) Rating Scale for Evidence Quality

Good: Evidence included consistent results from well-designed, well-conducted studies in representative populations that directly assess effects on health outcomes.

Fair: Evidence is sufficient to determine effects on health outcomes, but the strength of the evidence is limited by the number, quality, or consistency of the individual studies; generalizability to routine practice; or the indirect nature of the evidence on health outcomes.

Poor: Evidence is insufficient to assess the effects on health outcomes because of limited number or power of studies, important flaws in their design or conduct, gaps in the chain of evidence, or lack of information on important health outcomes.

Available at http://www.ahrq.gov/clinic/3rduspstf/ratings.htm.

The ratings allow practitioners to accept or reject recommendations on the strength of the evidence used in creating the guidelines.

One challenge for nursing is mastering the incorporation of qualitative information into evidence-based practice frameworks. Mulhall (1998) issued a plea for ensuring that nursing research not abandon its diverse approach to research and rely solely on quantitative methodology for evidence. In fact, many nursing questions address patients' emotional and spiritual response to therapy; quantitative models are inferior to qualitative paradigms in addressing these concepts. Nurse scientists must be diligent in ensuring that the humanistic perspective of nursing is not lost in the desire to base practice on evidence.

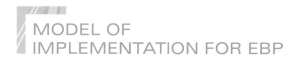

MODEL OF IMPLEMENTATION FOR EBP

Inasmuch a number of excellent models of EBP exist (Rosswurm & Larrabee, 1999; Stetler, 1994; Goode & Piedalue, 1999), this text will

Table 7.2 The U. S. Preventive Services Task Force (USPSTF) Strength of Recommendation Guidelines

A.—The USPSTF strongly recommends that clinicians provide [the service] to eligible patients. The USPSTF found good evidence that [the service] improves important health outcomes and concludes that benefits substantially outweigh harms.

B.—The USPSTF recommends that clinicians provide [this service] to eligible patients. The USPSTF found at least fair evidence that [the service] improves important health outcomes and concludes that benefits outweigh harms.

C.—The USPSTF makes no recommendation for or against routine provision of [the service]. The USPSTF found at least fair evidence that [the service] can improve health outcomes but concludes that the balance of benefits and harms is too close to justify a general recommendation.

D.—The USPSTF recommends against routinely providing [the service] to asymptomatic patients. The USPSTF found at least fair evidence that [the service] is ineffective or that harms outweigh benefits.

I.—The USPSTF concludes that the evidence is insufficient to recommend for or against routinely providing [the service]. Evidence that the [service] is effective is lacking, of poor quality, or conflicting and the balance of benefits and harms cannot be determined.

Available at http://www.ahrq.gov/clinic/3rduspstf/ratings.htm.

WRITING EXERCISE 7.2

Using writing exercise 7.1: review the evidence-based protocol or clinical-practice guideline. Using the USPSTF rating scale, what was the level of evidence used to develop the protocol guideline? Explain your choice.

CASE SCENARIO 7.1

In a study by Roland, Russell, Richards, and Sullivan (2001), the nurses in a critical-care unit (CCU) disagreed about visitation policy. Some of the nurses were in favor of a completely unrestricted visitation policy whereas others believed strongly that restrictions on visitation facilitated patient recovery as well as completion of nursing responsibilities during the shift. A committee of nurses chose to review the evidence in the literature regarding visitation in order to make the best decision for the patients, families, and staff. The first step involved a poll of the nursing staff on the unit as well as the physicians and ancillary staff such as respiratory therapy and social workers. The patients and families also answered questions regarding their perceptions of current visitation policies. The investigators also sent a poll to 114 comparable hospitals within the network as well as 7 other local facilities. Meanwhile, the members of the committee conducted a literature search for evidence regarding visitation in CCUs.

Most nursing staff members expressed satisfaction with the current policy, however patients and families wanted more visitations. Ancillary personnel agreed with the patients and families. The literature did not support most nursing concerns regarding the physical effect of visitation. After obtaining administrative approval and support,

the investigators implemented a more liberal policy. Patient and family satisfaction increased significantly ($p < .05$), and nursing satisfaction with the policy was unchanged. Reference used in this case scenario: Roland, P., Russell, J., Richards, K., & Sullivan, S. (2001). Visitation in critical care: Processes and outcomes of a performance improvement initiative. *Journal of Nursing Care Quality (15)*2, 18–26.

1. Many of the nurses on this unit had anecdotal experiences of deterioration in the client's physical condition during a visitation. This provided a major barrier to implementation of an evidence-based protocol. List some effective ways that evidence can be used to counter such barriers.

2. What database would be most effective in searching the literature for evidence regarding visitation in critical care? Search both Medline and CINAHL using the same search terms, and compare your results.

3. Does the American Association of Critical Care Nurses have a policy or position statement on visitation? If so, locate it, and determine the level of evidence based on the USPSTF criteria.

focus on the ACE Star Model of Knowledge Transformation.

ACE Star model of Knowledge Transformation

At the Academic Center for Evidence-Based Nursing, based at the University of Texas Health Science Center in San Antonio, K. R. Stevens (2004) developed the ACE Star Model to describe the transformation of knowledge from discovery to implementation in practice (see Figure 7.2). Each point of the star depicts a point in the transition of knowledge from research through synthesis of the evidence, creating recommendations for practice, integration of these recommendations into practice, and evaluation of the outcomes based on the recommendations.

The Discovery stage incorporates the research process as new knowledge is developed and disseminated. The Summary stage attempts to synthesize all extant knowledge on a particular intervention or concept. It is in this stage that meta-analysis occurs. The Translation stage incorporates the process of creating clinical-practice guidelines or protocols for practitioners. Integration of these guidelines is the

next step, and this stage requires an understanding of change theory and often salesmanship to encourage others to "buy into" the new protocol. Finally, the protocol must actually work to solve the problem in a cost-efficient manner; thus, an Evaluation of the outcomes of the new guidelines by health-services research methods is required.

This framework also provides a map for those interested in implementing EBP. For example, if a general oncology unit is interested in nonpharmacological methods of pain relief, they could create or obtain a summary of the known evidence on these techniques. Based on the outcomes of the studies summarized, they would create policies and procedures to guide practice on the unit. After educating the staff on the techniques, the staff would implement the new recommendations for a time and evaluate patient pain relief for efficacy.

IMPLEMENTING EBP

It certainly seems appropriate for major urban medical centers associated with research universities to consider the use of EBP in their facilities. However, for the rest of the world, how practical is EBP? Can it be implemented in smaller facilities or in non-hospital settings?

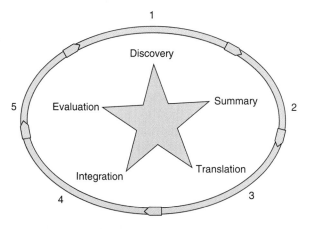

Figure 7.2 ACE Star model of Knowledge Transformation.
Reprinted with permission by Dr. K. R. Stevens.

Practice

Following the desire to utilize EBP in a particular facility, the most important thing needed for implementation of EBP is managerial support. Omery and Williams (1999) surmise that unless the nursing leadership actively supports implementation practices based on the available evidence and creates a climate in which such nursing practice is supported, using the evidence will not be a valued part of nursing. The literature (Stetler, et al., 1998; Rutledge & Donaldson, 1995) suggests three steps

RESEARCH APPLICATION ARTICLE

Gerrish, K., & Clayton, J. (2004). Promoting evidence-based practice: An organizational approach. *Journal of Nursing Management, 12*, 114–123.

Gerrish and Clayton (2004) evaluated the implementation of EBP in a British teaching hospital. The authors surveyed 330 clinical nurses asking to what extent the nurses used differing types of information in determining patient care, anticipated barriers to EBP, and evaluation of their personal skills in using EBP. They found that these nurses depended on their clinical experiences as well as peer advice, physician advice, and patient information. Policy and procedures were reviewed more frequently than were research reports. Reported barriers included insufficient time, insufficient resources, and insufficient power in changing practice. The authors suggest that managerial support, ensuring that evidence-based information is readily available to practicing nurses to read in an easily understandable form, and administrative openness to organizational change would promote adaptation of EBP.

for nursing leaders in promoting this change: establishing a new culture, creating the capacity for organizational change, and sustaining the change through revision of the system's infrastructure. Changes in daily language patterns create a new culture by exemplifying the newly adopted belief patterns. For example, a nurse manager would no longer explain policy revisions by simply stating that the administration ordered it. A brief and simplified explanation of the evidence more effectively justifies the new policy. Creating the capacity for change relies heavily on educating the staff not only regarding new policies but how to find the evidence themselves. Further, making sure staff have the capacity to access the information is crucial. Stetler and colleagues (1998) suggest work groups, forums, and support for research review. Rutledge and Donaldson (1995) further suggest journal clubs, research posters covering current literature on topics selected by the nursing staff, and mailing selected articles to key personnel throughout the institution. Finally, sustaining the change is supported by such items as clinical-ladder recognition for participation in EBP work groups and adjustments in job descriptions or committee expectations. Several years after these studies, Gerrish and Clayton (2004) found little difference in the perceived needs of nurses to effect the change of EBP.

Clearly, without administrative and managerial support, any such effort is unlikely to succeed. However, the individual nurses must also be committed to the undertaking of implementing EBP. Goode and colleagues (2000) found a change in provider behavior following implementation of an EBP guideline, suggesting that the participants valued EBP due to the potential to improve quality and thus patient outcomes. This can only come about when nurses are aware of what EBP is, how it functions, and the potential benefits as well as pitfalls.

There are a number of barriers to EBP identified by nurses in several studies. Cooke and colleagues (2004) summarized these to include lack of time, literature not readily available, uncertain of personal ability to use research, critical colleagues, lack of organizational support, and lack of perceived power to effect change. U.K. nurses identified lack of time, cost, patient issues, and lack of "incentive" as barriers (McKenna, Ashton, & Keeney, 2004). Additional U.K. concerns included conflicting research findings and the volume of literature for review.

With the current international nursing shortage, lack of time will continue to be an issue. Managers will either need to pay for research-related efforts or hire nurses specifically for this task. With the Internet, fewer Americans are isolated from the literature; however, this is not true globally. Education regarding the research process should be mandatory for all registered nurses. Other issues are relative to organizational matters as previously discussed.

Populations

Two recent studies have highlighted the particular barriers specific provider populations encounter when attempting to implement EBP. Olade (2004) studied EBP and research utilization practices among rural nurses in the southwestern United States. This study found merely 20 percent of these nurses were active in use of research. More strikingly, 42 percent had never "participated in nursing utilization in their entire nursing career" (p. 222). Over 75 percent of the nurses polled, however, stated they would like to participate in nursing research utilization ventures in the future. A major barrier identified by these nurses, in addition to barriers common to all nurses, included their lack of access to nurse researchers or other nurses capable of modeling EBP. One possible explanation for the lack of confidence in their personal ability to use research is that only 32 percent had bachelor's degrees (research is required in bachelor's programs whereas it is not consistently required of associate degree or diploma graduates). Of the associate-degree nurses, only 26 percent had received formal instruction regarding nursing research.

Nurses in the United Kingdom varied on their concerns regarding EBP implementation (McKenna, et al., 2004). The researchers contrasted community-based nurses (such as district nurses) with general practitioners (such as practice nurses). Of the 462 participants, 83 percent had no formal research education and 29 percent had been involved in a research project at some time in their career. Only 44 percent had Internet access, with the majority (64 percent) being general practitioners, who identified their barriers to EBP as lack of relevance of current research to their personal practices, the

difficulty in staying current, and limited ability to seek out evidence-based information. However, the community nurses were more concerned about computer access, patient compliance with changes in regimen, and the ability to influence and effect change in their practice.

Education

The previous sections clearly identify a need for inclusion of the research process into education curricula across all levels of preparation as well as internationally. Price (2005) encourages educators to weave EBP principles throughout the curricula, enabling students and new practitioners to value the concepts inherent in EBP. Price suggests the PPIE model for integration of EBP into the curriculum, which includes a preparatory phase, a planning phase, implementation phase, and an evaluation phase. Price further identifies five steps of the EBP process that students must understand in order to ensure their personal practice is evidence-based:

1. Develop a researchable practice question.
2. Design and implement an evidence search.
3. Retrieve and appraise evidence.
4. Integrate clinical evidence in order to implement an evidence-based decision.
5. Evaluate clinical practice and EBP process outcomes.

CHAPTER SUMMARY

Economic trends and health care initiatives have combined to encourage health care practitioners to seek out an evidentiary basis for practice. A number of consortiums exist internationally to support the search for evidence-based practice, including the Cochrane Collaboration. Further, health care practitioners can find clinical practice guidelines, based on synthesis of extant literature, on the Internet or may develop their own for their practice area.

Although legitimate concerns exist regarding EBP, the mandate is clearly urgent, and the U.S. government has linked EBP with safety initiatives. Barriers to implementation include the nursing shortage and lack of time in the workplace, access to the literature, understanding the process of EBP, and lack of formal education in research methods. Differing barriers exist depending on one's area of practice, so differing strategies will be required to overcome these constraints. Nursing educators must begin to adapt EBP principles into curricula in order to prepare the workforce to function in this new method of health care.

> *The fact that an opinion has been widely held is no evidence whatever that it is not utterly absurd.*
> —Bertrand Russell

REFERENCES

Agency for Healthcare Research and Quality (2002). *Systems to rate the strength of scientific evidence, summary.* March 2002 (No. 47). Washington, DC: Author. Accessed April 20, 2005, from http://www.ahrq.gov/clinic/epcsums/strengthsum.pdf.

Alspach, G. (1999). When the "evidence" in evidence-based practice is ignored: A time for advocacy. *Critical Care Nurse, 19*(4), 10, 12, 14.

American Journal of Critical Care (2002). Research evaluation checklist. *American Journal of Critical Care, 11*(5), 438–440.

Ciliska, D., DiCenso, A., & Cullum, N. (1999). Centres of evidence-based nursing: Directions and challenges. *Evidence-Based Nursing, 2*(4), 102–104.

Cochrane, A. (1979). *Effectiveness and efficiency: Random reflections on health services.* London: Nuffield Provincial Hospitals Trust.

Colyer, H., & Kamath, P. (1999). Evidence-based practice. A philosophical and political analysis: Some matters for conisdertaion by professional practitioners. *Journal of Advanced Nursing, 29,* 188–193.

Cooke, L., Smith-Idell, C., Dean, G., Gemmill, R., Steingass, S., Sun, V., Grant, M., & Borneman, T. (2004). "Research to practice": A practical program

to enhance the use of evidence-based practice at the unit level. *Oncology Nursing Forum, 31*(4), 825–832.

Davis, B. R. (2000). Major cardiovascular events in hypertensive patients randomized to doxazosin vs chlorthalidone. *Journal of the American Medical Association, 283*(15), 1967–1975.

DiCenso, A., Ciliska, D., Marks, S. et al. (2004). *Evidence-based nursing —An introduction. Syllabus for evidence-based nursing.* Accessed July 21, 2005, from http://www.cebm.utoronto.ca/syllabi/nur/print/intro.htm.

DiCenso, A., Cullum, N., & Ciliska, D. (1998). Implementing evidence-based nursing: Some misconceptions. *Evidence Based Nursing, 1,* 38–39.

Dracup, K. A., & Breu, C. S. (1978). Using nursing research findings to meet the needs of grieving spouses. *Nursing Research, 27,* 4, 212–216.

Fain, J. (1999). *Reading, understanding, and applying nursing research: A text and workbook.* Philadelphia: F. A. Davis.

Gerrish, K., & Clayton, J. (2004). Promoting evidence-based practice: An organizational approach. *Journal of Nursing Management, 12,* 114–123.

Goode, C. J., Tanaka, D. J., Krugman, M., O'Conner, P. A., Bailey, C., Deutchman, M., & Stolpman, N. M. (2000). Outcomes from use an evidence-based practice guideline. *Nursing Economics, 18*(4), 202–207.

Goode, C. J., & Piedalue, F. (1999). Evidence-based clinical practice. *Journal of Nursing Administration, 29*(6), 15–21.

Grahame-Smith, D. (1995). Evidence based medicine: Socratic dissent. *British Medical Journal, 310,* 1126–1127.

Horsley, J., & Crane, J. (1981). New York: Grune & Stratton.

CURN Project:
Includes: Structured preoperative teaching. (1981). Intravenous cannula change. (1981). Pain: Deliberative nursing interventions. (1982). Preventing decubitus ulcers. (1981). Reducing diarrhea in tube-fed patients (1981). Using Research to improve nursing practice: A guide. (1983). Mutual goal setting in patient care. (1982). Clean intermittent catheterization. (1982). Preoperative sensory preparation to promote reocovery. (1981).

Institute of Medicine, Committee on Quality of Health Care in America. (2001). *Crossing the quality chasm: A new health system for the 21st century.* Washington, DC: National Academies Press. Accessed July 18, 2005, from http://www.iom.edu/file.asp?id=27184,

Institute of Medicine of the National Academy of Sciences (1990). In M. J. Field, & K. Lohr, (Eds.), *Clinical practice guide-lines: Directions for a new program.* Washington, DC: National Academy Press.

Jones, C. I. (2005). More life vs. more goods: Explaining rising health expenditures. *FRBSF Economic newsletter,* 2005–2010. Accessed July 11, 2005, from http://www.frbsf.org/publications/economics/letter/2005/el2005-10.html,.

McKenna, H. P., Ashton, S., & Keeney, S. (2004). Barriers to evidence-based practice in primary care. *Journal of Advanced Nursing, 45*(2), 178–189.

McPheeters, M., & Lohr, K. (1999). Evidence-based practice and nursing: Commentary. *Outcomes Management for Nursing Practice, 3*(3), 99–101.

Muir-Gray, J. A. (1997). *Evidence based healthcare.* New York: Churchhill Livingstone.

Mulhall, A. (1998). Nursing, research, and the evidence. *Evidence-Based Nursing, 1,* 4–6.

Murdaugh, C. L. (1999). Relationship of research perspectives to methodology. In A. S. Hinshaw, S. L. Feetham, & J. L. F. Shaver (Eds.), *Handbook of clinical nursing research,* (pp. 61–73). London: Sage Publications.

Noblit, G. W., & Hare, R. D. (1988). *Meta-ethnography: Synthesizing qualitative research studies.* London: Sage.

Olade, R. (2004). Evidence-based practice and research utilization activities among rural nurses. *Journal of Nursing Scholarship, 36*(3), 220–225.

Polit, D. F., & Beck, C. T. (2004). *Nursing research: Principles and methods* (7th ed.). Philadelphia: Lippincott Williams & Wilkins.

Price, S. (2005). Integrating evidence-based practice into nursing curricula. In M. Oermann & K. Heinrich (Eds.), *Annual review of nursing education: Strategies for teaching, assessment, & program*

planning (Vol. 3). New York: Springer Publishing Company.

Roland, P., Russell, J., Richards, K., & Sullivan, S. (2001). Visitation in critical care: Processes and outcomes of a performance improvement initiative. *Journal of Nursing Care Quality, (15)*2, 18–26.

Rosswurm, M. A., & Larrabee., J. H. (1999). A model for change to evidence-based practice. *Image: Journal of Nursing Scholarship, 31*(4), 317–322.

Rutledge, D. N., & Donaldson, N. E. (1995). Building organizational capacity to engage in research utilization. *Journal of Nursing Administration, 25*(10), 12–16.

Rycroft-Malone, J., Seers, K., Titchen, A., Harvey, G., Kitson, A., & McCormack, B. (2004). What counts as evidence in evidence-based practice? *Journal of Advanced Nursing, 47*(1), 81–90.

Sackett D. L., Rosenberg W., Muir-Gray, J. A., Haynes R. B., & Richardson, W. S. (1996). Evidence-based medicine: What it is and what it isn't. British Medical Journal *312,* 71–2.

Stetler, C. B., Brunell, M., Giuliano, K. K., Morsi, D., Prince, L., & Newell-Stokes, V. (1998). Evidence-based practice and the role of nursing leadership. *The Journal of Nursing Administration, 28*(7–8), 45–53.

Stetler, C. B. (1994). Refinement of the Stetler/Marram model for application of research findings to practice. *Nursing Outlook, 42*(1), 15–25.

Stevens, K. R. (2004). *ACE Star Model of EBP: Knowledge transformation.* Academic Center for Evidence-based Practice. www.acestar.uthscsa.edu.

The Cochrane Collaboration. (nd). *The name behind the Cochrane collection.* Accessed July 18, 2005, from http://www.cochrane.org/docs/archieco.htm.

Tod, A., Harrison, H., Morris-Docker, S., Black, R., & Wolstenholme, D. (2003). Access to the Internet in the clinical area: Expectations and experiences of nurses working in an acute care setting. *British Journal of Nursing, 12,* 425–434.

TWO

Environment
of the Profession

CHAPTER 8

Health Services in the United States

Theresa Perfetta Cappello

By keeping costs under control, expanding access and helping more Americans afford coverage, we will preserve the system of private medicine that makes America's health care the best in the world.
—President G.W. Bush (Bush, 2004)

LEARNING OBJECTIVES

At the completion of the chapter, the learner should be able to do the following:

1. Compare and contrast outpatient and inpatient care.
2. Compare the four types of health care services.
3. Identify the multiple members of the health care team.
4. Describe the systems of health care financing in the United States.
5. Discuss health care demands and changing trends.

KEY TERMS

Advanced-practice nurse	Inpatient health care settings	Primary care
Allied health care practitioner	Long-term care	Private health insurance
Baby boomer	Medicaid	Secondary care
Community-based care	Medicare	Social worker
DRG	Outpatient health care settings	Tertiary care
Emergency care	Pharmacist	Worker's compensation
HMO	Physician assistants	
Hospice care	PPO	

INTRODUCTION

In 1993 President Clinton proposed the first far-reaching health reform proposal since the institution of Medicare and Medicaid in 1965. This plan would have provided government-sponsored health insurance through contracts with insurers and included regulated pricing for a standard set of benefits for all those under the age of 65. The Clinton plan would have effectively providing government control over health care for everyone in the country (Feldman, 2000). This plan failed to pass Congress in 1994 primarily because governmental control over the health care industry would hinder the free market system (Zerwekh & Clayborn, 2003). Since 1994 free-market forces have dominated the health care system with competition among insurance companies, managed care, the rise of for-profit hospital corporations, and an increase in physicians' group practice.

Today the health care system in the United States is shaped by many and competing forces such as the changing demographics of the population; health insurance or the lack thereof; managed care; shortages in health care personnel, particularly nurses; medical technological advances; and information technology. The system for providing health care services has endured rapid and continuous change over the last quarter century with the expectation that changes will continue at an even more rapid pace in the future. Today there remains considerable discussion regarding the escalating costs of health care, the baby boomers reaching retirement age, and the large number of people in the United States with inadequate or no health care insurance.

This chapter describes the present health care system, including current settings, services, financing, and providers. Future trends in health care including increased personal choice in health care decisions, increased use of technology, and a growing emphasis on primary prevention will be discussed.

HEALTH CARE SETTING

Health care services are delivered in settings that provide care on a continuum from outpatient preventive care for those who are well to inpatient settings for those critically ill. Health care agencies may be government sponsored, private for-profit, or not-for-profit agencies. **Inpatient health care settings** are those that require an overnight stay. These include hospitals, including specialty hospitals such as psychiatric or orthopedic hospitals; hospice; long-term care facilities such as nursing homes; and rehabilitation centers. **Outpatient health care settings** provide services that do not require an overnight stay. These include physicians' offices, school health clinics, occupational health services, hospitals, freestanding emergency centers or those associated with a hospital, family-planning centers, clinical laboratories, clinics, ambulatory-care centers, outpatient surgical centers, and a variety of community settings, including adult daycare, home health care services, and respite care.

Inpatient

Hospitals are complex institutions that bridge the span of services from outpatient diagnostic to inpatient chronic care and that range from government sponsored to for- profit agencies. Hospitals provide nursing, medical, and surgical care to those needing emergency, obstetric, psychiatric, recuperative, and rehabilitative services. Modern hospital organization and administration has endured continuous change since the early 1940s when the federal government provided funds for hospital construction. The advent of Medicare and Medicaid in the 1960s, coupled with advances in technology, and pharmaceuticals increased the demand for hospital care, consequently increasing costs. By the late 1960s the spiraling costs of health care began to decline as corporations and state governments began to control the rates charged by hospitals. By the early 1980s the federal government implemented the prospective payment system for Medicare patients. Private and federal controls on health care payments resulted in a decline in the number of patients admitted to hospitals and, therefore, a decline in needed hospital beds. Today hospitals are competing for patients while health payers carefully evaluate the efficacy and quality of services provided (Raffel & Barsukeiwicz, 2002).

Hospitals may be classified in several different ways: by specialty services provided such as pediatrics, orthopedics, psychiatric, and other specialties, and by their location, such as general, community, or rural, urban, and tertiary-care centers. Community and rural hospitals are usually nonfederal, short-stay general, and specialty-care facilities that provide the public with a more limited scope of service than urban hospitals, which generally offer a wider range of services including up-to-date technological care provided by specialists. Tertiary-care centers are large medical centers that draw patients from a large geographical area. They provide cutting-edge care and are almost always associated with teaching and research programs (Harkreader & Hogan, 2004). Hospitals are also classified by ownership. The major categories are nonprofit, for-profit, and government owned. Whereas these categories are meaningful, today there is a wide range of integrated systems for owning hospitals. For example, a community hospital may be owned in part by the community and in part by a for-profit organization.

Although confusing, nonprofit hospitals are not prohibited from making a profit; however, any profits made must be returned to the hospital's operation or used to benefit the community. Nonprofit hospitals are exempt from paying taxes and generally have a board of trustees as their governing body. Conversely, for-profit hospitals operate with the goal of making a profit. These organizations have shareholders or owners who usually elect a board of trustees whose responsibilities are similar to those of nonprofit organizations. For-profit hospitals operate under corporate structures in competitive environments. Government hospitals may be federal, state, or community owned. Federal hospitals owned by the Department of Defense (DOD) are Army, Navy, and Air Force hospitals. The DOD is currently working to consolidate and decrease the number of military hospitals. The Veterans Administration has over 100 hospitals throughout the country, and the Indian Health Services in the U.S. Public Health Service owns hospitals on various reservations. State, county, and city hospitals exist in many parts of the country. Government hospitals tend to be political and serve the poor and uninsured. Often state and local hospitals serve the mentally ill.

Other inpatient services are provided in long-term care facilities. **Long-term care** refers to a large range of housing and health services provided to people who are unable to care for themselves independently or who need assistance with daily living. Although long-term care facilities are generally associated with nursing homes for senior adults, they also offer services to any age of people who have functional disabilities. For example, people with mental or neurological impairment, spinal cord injuries, birth defects, and other chronic debilitating conditions may be cared for in long-term care facilities. Many individuals, following inpatient hospitalization, require a short stay in a long-term facility until they are able to return to independent living. Some patients, following discharge from acute-care hospitals, are admitted to rehabilitation hospitals that offer specialized restorative services to chronically ill or disabled patients. Generally rehabilitation hospitals provide short-term nursing care, physical therapy, occupational therapy, and social and vocational services.

Hospice care is a specialized service available to those who are terminally ill and their families. Most hospice-care facilities use an interdisciplinary-team approach to provide palliative and supportive care to meet the physical, emotional, social, spiritual, legal, and financial needs that occur during end of life and bereavement. Hospice services are provided in inpatient as well as outpatient settings.

OUTPATIENT SETTINGS

Emergency care for victims of accidents and acute illnesses is most often provided by emergency medical technicians (EMTs) who work from mobile units based in local fire departments or specialized medical centers. EMTs are trained to provide first-aid and life-saving early treatment onsite and enroute, via ambulance or helicopter, to nearby hospitals or to regional trauma centers that provide a full range of complex services.

Community-based care is provided in ambulatory-care centers, physicians' offices, adult daycare settings, school health clinics, and centers for respite-care services, home health care, and hospice services. Ambulatory-care centers include freestanding walk-in emergency centers, same-day surgical centers, mobile health units, health-promotion centers, health department and community free clinics, community mental health centers, and in some cases, prison health centers. These are centers where patients can walk in and be seen by a physician and receive testing, diagnosis, treatment, and possibly physician referral. Physicians in their offices provide similar services. School health clinics provide first-aid and emergency treatment and referral. Health-promotion centers provide health assessments, health education, and programs for promoting or sustaining health such as smoking-cessation classes. Adult daycare centers offer daytime programs to individuals, usually older adults, who require supervision and care while their primary caregivers are at work. Respite-care programs offer temporary in-home assistance to those who care for older adults or others requiring in-home supervision. Home health care services, such as skilled nursing care; home health aids; physical, speech or occupational therapy; homemaker services; and social services, may be provided to patients who are unable to leave their homes.

Major types of health care services

In the United States, the health care system has traditionally been illness oriented with little attention to disease prevention. While the U.S. government has no definitive national health policy, an important first step was taken in 1980 when the U.S. Public Health Service established the goals and objectives for improving the health of citizens by the year 2000. The result of this work was *Healthy People 2000: National Health Promotion Objectives*. These objectives were revised in 2003 in the latest iteration of the objectives, *Healthy People 2010: Healthy Communities* (Chitty, 2005).

WRITING EXERCISE 8.1

1. Given the brief introduction to heath care settings in this chapter, what are the differences and similarities in the role of the nurse in each of the health care agencies described above?

2. Because many of the services provided in health care agencies seem to overlap, describe the different services provided in a community health department as opposed to a community health center at a hospital. What services are different and what services are the same?

3. Discuss the role of the nurse as a gatekeeper in introducing the patient to the health care system and in moving the patient from one health care agency to another. Is this a proper role for the nurse?

Mindful of the types of settings where health care is provided, there are three major types or categories of health care services: primary, secondary, and tertiary. **Primary care** refers to those services that promote health, such as those specific to preventing disease and illness and promoting healthy lifestyles. Keeping people healthy is the concern in primary care. Illness prevention includes identifying risk factors for disease and illness. A goal of health promotion is to modify a patient's knowledge, attitude, skills, and behavior in order to achieve wellness and prevent illness. Health education is essential in primary care; however, education alone is not sufficient in promoting healthy behaviors, patient motivation is also an essential element. Health-promotion services assume that persons who participate in healthy lifestyles will avoid certain diseases such as lung cancer and heart attacks; avoid certain pulmonary diseases, diabetes, motor-vehicle accidents, and other risk-taking behaviors; and will decrease infant mortality. There remains a controversy regarding legislating healthy behaviors. For example, wearing a seat belt while riding in a motor vehicle as well as smoking in public places remain controversial, although there are laws regarding both in most states. Primary care includes but is not limited to nutritional awareness for children and adults, prenatal care for all pregnant women, well-baby care including immunizations, adult immunizations, aerobic exercise for all ages, smoking-cessation classes, decreasing obesity, asthma prevention, worksite wellness, and occupational safety programs.

Secondary care focuses on detection of disease in the early stages when treatment may be less costly and lead to positive outcomes and the treatment of disease and injury. These services also require active participation by patients. Examples of secondary care include the use of mammograms, cholesterol screening, blood glucose screening, cervical pap smears, osteoporosis screening, prostate-specific antigen screening, vision and hearing screening as well as high-tech computerized tomography (CT) scans and three-dimensional ultrasonograhpy. Secondary care includes treatment of illness and disease and usually takes place in inpatient and outpatient settings. This major component of the health care system continues to improve as technological and pharmacological advances allow earlier diagnosis and more efficient treatment of disease and illness.

Tertiary care is rehabilitative and restorative care that may be provided in outpatient and inpatient settings. Tertiary care usually requires practitioners with highly specialized skills, support, and technology. The goal of tertiary care is to bring each patient to his or her highest level of functioning. This includes managing chronic illness, disability, or terminal illness when restoration or rehabilitation is not a realistic goal (Harkreader & Hogan, 2004). Disease management is a relatively modern phenomenon that belongs under tertiary care. The concept of managing disease is directly related to the aging population in the United States and the chronic diseases suffered by this population. Chronic diseases such as arthritis, diabetes, congestive heart disease, coronary artery disease, hypertension, asthma, and chronic obstructive pulmonary diseases decrease quality of life and require symptoms prevention and management. Disease-management specialists provide information, coaching, and education along with national guidelines, medication lists, and alternative therapies not normally available to patients (Chitty, 2005).

THE HEALTH CARE TEAM

The U.S. health care industry employs more individuals than any other industry in the nation (Shi & Singh, 2004). For an indefinite future, there is a severe shortage of health care workers across the entire United States. It affects most disciplines including nursing, pharmacy, medical coders, physicians, radiology technicians, laboratory technicians, and respiratory therapists. It is predicted that the health care industry will grow at a rate of 30 percent between 2002 and 2012, adding 3.5 million new jobs (U.S. Bureau of Labor Statistics, 2004).

Table 8.1 **Employment of Wage and Salary Workers in Health Services by Occupation, 2004 and Projected Change, 2004–14. (Employment in Thousands)**

| Occupation | Employment 2004 | | Percent change 2004–14 |
	Number	Percent	
Total, all occupations	13,062	100.0	27.3
Management, business, and financial occupations	574	4.4	28.3
Top executives	101	0.8	33.3
Medical and health services managers	175	1.3	26.1
Professional and related occupations	5,657	43.3	27.8
Psychologists	33	0.3	28.1
Counselors	152	1.2	31.8
Social workers	169	1.3	29.3
Health educators	17	0.1	27.0
Social and human service assistants	99	0.8	38.6
Chiropractors	21	0.2	47.8
Dentists	95	0.7	18.5
Dietitians and nutritionists	32	0.2	20.1
Optometrists	18	0.1	29.6
Pharmacists	63	0.5	17.3
Physicians and surgeons	417	3.2	28.7
Physician assistants	53	0.4	54.8
Podiatrists	7	0.1	22.2
Registered nurses	1,988	15.2	30.5
Therapists	358	2.7	32.8
Clinical laboratory technologists and technicians	257	2.0	22.7
Dental hygienists	153	1.2	43.7
Diagnostic-related technologists and technicians	269	2.1	26.4
Emergency medical technicians and paramedics	122	0.9	27.8
Health diagnosing and treating practitioner support technicians	226	1.7	18.0
Licensed practical and licensed vocational nurses	586	4.5	14.2
Medical records and health information technicians	134	1.0	30.0

NOTE: May not add to totals due to omission of occupations with small employment.
Occupational Outlook. Retrieved March 30, 2006 from www.bls.gov/emp/home.htm

The accelerated employment growth and the current shortage of health care personnel guarantee employment for those participating in the multidisciplinary health care team.

Registered Nurses

Nurses comprise the largest number of health care providers. The U.S. Census Bureau reports that there are 2.4 million registered nurses in the United States, with a projected growth of 623,000, by 2012, the largest job growth of any occupation (U. S. Dept. of Labor, 2004). A registered nurse is a graduate of a two to four year formal program of nursing that is state approved, and who is licensed by the appropriate state as defined by the Nurse Practice Act of that state. Licensure requires successfully completing a national examination, the National Council Licensure Examination-RN, (NCLEX-RN) developed by the National Council of State Boards of Nursing.

Although the American Nurses Association recommends that states require a baccalaureate degree to practice nursing, there are several educational entry paths to RN licensure. These include a limited number of two- to three-year diploma programs associated with hospitals, associate-degree programs found frequently in community colleges, and baccalaureate-degree programs most often found in comprehensive colleges or universities. The shortage of nurses throughout the country has prompted the development of fast-track programs for acquiring a degree in nursing. For example, many colleges offer a 15-month program in nursing to those who hold a baccalaureate degree in another discipline.

Nurses are the major caregivers in health care agencies. They provide holistic care to patients in inpatient and outpatient settings. Nurses provide health teaching, case finding, health counseling, supportive care, and implement regimens prescribed by licensed physicians. Increasingly, nurses are employed in supportive positions such as case management, quality assurance, and utilization review. The increasing use of technology in health care offers opportunities for nurses in this field, while a growing older population, demanding primary preventive care, offers additional opportunities for nurses. The professional practice of nursing is based on theoretical frameworks. Most nursing theory is evolving; however, theorists such as Martha Rogers, Sister Callista Roy, Dorothea Orem, and Betty Neuman have contributed to theory-based nursing science (Zerwekh & Clayborn, 2003).

Advanced-Practice Nurses

Advanced-practice nurses are registered nurses. These recently trained nurses have at least a master's degree and clinical practice beyond the 4-year graduate. *Nurse practitioners* and *clinical nurse specialist* are terms used to describe advanced-practice nurses.

Nurse practitioners (NP) generally have a specialty area such as adult, family, or pediatrics. NPs diagnose and treat common illnesses and injuries, counsel and educate patients, and in most states prescribe medications. Some states allow NPs independent practice status that is reimbursed by Medicare and Medicaid. Most NPs are certified by national organizations or the American Nurses Association. The latest available number for currently licensed nurse practitioners in the U.S. is around 141, 209 with the number to continually increase in the upcoming year (http://www.acnpweb.org/files/public/FAQ_about_NPS_May06.pdf).

Clinical nurse specialists (CNS) are registered nurses with a minimum of a master's degree, who are experts in a specialized clinical practice area such as critical care, mental health, gerontology, cardiac care, cancer care, neonatal care, and community health. There are approximately 58,185 CNSs in the United States. In addition to providing patient care, CNSs conduct health assessments; conduct or participate in research, education and administration; and develop quality-control methods. They work in all health care settings from acute-care hospitals to private practice, and most are eligible for reimbursement from Medicare and Medicaid. (www.nursingworld.org/readroom/fsadvprc.htm.)

Advanced-practice nurses are capable of providing preventive and primary health care that is cost-effective and convenient to a vast majority of patients who may lack basic care. Other categories of advanced practice include Certified Nurse Midwife (CNM), who provide well-women, gynecological and low-risk obstetrical care; and Certified Registered Nurse Anesthetist (CRNA), who administer more than 65 percent of all anesthetics given to patients each year. (www.nursingworld.org/readroom/fsadvprc.htm.)

Physicians

Physicians have the major responsibility of evaluating, diagnosing, and prescribing treatment for patients. They are primarily responsible for admitting patients to health hospitals, ordering tests, and referring patients to therapists. Increasingly, physicians are providing primary and culturally competent care. A physicians is a graduate of a medical school or school of osteopathy and has participated in a one- or two-year internship. They must be licensed by the state in which they practice, diagnose, and treat patients according to the medical-practice act for that state. They work in a variety of settings, but most are in private or group practices. Many specialize in particular areas that require additional years of education and training and specialty board certification. Common specialties include medicine, surgery, obstetrics, gynecology, pediatrics, psychiatry, and radiology (Harkreader & Hogan, 2004).

Physician Assistants

The American Academy of Physicians Assistants (2005) defines **physician assistants** (PA) as "health care professionals licensed to practice medicine with physician supervision." Eugene Stead of Duke University Medical Center, recognizing the shortage of primary-care physicians at the time and the number of corpsmen who were returning from the Vietnam War, put together the first class of PAs in 1965. Following defined courses of study usually leading to a baccalaureate degree, PAs may be certified by the National Commission on Certification of Physician Assistants. According to Harkreader and Hogan (2004, p. 60), "PAs practice only under the supervision of a physician and are not meant to be a separate profession such as nursing."

Pharmacists

A **pharmacist** is a graduate of an accredited program in pharmacology, usually at the doctoral level, licensed to prepare and dispense drugs when presented with a prescription from a licensed practitioner. Today pharmacists are taking an active role in assisting practitioners in making appropriate drug choices for patients and in counseling patients regarding medication administration and expected results.

Social Workers

A **social worker** is usually a graduate of a master's program in social work whose scope of practice is licensed and regulated in most of the United States. On their Web site, the International Federation of Social Workers defines social work as "The social work profession promotes social change, problem solving in human relationships, and the empowerment and liberation of people to enhance well-being. Utilizing theories of human behavior and social systems, social work intervenes at points where people interact with environments. Principles of human rights and social justice are fundamental to social work." Social workers are engaged in counseling, family therapy, and in assisting people in obtaining services and resources in the community. They often work in managed care and in clinical settings to facilitate appropriate discharge planning and follow-up for patients.

Allied Health Practitioners

Allied health practitioners range from those who have some college education, often an associate degree, and on-the-job training, to those who have doctoral-level preparation. This broad category of workers includes technologists; technicians such as dietary, respiratory, radiology, rehabilitation, and sonography technicians; and nursing assistants, also called unlicensed assistive personnel (UAP). Allied health providers are the fastest growing occupations in the United States and constitute approximately 60 percent of the U.S. health care work force (Shi & Singh, 2004 p. 140).

HEALTH CARE FINANCING

Health care in America is more expensive than in any other developed country. Over the past 35 years, financing health care in the United States has evolved and continues today as a blend of public and private responsibilities. Restructuring of health care reimbursement began in the 1980s, and since that time change has been continuous. No description of health care financing is complete without Medicare, Medicaid, private health insurance, and managed care.

Medicare

Medicare is a federally funded health insurance program, initiated in 1965 as Title XVIII of the Social Security Act. It was originally intended for persons over age 65, but in 1973 benefits were extended to younger persons with chronic illnesses who were entitled to Social Security benefits and for those with end-stage renal disease. Medicare has two parts, A and B. Americans over the age of 65 receive Medicare part A free of premiums if they or a spouse paid taxes while they worked, and for a fee for those who never paid taxes. Part A pays for some costs for inpatient hospital care, skilled nursing facilities, hospice care, and home health care. These services are not free with Part A; beneficiaries are required to pay deductibles and coinsurance premiums. Medicare part B was available for a premium of approximately $78.60 a month in 2005. Part B pays some

physicians' fees, outpatient hospital care, physical and occupational therapy, and some home health care fees.

In 1983 the Medicare fee system changed to help contain escalating costs. Hospital reimbursement became prospective using a system based on diagnosis-related groups (DRGs). A **DRG** is a group of diagnoses that cause a similar length of stay in a hospital. Length of stay for each classification of DRG became the standard for calculating reimbursement for hospitals. Private insurers quickly followed the Medicare system reimbursing prospectively based on DRG rather than retrospectively after the care was delivered. When initiated, Medicare payments were based on the amount physicians charged. The Omnibus Budget Reconciliation Act of 1989 changed Medicare payments to physicians. The new system is a national fee schedule that pays for services based on time, skill, and intensity. The Balanced Budget Act of 1997 again changed Medicare funding. This plan increased the number of health plans that were eligible for Medicare payments and increased Medicare benefits to include screening and preventative services (Kovner & Jonas, 2002).

One serious problem with medical costs for seniors in the United States remained unanswered, the cost of medications. On November 15, 2005, nearly 40 million Americans eligible for Medicare were offered Medicare Part D, prescription drug insurance. The Prescription Drug Improvement Act of 2003, PL108-173, passed through Congress after a highly political battle and amended Title XVIII of the Social Security act to establish the prescription drug benefit program. The Act established the initial standards to be used in a pilot project in the year 2006. A report on the pilot is due to Congress in April 2007, and the final standards must be in place by April 2008. The plan provides insurance coverage to seniors who have no medication insurance and to those who have insurance that is substandard to Medicare Part D. Those who have medication insurance through employers or a retiree plan that provides as good as or better insurance than Medicare Part D should remain in their current plan.

Medicare is working to provide subsidies to support good quality medication retiree coverage. The first beneficiaries of this plan are those who enrolled by December 30, 2005. Their coverage began on January 1, 2006. Those eligible for coverage were able to enroll until May 15, 2006 without penalty and their coverage began the first day of the month after enrollment. After May 15, 2006, those who wanted to enroll in Medicare Part D were subject to a penalty of 1 percent of the average monthly payment for the time they delayed enrollment for the life of the program. The average monthly premium cost for an individual is approximately $37.00, and this may be deducted from Social Security Benefits. The monthly premium cost decreases for those with low income and few savings or assets; for example, someone with an annual income of $8700 would pay no monthly premium. Prescription medications are not free for those who participate in Plan D. The plan is complicated and has four parts: (1) a monthly premium and deductible, usually $250; (2) a co-insurance of up to $2000, insurance pays 75 percent, insured pays 25 percent; (3) after receiving medications worth up to $2000, Gap insurance pays 0 percent, insured pays 100 percent up to $2800; (4) The plan pays 95 percent of all eligible drug costs for the remainder of the calendar year. The government has an approved list of drugs it covers called a formulary. Before choosing a plan, those eligible for Part D should speak with their health care provider about the medications covered by various plans. Table 8.2 illustrates medical enrollee costs.

Medicaid

Medicaid is a federally and state funded program specifically for the aged poor, and those blind and disabled who have limited income. Medicaid is also available to families with dependent children who have only one parent who is unemployed or unable to work. Low-income pregnant women and teenagers may be eligible for Medicaid. The rules for eligibility and for services vary by state. Federal funds for Medicaid also vary by state and are dependent on the state's per-capita income. Title XIX of the Social Security Act requires that the following services must be available under Medicaid in order for states to receive Federal funds: inpatient and outpatient hospital services; physician medical, surgical, and dental services; nursing-home care and nursing facility services; family planning services; rural health and clinic services; laboratory and x-ray services; pediatric and family nurse practitioner and nurse midwife services; health center and ambulatory-care services; screening, diagnostic, and treatment services for those under 21 years of age. Some states provide additional services that may include prenatal care; home health and nursing facility services; services for the mentally challenged; optometrist care and eyeglasses; prescription drugs; tuberculosis testing and services; prosthetic and dental services.

Worker's Compensation

An additional health payment system provided by states is the **worker's compensation** insurance system. This provides some financial assistance to those who incur medical costs and loss of income due to work-related injuries or illness.

Private Insurance

Insurance is defined as an agreement or contract in which an agent agrees to pay for another party's financial loss. Health insurance pays the expenses for medical care needed as a result of sickness or injury. **Private health insurance** refers to many different types of plans provided by large and small insurance companies such as Blue Cross and Blue Shield, Aetna, Cigna, and many others. Most individuals obtain health insurance in a group plan through their employers. Insurance agencies, using sophisticated actuarial statistics, assign a risk factor to the group based on individual member characteristics. For example, young adults in the United States are generally considered healthy and, aside from childbirth, use the health care system sparingly. Compare this with a group of senior citizens aged 70 to 80, and the risk of using the health care system increases significantly. The assigned risk determines the fee charged for insurance that is distributed among all members

Table 8.2 **Medical Enrollee Costs (in 2003)**

Medicare part A enrollee costs

Hospital stays for each benefit period

- A total of $840 for a hospital stay of 1–60 days.
- $210 per day for days 61–90 of a hospital stay.
- $420 per day for days 91–150 of a hospital stay.
- All costs for each day beyond 150 days.

Skilled nursing facility care for each benefit period

- Nothing for the first 20 days.
- Up to $105 per day for days 21–100.
- All costs beyond the 100th day in the benefit period.

Home health care

- Nothing for home health care services.
- 20% of the Medicare-approved amount for durable medical equipment.

Hospice care

A copayment of up to $5 for outpatient prescription drugs and 5% of the Medicare-approved amount for inpatient respite care (short-term care given to a hospice patient so that the usual caregiver can rest). Medicare generally does not pay for room and board except in certain cases. For example, room and board are not covered for general hospice services while a patient is a resident of a nursing home or a hospice's residential facility. However, room and board are covered for inpatient respite care and during short-term hospital stays.

Medicare part B enrollee costs

Medical and other services each year

- $100 deductible (once per calendar year).
- 20% of Medicare-approved amount after the deductible.
- 20% for all outpatient physical, occupational, and speech/language therapy services. (No coverage limit for these therapy services provided by a hospital outpatient facility. If provided at another type of outpatient setting, $1,590 coverage limit per year for occupational therapy services, and $1,590 limit per year for physical and speech/language therapy services combined).
- 50% for outpatient mental health care.

Clinical laboratory services

No enrollee payments for Medicare-approved services.

Home health care

- Nothing for Medicare-approved services.
- 20% of the Medicare-approved amount for durable medical equipment.

Outpatient hospital services

A coinsurance or copayment amount, which may vary according to the service

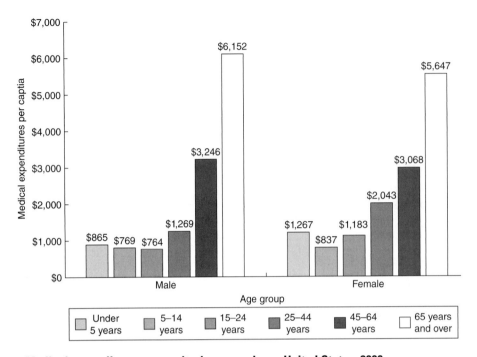

Figure 8.1 **Medical expenditures per capita, by age and sex, United States, 2000.**

SOURCE: *Household Component Analytical Tool* (*MEPSnet/HC*). August 2003. Agency for Healthcare Research and Quality, Rockville, MD http://www.meps.ahrq.gov/mepsnet/HC/MEPSnetHC.asp (accessed on October 8, 2003).

of the group. If one is in an insurance group with those who are fairly healthy and who use the health care system sparingly, the assigned risk will be low, and the amount each member pays for insurance will be less than those who are in a group with individuals who frequently use the health insurance benefits.

Many employers pay a portion of the health insurance premium as a benefit to employees. Individual private health insurance may be available to those who are self-employed or to those who work for employers that do not provide insurance benefits. Unlike group insurance wherein the group determines the risk, individual insurance risk is determined by the health status and demographics of each individual, often making costs prohibitively high.

Health insurance for those under age 65 remains a critical issue in the United States. National statistics confirm that as of 2003, 17 percent of those under age 65 have no health insurance, with those ages 18 to 24 and those with incomes below or near the poverty level the least likely to have insurance. The growing number of Hispanic immigrants is expected to further increase the percentage of the population without insurance. Figure 8.1 illustrates the medical expenditures per capita, by age and sex, in the United States. Figure 8.2 illustrates the number of persons without health insurance coverage.

MANAGED CARE

The evolution of the health care system, the Federal system of Medicare and Medicaid, and the escalation of health care costs brought dramatic changes in the private health insurance market. The most notable change occurred in the 1980s with the advent of managed care. Insurance companies began charging employers or individuals annual premiums based on a fee for service. This system provides a certain fixed fee for service that is negotiated

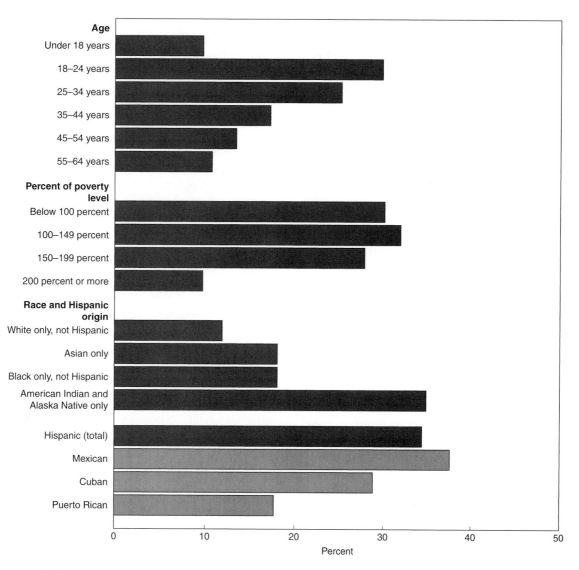

Figure 8.2 **No health insurance coverage among persons under 65 years of age by selected characteristics: United States, 2003.**

NOTES: Persons of Hispanic origin may be of any race. Asian and American Indian and Alaska Native races include persons of Hispanic and non-Hispanic origin. See Data Table for data points graphed, standard errors, and additional notes.

SOURCE: Centers for Disease Control and Prevention, National Center for Health Statistics, National Health Interview Survey.

between insurers and the providers and is paid by the insurer each time a service is provided.

A rapidly growing managed-care approach that began in the early 1980s and continues to grow in popularity in the United States is Health Maintenance Organizations (HMOs). HMOs provide health care on a capitated basis not on a fee-for-service basis. That is, payers pay a flat rate for each person per year regardless of the number of times the insured uses the health care system. Different types of HMOs provide services by hiring physicians as employees of the HMO, by contracting with physicians for services, or by contracting with a range of private office-based physicians. Preferred provider organizations (**PPOs**) require insured members to use a set list of physicians who generally offer discounts to insurance providers (Kovner & Jonas, 2002). The dollars spent on health care in the United States is a direct result of payments made by consumers. Whether through tax dollars eventually resulting in Medicare and Medicaid payments, public or private health insurance premiums, or in private pay-for-services fees, health care dollars come from consumers.

Chartbook on Trends in the Health of Americans, (National Center for Health Statistics, 2005) reported that in 2003, the United States spent $1.7 trillion on health care. This is on average $5,671 per person, with private insurance paying for 36 percent of the total, the federal government paying 33 percent, state and local governments 11 percent, and out of pocket was 16 percent. Approximately one-third of this total amount was for hospital care, one-quarter for physician care, one-eighth for prescription drugs, and one-fifth for other personal health care such as visits to nonphysician medical providers, medical supplies, and other services.

Over the last twenty years, managed care had slowed the escalation of health care costs. However, discounted fees, restricted paths to specialty providers, prior authorization for services, and physician networks have created controversy regarding patient rights, access to care, and quality of care. The controversy has become a major political and legislative issue along with the fact that in 2005, 45 million Americans had no health insurance, this includes 8.4 million children. (U.S. Census Bureau News, August, 2004a).

The quality of health care in the United States should not be confused with the quantity of health care. In trying to measure quality, the use of computerized records, interviews, observation, and individual record review are data sources. Regardless of the methods of assessment, quality assurance methods that have been used are licensing, accreditation, and Professional Standards Review Organizations (PSRO). Continuous Quality Improvement (CQI) is an industrial concept that uses statistical methods to encourage change and growth in order to raise the norm of performance. CQI does not seek to identify errors, but assumes that a faulty system is responsible for error. CQI measures provide analysis of systems that can be used by managers to enhance care. CQI has the potential to transform the health care delivery system (Kovner & Jonas, 2002).

HEALTH CARE DEMANDS AND CHANGING TRENDS

To make our economy stronger and more productive, we must make health care more affordable and give families greater access to good coverage and more control over their health decisions. I ask Congress to move forward on a comprehensive health agenda with: Credits to help low-income workers buy insurance, a community health center in every poor county, improved information technology to prevent medical error and needless costs, association health plans for small business and their employees. Expanded health savings accounts, and medical liability reforms that will reduce health care costs and make sure patients have the doctors and care they need (George Bush, State of the Union Speech, Feb 2, 2005).

Major changes in the health care delivery system will continue as societal influences have a major impact on the medical profession as a whole. Changes in demographics, environmental changes related to public health disasters, unhealthy lifestyles, government regulations, the insurance industry, scientific and technological advances, and standardization and regulation of health care will no doubt influence health care delivery in the future.

WRITING EXERCISE 8.2

Evaluating the cost of health care delivery in the United States in many ways connects access to health care.

1. Investigate the Medicare, Medicaid, and insurance reimbursement for a common admission diagnosis using DRG length of stay.

2. Identify any differences in cost per day for a nursing home resident under Medicare, public assistance, private long-term-care insurance, and private pay.

3. Identify and evaluate the services available to those in your community who have no health care insurance. Consider emergency care, wellness care, and routine-illness care as well as the age of the patient. Are available services different for children and older adults?

4. Visit a health care agency in your community. Identify changes in the facility, management, organizational structure, or services provided in the last three years.

5. Evaluate the differences in services provided by a health insurance plan and a health maintenance plan in your community. Describe any differences in choice and accessibility and how these differences affect primary, secondary, and tertiary care.

Changing Demographics: The Aging Population

The single most important issue facing the health care system in the next century is dealing with the aging **baby boomers,** those 76 million Americans born between 1946 and 1964 (Strying & Jonas, 1999). The retirement age in the United States is around 62 to age 65. By 2010 the first of the boomers will have reached retirement age, and over the next 20 years all will. It is generally agreed that the most productive working years are from ages 25 to 64. The ratio of those 25 to 64 and those over 65 has remained at about 4:1 for decades. When the boomers reach retirement age, this ratio will fall to 3:1 by 2020, and 2:1 by 2030 (Strying & Jonas, 1999).

Table 8.3 **Projected Population of the United States by Age from 2000 to 2050**

	(In Thousands) YEAR AGE and % of Population in each Age Group			
	20–44	45–64	65–84	85+
2000	36.9	22.1	10.9	1.5
2010	33.8	26.2	11.0	2.0
2020	32.3	24.9	14.1	2.2
2030	31.6	22.6	17.0	2.6
2040	31.0	22.6	16.5	3.9
2050	31.2	22.2	15.7	5.0

SOURCE: U.S. Census Bureau 2004.

The rising tide of older Americans will have a profound effect on the health insurance industry, Medicare, and the health care system in general. Health care spending is projected to account for 15.9 percent of the gross domestic product (GDP) by 2010, up from 13.9 percent in the year 2000. Medicare spending will account for 16.8 percent of national health spending, up from 15.4 percent in 1999 (Heffler, Levit, Smith, C., Smith, S., Cowan, Lazenby, & Freeland, 2001).

Today approximately 47 percent of all hospital admissions in the U.S. are by those 65 years or older. Over the next 25 years this population will double as demands for health care services, especially for chronic care conditions escalate (Kovner & Jonas, 2002). As the population ages, geriatrics and a focus on chronic care and the frail elderly will pervade the health care system. Physicians will develop better systems for managing chronic illnesses using evidence-based practice, and technological advances for tracking symptoms and for data management. Multidisciplinary health care teams will provide services to patients who are motivated to manage their own care.

As Americans influence managed care by making informed decisions about their health care providers and payers, the health care payment system will change to accommodate their needs. The evolution of managed care will result in decreased hospitalizations and focus on primary and tertiary care. Statistical data from disease management protocols and from clinical pathways will contribute to financial and administrative health system decisions. Specialty and tertiary care services will increase as the length of stay in hospitals decreases and the need for skilled nursing care facilities increases (Simonet, 2005).

Technology

The health care industry began using information technology (IT) as a tool for administration in billing and finance. Increasingly, IT is now used for data collection, medical records, and documenting quality of care. The information gathering capabilities of IT is providing data that is used by physicians in diagnosis and treatment protocols, and in documenting standards of care. Computerized patient records will result in information standardization across health care providers and health care settings. From primary physicians to specialists, physicians' offices to long-term care, patient records will be standardized and available. The possibility of computerized records on drivers' licenses, military dog tags, or other cards embedded with computerized chips is a reality, not an innovation of the future. Public health nurses working in rural areas are using sophisticated robotic monitoring equipment in patients' homes to continuously or periodically monitor vital signs and communicate with patients. Hospitals employ physicians and nurses who monitor those in intensive care units from remote sites, and digital x-rays taken in emergency rooms are read by physicians in far away countries.

Technological Innovations and Genetics

The Human Genome project is a federally funded research effort that has mapped each human gene in order to better understand human genetic makeup. This project has enormous implications for medical care in the future. It is likely that as a result of this project, many traditional diseases as well as genetically transmitted and genetically predisposed diseases will be prevented. This project sparked the development of very large long-term studies of particular groups or entire populations to establish "biobanks" for the discovery of genes and other factors such as chemical, physical, infectious, and social factors that either singly or in combination increase or decrease the risk of common diseases (Knoppers, 2005). The idea of studies that evaluate genetic predisposition is laden with ethical questions. It may be necessary to shed the ethical principles of individual autonomy so prevalent in the United States today in order to focus on ethical and legal principles that are based on the concept of the "common good." Pharmacogenomics will make possible the production of individualized medications to treat patients based on their genetic makeup. These advances will no doubt change

CASE SCENARIO 8.1

Gina is an experienced intensive care nurse and is working with a novice nurse just hired on the unit. Gina is caring for a patient who has a severe head injury and was recently admitted to the unit. The patient is on a cardiac monitor, a ventilator, has several central venous lines connected to pumps, and has a Foley catheter, a cranial shunt, and other monitoring devices connected with various wires and tubes on his body. The new nurse in impressed with Gina's skill in monitoring the patient and in providing for the patient's physical needs. She comes to you to report how skillful Gina is in her work but then asks if anyone ever talks to patients or the patients' families on this unit.

1. As nurses use technology to improve information for decision making, how can they guard against ignoring the human interaction necessary when caring for patients?

2. Technological advances are introduced into health care continually. Should nurses automatically accept technology as enhancements to care?

3. What measures can the nurse take to ensure the proper use of technology in health care settings that require high tech?

4. How can the nurse meet the combined needs for high tech and still provide for the emotional and spiritual needs of the patient?

health care and will require a further restructuring of the health care reimbursement system (Chitty, K. K. 2005; Kovner & Jonas, 2002).

Natural Disasters and Terrorism

The aftermath of September 11, 2001 revolutionized disaster preparedness in the United States. According to Chitty (2005), a disaster is an event or situation that is of greater magnitude than an emergency which disrupts essential services including but not limited to housing, transportation, communication, sanitation, water, and health care, and requires the response of people outside the affected community. Disasters can be manmade, such as water or food contamination; transportation accidents; chemical, biological, or nuclear accidents; or group violence, such as riots or acts of terrorism. Examples of natural disasters are earthquakes, mudslides, influenza, such as bird flu, epidemics, floods, tornadoes, tsunamis, and hurricanes, such as Hurricane Katrina that devastated the city of New Orleans and the surrounding gulf area in August 2005. The effects of Hurricane Katrina brought to light a public

sense of insecurity and a general lack of confidence in local, regional, and national leaders when faced with a major disaster. Generally, health care agencies have disaster or emergency plans in place that address natural disasters. It wasn't until September 11th that planning for human-generated disasters became necessary. Even today, many health care personnel, especially those in rural areas, do not feel vulnerable to human-generated attacks. Each health care provider should be prepared to answer the following: Do you know where your agency's disaster plan is and are you prepared to execute the plan as conceived? In addition, are you and your colleagues prepared for the physical, emotional, spiritual, and other demands that accompany a major disaster such as Hurricane Katrina? (Miller, 2005; Lach, Langan, & James, 2005).

Bioterrorism is the use of a biological or chemical agents as a weapon. All health care providers and especially physicians and nurses must recognize the symptoms associated with biological agents such as anthrax, smallpox, ricin, and others. A critical role for nurses is the notification of the proper authorities and assistance with the diagnosis, postexposure prophylaxis, and treatment of biological exposure. Gebbie and Qureshi (2002), described the following competencies each nurse should have in order to be prepared for and emergency or disaster.

Core Competencies for Nurses:

- Describe the agency's role in responding to a range of emergencies that might arise. (This is specific to your place of work.)
- Describe the chain of command in emergency response. (Know who reports to whom.)
- Identify and locate the agency's emergency response plan (or pertinent portion of it).
- Describe emergency response functions or roles and demonstrate them in regularly performed drills.
- Demonstrate the use of equipment (including personal protective equipment) and the skills required in emergency response during regular drills.
- Demonstrate the correct operation of all equipment used for emergency communication.
- Describe communication roles in emergency response (within our agency; with news media; the general public including patients and families; personal contacts such as one's own family, friends, and neighbors).
- Identify the limits of your own knowledge, skills, and authority, and identify key systems resources for referring matters that exceed those limits.
- Apply creative problem-solving skills and flexible thinking to the situation within the confines of your role, and evaluate the effectiveness of all actions taken.
- Recognize deviations from the norm that might indicate an emergency and describe appropriate action.
- Participate in continuing education to maintain up-to-date knowledge in relevant areas.
- Participate in evaluating every drill or response, and identify necessary changes to the plan.
- Ensure that there is a written plan for major categories of emergencies.
- Ensure that all parts of the emergency plan are practiced regularly.
- Ensure that identified gaps in knowledge or skills are filled.

Unhealthy Lifestyle and Health Behavior

An overwhelming fact is that approximately one half of all deaths in the United States are attributable to individual behaviors and environmental factors including smoking, obesity, alcohol and other drugs, inactivity, and motor-vehicle accidents (Kovner & Jonas, 2002). Year after year, public health officials report increases in obesity among all age groups in the United States. In a study reported in the *Archives of Internal Medicine* (2003) Roland Sturm reports that the number of extremely obese Americans, those at least 100 pounds overweight, has quadrupled to about 1 in every 50 adults since 1980. In the United States approximately 13 percent of children and adolescents aged 6 to 9 are overweight. Obesity in this age group is 3 times more prevalent than in 1960. Another 10 percent of children and adolescents, particularly those 4 to 6 years old, are affected by an increased prevalence of this trend (Eckel, York, Rossner, Hubbard, Caterson, St. Jeor, Haymen, Mullis, & Blair, 2004). It is interesting to note that type 2 diabetes mellitus has been increasingly diagnosed in children, and that in some parts of the world, malnutrition and obesity coexist in the same community (Eckel et al., 2004). There is a worldwide increase in obesity, possibly related to socioeconomic status; however, other factors such as urbanization, increased levels of dietary fat, inactivity, and lack of physical exercise are implicated in this trend. It is estimated that 280,000 to 325,000 deaths in the United States annually are caused by obesity (Eckel et al., 2004). Treating obesity begins with recognition and prioritizing the problem. The U.S. health care community currently lacks tools to deal with this pervasive problem, and obese patients are often stigmatized in society and by those in the health care setting. It is unfortunate that the health problems associated with

RESEARCH APPLICATION ARTICLE

The Agency for Healthcare Research and Quality reviewed 60 studies to determine the most useful training of health care providers in the event of bioterrorism. Infectious disease outbreak models and hospital disaster-drill training were evaluated for effectiveness. While hospital disaster drill training appears to prepare health care workers to identify problems that may occur during a disaster, there are too few studies to determine the effectiveness of bioterrorism preparedness training. One method that is effective in teaching bioterrorism preparedness is using teleconferences. This method reaches large numbers of health care providers and allows for standardization of information.

The U.S. Department of Health & Human Services Agency for Healthcare Research and Quality, www.ahrq.gov, lists the latest studies in Public Health Preparedness and Bioterrorism Planning and Response. This is an excellent resource for health care providers. Other Web sites include the following:

www.bt.cdc.gov/disasters
www.dhs.gov/dhspublic
www.redcross.org
www.hospitalconnect.com/aha/keyissues/disaster-readiness/resources
www.hhs.gov/disasters/index.shtml
www.ready.gov
www.fema.gov/areyouready/
http://palimpsest.stanford.edu/bytopic.disasters/

---

obesity, including heart disease, diabetes, high blood pressure, and arthritis, will create a much greater need for physicians and health care agencies in the future. According to Eckel and colleagues (2004), prevention of obesity will require lifestyle changes in society that include the following:

- Families need to implement healthy food choices and better menu planning.
- Schools should provide highly nutritious meals in lunch programs and provide nutrition education and physical education programs for regular physical activity.
- Work sites could provide opportunities for regular exercise and promote healthy eating through education.
- Communities could promote healthy living by providing access to outside and inside recreational facilities and provide healthy eating programs.
- Health care professionals must treat obesity as an epidemic.

- The government should support healthy lifestyle programs that focus on mass behavioral change.
- Exercise should become expected in all age groups and in all settings.

Primary prevention of obesity will require massive efforts and discoveries not only in health care but in all of society. Figure 8.3 illustrates current overweight and obesity rates by age.

Lung cancer is the leading killer of both men and women in United States. It is well known that smoking is a leading cause of lung cancer, emphysema, and other chronic lung diseases as well as a host of other health problems. Smoking continues to increase in the young, females, and minorities, insuring that tobacco-related deaths will continue in the future (Chitty, 2005).

Trends in physical activity among adults in the United States have been stable over the last few years with 3 in 10 adults engaging in regular leisure time activity. The benefits of regular physical exercise are numerous and include a decreased

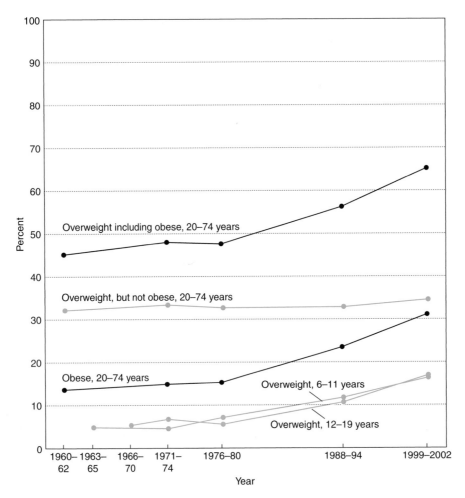

Figure 8.3 **Overweight and obesity by age: United States, 1960–2002.**

NOTES: Percents for adults are age adjusted. For adults: overweight including obese is defined as a body mass index (BMI) greater than or equal to 25, overweight but not obese as a BMI greater than or equal to 25 but less than 30, and obese as a BMI greater than or equal to 30. For children: overweight is defined as a BMI at or above the sex- and age-specific 95th percentile BMI cut points from the 2000 CDC.

Growth Charts: United States. Obese is not defined for children. See Data Table for data points graphed, standard errors, and additional notes.

SOURCES: Centers for Disease Control and Prevention, National Center for Health Statistics, National Health Examination Survey and National Health and Nutrition Examination Survey.

risk of coronary heart disease, colon cancer, osteoporosis, hypertension, diabetes, depression, and prevention of obesity (National Center for Health Statistics, 2005). It is recommended that adolescents exercise for at least 60 minutes a day and for adults to exercise for 30 minutes each day. Figure 8.4 illustrates the physical activity rates for HS students.

Figure 8.5 illustrates the seatbelt usage and under age drinking of high school students. One-third of

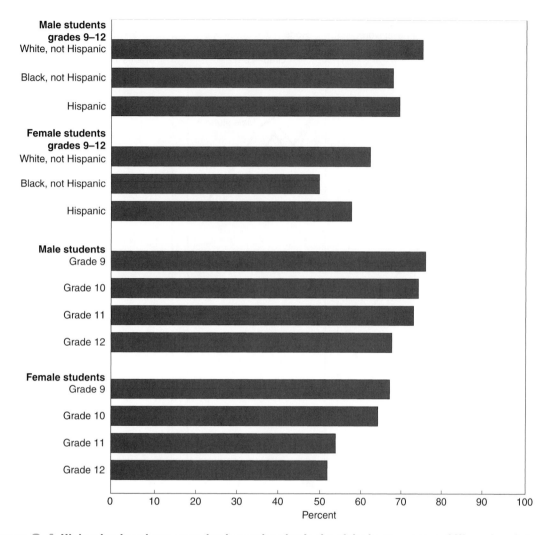

Figure 8.4 **High school students engaging in regular physical activity by sex, race and Hispanic origin and grade: United States, 2003.**

NOTES: Regular physical activity is at least 20 minutes of vigorous activity on 3 or more days or 30 minutes of moderate activity on 5 or more days during the past 7 days. See Data Table for data points graphed, standard errors, and additional notes.

SOURCE: Centers for Disease Control and Prevention, National Center for Chronic Disease Prevention and Health Promotion, Youth Risk Behavior survey.

deaths in people 15 to 24 years old are due to motor-vehicle accidents. Seat belt use can reduce the rate of injury in accidents by up to 45 percent, yet approximately 18 percent of high-school students rarely or never used seat belts in 2003 (National Center for Health Statistics, 2005). Although this figure may seem staggering, 30 percent of high-school students reported in 2003 that they rode in a car with a driver who had been drinking alcohol.

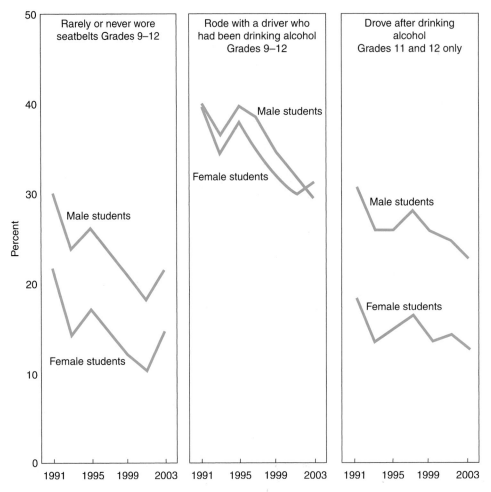

Figure 8.5 **Seatbelt use and drinking and driving among high school students by sex: United States, 1991–2003.**

NOTE: See Data Table for data points graphed, standard errors, and additional notes.

SOURCE: Centers for Disease Control and Prevention, National Center for Chronic Disease Prevention and Health Promotion, Youth Risk Behavior Survey.

Primary Care

As the health care industry continues to evolve, primary care will increase as the focus moves from illness to wellness. Primary-care physicians and nurse practitioners will receive resources to develop early-detection, preventive-care, and ambulatory-care programs in community clinics that will serve the poor as well as those with health care insurance. Increasingly, employers will seek primary-care insurance for employee health, and the growing number of baby boomers interested in wellness will take charge of their health through primary-care providers.

FUTURE TRENDS

The system will change to accommodate primary care offered on an ambulatory-care basis in non-hospital environments; hospital care will be for the most part short stay; there will be residential nursing and therapeutic programs for chronic diseases, nonacute illnesses, and behavioral problems; there will be in-home nursing and support services along with medical equipment, diagnostic and therapeutic services, drugs, and devices using telecommunication (Simonet, 2005).

Human life will be extended through technological advances that include cloning cells, gene replacement, bionics, transplants, and pharmacogeonomics. There will be noninvasive diagnostic tools and robotic surgical procedures controlled by physicians miles or continents away. Alternative medicine for health problems that traditional medicine cannot resolve will continue to grow. Acupuncture, massage therapy, biofeedback, chiropractic, hypnosis, herbal medicine, meditation, and other nontraditional practices are gaining acceptance by the general population. Academic medical centers and the Center for Complementary and Alternative Medicine at the National Institute of Health have brought credibility to many alternative approaches. Alternative medicine is gaining acceptance by some insurance plans.

CHAPTER SUMMARY

The health care delivery system in the United States continues to change because many contributing and often opposing forces compete for access and market share. The number of health care providers in the future will be a major contributor to changes that may occur in health care. Other influences on the future of health care are technological advances unimagined at this time. For today the health care delivery system in the United States is the most sophisticated, complicated, expensive, wasteful, and often dysfunctional system in the world (Kovner & Jonas, 2002).

REFERENCES

American Academy of Physician Assistants (2005). *Information about PAs and the PA profession.* Retrieved August 28, 2005, from http://www.aapa.org/geninfo1.html

American College of Nurse Practitioners (2006). Frequently asked questions from http://www.acnpweb.org/files/public/FAQ_about_NPS_May06.pdf.

Bush, G. W. (2004). [address] *2004 State of the Union address.* [Transcript]. Retrieved September 19, 2005, from http://www.whitehouse.gov/news/releases/2004/01/print/20040120-7.html

Centers for Medicare and Medicaid Services (2004). *Medicaid services.* Retrieved September 1, 2005, from http://www.cms.hhs.gov/medicaid/mservice.asp

Chitty, K. K. (2005). *Professional nursing: Concepts & challenges* (4th ed.). St. Louis, MO: Elsevier Saunders.

Eckel. R. H., York, D., Rossner, S., Hubbard,V., Caterson, I., St. Jeor, S. T., Haymen, L. L., Mullis, R. M., & Blair, S. N.(2004). Prevention conference VII: Obesity, a worldwide epidemic related to heart disease and stroke executive summary. *American Heart Association, Inc. 110*(18), 2968.

Feldman, R. D. (2000). *American health care: Government, market processes, and the public interest.* New Brunswick, NJ: Transaction Publishers.

Gebbie, K. M., & Qureshi, K. (2002). *American Journal of Nursing. 20*(2), 46.

Harkreader, H. C., & Hogan, M. A. (2004). *Fundamentals of nursing: Caring and clinical judgement* (2nd ed.). St. Louis, MO: Saunders.

Heffler, S., Levit, K., Smith, S., Smith, C., Cowan, C., Lazenby, H., & Freeland, M. (2001). Health spending growth up in 1999; faster growth expected in the future. *Health Affairs, 20*(2), 193.

Knoppers, B. M. (2005). Of genomics and public health: Building public "goods"? *Canadian Medical Association Journal: 173*(10), 1185.

Kovner, A. R., & Jonas, S. (2002). *Jonas and Kovner's health care delivery in the United States* (7th ed.). New York: Springer Pub.

Lach, H. W., Langan, J. C., & James O. C. (2005). Disaster planning: Are gerontological nurses prepared? *Journal of Gerontological Nursing, 31*(11), 21–27.

Miller, E. (2005). Disaster preparedness: Are you ready? *Rehabilitation Nursing. 30*(6), *214.*

National Center for Health Statistics (2004). *Fact sheets: National health care survey.* Retrieved August 27, 2005, from http://www.cdc.gov/nchs/data/factsheets/nhcs.pdf

National Center for Health Statistics. (2005). *Health United States 2005, with chartbook on trends in the health of Americans.* Hyattsville MD. Retrieved January 4, 2006, from http://www.cdc.gov/nchs/data/hus/hus05.pdf

Raffel, M. W., & Barsukiewicz, C. K. (2002). *The U.S. health system: Origins and functions* (5th ed.). Albany, NY: Delmar Thomson Learning.

Shi, L., & Singh, D. A. (2004a). *Delivering health care in America: A systems approach* (2nd ed.). Gaithersburg, MD: Aspen Publishers.

Shi, L., & Singh, D. A. (2004b). *Delivering health care in America: A systems approach* (3rd ed.). Boston, MA: Jones and Battlett.

Simonet, D. (2005). Where does the U.S. experience of managed care currently stand? *The International Journal of Health Planning & Management, 20*(2), 137.

Sturm, R. (2003). Increases in clinically severe obesity in the United States, 1986–2000 [Abstract]. *Archives of Internal Medicine, 163*(18), 2146. Abstract retrieved September 3, 2005, from the PubMed database.

Styring, W., & Jonas, D. K. (1999). *Health care 2020: The coming collapse of employer-provided health care.* Indianapolis, IN: Hudson Institute.

U.S. Census Bureau (2004a). *Income stable, poverty up, numbers of Americans with and without health insurance rise, Census Bureau reports.* Retrieved August 27, 2005, from http://www.census.gov/Press-Release/www/releases/archives/income_wealth/002484.html

U.S. Census Bureau. (2004b). *U.S. Interim projections by age, sex, race, and Hispanic origin.* Retrieved November 26, 2005, from http://www.census.gov/ipc/www/usinterimproj/

U.S. Department of Health & Human Services (2001). *Preliminary findings from the National Sample Survey of Registered Nurses 2000.* Retrieved September 19, 2005, from ftp://ftp.hrsa.gov/bhpr/nursing/sampsurvpre.pdf

U.S. Department of Labor, & U.S. Department of Education (2004). *High-growth industry profile: Health care.* Retrieved August 28, 2005, from http://www.careervoyages.gov/pdf/healthcare-profile-504.pdf

Zerwekh, J. G., & Clayborn, J. C. (2003). *Nursing today: Transitions and trends* (4th ed.). St. Louis, MO: Saunders.

CHAPTER 9

Professional Accountability: Credentialing and Accreditation

Lillian Wise and Amy Spurlock

Regulation is the major vehicle ensuring our accountability to the public.
—Dr. Margretta Madden Styles

LEARNING OBJECTIVES

At the completion of the chapter, the learner should be able to do the following:

1. Analyze the issues related to professional accountability in the profession of nursing.
2. Explain current accreditation and approval trends in nursing education.
3. Identify current licensure requirements and trends in nursing.
4. Discuss the mutual recognition model for nurse licensure and identify Nurse Licensure Compact states.
5. Analyze mandatory continuing education issues in the nursing profession.
6. Differentiate certification and credentialing in nursing practice.
7. Identify the purpose of JCAHO in the regulation of nursing practice.

KEY TERMS

Accreditation

Certification

Credentialing

Licensure

Mandatory continuing education

Mutual recognition model of nurse licensure

Professional accountability

Regulation

In the twenty-first century a complex and shrinking world as well as rapid changes compels health care professionals to expand the focus on **professional accountability** in nursing. Decreasing resources, public demands for quality health care, the nursing shortage, report cards for health care agencies, telemedicine, and the explosion of the information available to the consumer on the Internet demand a clear emphasis on accountability and the related regulatory processes for the nurse (Miller, 2003; Styles, 1998). Professional accountability is defined as the responsibility that nurses assume for their nursing practice and the obligation to report or account for their actions to the profession, the public, and themselves.

Nursing is regulated through multiple processes that nurses should understand as they relate to their nursing practice. These processes may regulate individual nurses through licensure and certification or may regulate a school of nursing or health care service agency through approval and accreditation (Styles, 1998). These regulatory processes enhance the professional accountability in nursing by monitoring standards of practice, competency, and quality improvement (Styles, 1998; 2005). Professional accountability is a multileveled concept that may refer to the individual nurse; the institution, such as a school of nursing or health care agency; or the governmental agency, such as a state board of nursing. National, state, and local agencies guide the regulation of the profession of nursing to protect the public's health, safety, and welfare.

Watson stated that accountability is the "hallmark of professionalism" or a characteristic of professionalism (2004, p. 38). Styles (2005) identified five elements of a true profession: "(a) university education, (b) a distinct service or practice and discipline, (c) a research-based body of knowledge, (d) autonomy (self-governance) and accountability, (e) a code of ethics, and (f) an association to organize, serve, and speak for members and public welfare" (p. 81). These elements of a profession shape the development of the profession of nursing and guide the development of a professional accountability in nursing.

PROFESSIONAL ACCOUNTABILITY IN NURSING

How did accountability develop in the profession of nursing? It has evolved in an exciting way through historical champions who stepped forward

as nursing leaders and who made the profession accountable to the public. Early evidence of accountability can be traced to the 1850s and the Crimean War when Florence Nightingale organized the first nurses who set standards of care and introduced nursing care and support services to military hospitals. As a result of Nightingale's leadership and accountability for the profession, British military hospitals experienced an overall reduction in the mortality rate from 42 percent to 2.2 percent (Kalisch & Kalisch, 1995).

Another historical champion of accountability in nursing was Lillian Wald, a leader in public health nursing. In 1893 Wald and Mary Brewster established what evolved into the Henry Street Settlement on the Lower East Side in New York (Wald, 1935). Through Wald's leadership, public health nursing became accountable to the public in the community setting as she led the march to improve health conditions for immigrants, children, women, and workers in industry. Wald and her nurses increased access to health care through the formation of the Nurse Service and advocated for improved tenement living and food laws. Many of these changes occurred during a time before women had the right to vote, yet Wald's leadership enabled nurses to step forward and initiate great changes in the health care industry. These are remarkable actions when one considers that many physicians of the late 1800s thought that nurses did not need training because their work was equated to the work of housemaids (Kalisch & Kalisch, 1995).

What does the profession of nursing say about accountability? Bergman (1981) viewed accountability as the top of a pyramid that begins with the preconditions of ability, responsibility, and authority and that ends in accountability. Bergman states that all preconditions should be present for the nurse to be fully accountable for their actions and outcomes.

Lewis and Batey (1982) researched accountability through interviews with directors of nursing in nursing service. Lewis and Batey defined accountability as "the fulfillment of a formal obligation to disclose . . . the purposes, principles, procedures, relationships, results, income, and expenditures for which one has authority" (p. 10). They emphasize the importance in nursing to differentiate between terms that are often substituted for accountability such as responsibility, autonomy, or authority. Lewis and Batey point out the importance of accountability structure in nursing services.

Dr. Margretta Styles (2005), an international nursing leader and authority on regulation and credentialing in nursing, explained the role of regulation in profession building in nursing. She listed 11 powers of regulation and states that regulation is a major vehicle ensuring our accountability to the public ". . . regulation defines our scope of practice and sets standards and measures of competency" (p. 82). Styles identified that regulation in nursing may be either mandatory or voluntary.

Today nurses continue to be champions of accountability as they participate in projects across the United States in hospitals that are focused on reducing medical errors and related client mortality that have been attributed to 44,000 to 98,000 client deaths annually (Kohn, Corrigan, & Donaldson, 2000). Nurses have always asked challenging questions related to accountability in nursing, and today is no different. Dr. Linda Aiken is a nurse leader who has researched factors related to surgical client outcomes. Aiken and colleagues (2002) reported on the relationships between client workload of staff registered nurses and risk of death for the surgical client. Aiken, Clarke, Cheung, Sloane, and Silber (2003) also found significant relationships between the educational preparation of the registered nurse and surgical-client mortality and failure-to-rescue rates. These findings point to the fact that professional accountability in nursing is more important than ever as the profession improves strategies in health care to help protect the public from harm and to protect consumer confidence.

Professional accountability was advanced in 1897 with the creation of The Nurses Associated Alumnae of the United States and Canada, with the purpose of promoting ethical and education standards in nursing (ANA, 1996). The Nurses Associated Alumnae of the United States and Canada was later changed to the American Nurses Association (ANA). From the beginning the ANA has provided leadership in nursing by directing the high standards for

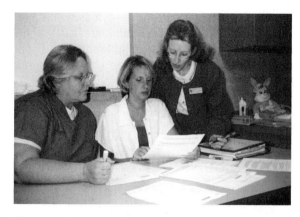

Figure 9.1 **One way nurses illustrate professional accountability is by ensuring that there is a smooth transition during shift changes.**

nursing practice that reflect professional accountability. Currently all 50 states as well as Washington, DC, Guam, the Virgin Islands, and the federal government are constituent members of ANA (ANA, 2005a). In the twenty-first century the ANA promotes the highest principles for the scope and standards of practice in nursing within 21 specialties in nursing (ANA, 2005a). The scope and standards of practice are utilized in practice, education, and research to elevate the quality of care and the health care environment. Today the ANA (ANA, 2005b) focuses on critical health care reform and other specific health care issues, such as safer needle devices and client's rights, that elevate quality of care and promote accountability in nursing practice.

Laschinger and Wong (1999) state that "Professional sources of accountability arise from the increasing scope of nursing practice, better educated nurses, and a valuing of the nurse-client relationship as a partnership" (p. 308). The profession of nursing has developed accountability in all areas of nursing, such as practice, education, and research. In 1994 the American Nurses Credentialing Center established the Magnet Recognition Program to recognize hospitals that meet rigorous standards in quality nursing practice and client care. In the twenty-first century many hospitals are striving for excellence in nursing care by focusing on improving client outcomes, such as reducing or eliminating infections among surgical clients. Instead of striving for minimal standards, health care is demanding excellence in client outcomes. Professional accountability continues to guide the profession of nursing to establish measurable standards that improve quality of nursing practice, nursing education, and the health care environment.

ACCREDITATION AND APPROVAL IN NURSING EDUCATION

One important aspect within professional accountability in nursing is **accreditation,** which is the regulatory process by which a nursing program is evaluated for educational quality and standards of performance. Nursing programs should meet or exceed these standards in order to receive accreditation, which is highly valued by educational institutions as well as students. Educational institutions value accreditation because federal funding and eligibility for grants are often dependent upon accreditation. Students should value accreditation because graduating from an accredited institution increases professional marketability and the ability to further one's education (Bellack, Gelmon, O'Neil, & Thomsen, 1999). Accreditation is rightly viewed as a hallmark of quality in educational programs and provides reassurance to the public that those institutions that prepare students in fields such as nursing, medicine, and law are guided by standards of excellence.

Until recently, nursing accreditation was the responsibility of the National League for Nursing (NLN), an organization founded in 1893 and devoted to advancing quality nursing education. The NLN was the sole accrediting body in nursing education with the exception of subspecialty accreditation for programs such as nurse midwifery, nurse anesthesia, and continuing nursing education. In the 1990s, however, the NLN was found by the U. S. Department of Education (DOE) to not fully comply with new criteria mandated by the Higher Education Act of 1992 for recognition of accrediting bodies (Bellack, et al., 1999). The NLN subsequently created an independent accrediting subsidiary, the National League for Nursing Accrediting Commission (NLNAC) and was renewed as an accrediting body by the DOE in 1999 (NLNAC, 2002).

Meanwhile, the American Association of Colleges of Nursing (AACN) created an autonomous agency, the Commission on Collegiate Nursing Education (CCNE), in order to coordinate specialized accreditation in nursing, especially those aimed at graduate nursing programs. The AACN was formed in 1969 as the only national nursing organization with the mission of furthering baccalaureate and higher education. The DOE has subsequently recognized the CCNE as another accrediting body for nursing (AACN, 2005b). Thus, accreditation for nursing programs may be granted by two separate organizations, the NLNAC or the CCNE. The debate over which accrediting agency to choose is as interesting as the debate over the entry degree level for professional nursing.

National League for Nursing Accrediting Commission (NLNAC)

The NLNAC was created in 1996 by the NLN Board of Governors with the aim of instituting core standards and criteria for accreditation in nursing. Today the NLNAC is the only body that accredits all five postsecondary- and higher-degree nursing programs, including practical nursing, diploma, associate-degree, baccalaureate-degree, and master's-degree programs. Accreditation has changed from its initial inception in 1938 from focusing on structural and process issues to outcomes, such as whether students are graduating from their school and passing the NCLEX licensure exam. NLNAC accreditation focuses on seven standards: mission and governance, faculty, students, curriculum, resources, program integrity, and program effectiveness, and involves program self-assessment and a strong peer-review component (Grumet, 2002). As of 2005, given estimates of total programs, NLNAC accredits approximately 40 percent to 45 percent of the master's- and baccalaureate-degree nursing programs in the United States and its territories, over 70 percent of the associate-degree nursing programs, 100 percent of diploma nursing programs, and 15 percent of practical nursing programs (C. Gilbert, personal communication, December 16, 2005). The annual fees involved in NLNAC accreditation range from $1,560 to $2,810, depending on whether the program is a NLN member, with additional fees required for accreditation reviews (NLNAC, 2004).

The NLN is also striving to promote standards of excellence in nursing with the development of 29 Hallmarks of Nursing Excellence through the work of the NLN's Task Force on Nursing Education Standards and Think Tank on Nursing Education. These Hallmarks of Excellence were developed through an extensive literature review and survey to create standards of excellence to which nursing programs should aspire (Anonymous, 2004). The NLN has also created Centers for Nursing Excellence, which recognize schools of nursing that have achieved distinction in one of the following areas: (a) creating environments that enhance student learning and professional development, (b) creating environments that promote ongoing faculty development, or (c) creating environments that advanced nursing education research (NLN, 2003).

Commission on Collegiate Nursing Education (CCNE)

The CCNE was created as an alliance formed in 1996 between the AACN and other nursing organizations interested in accrediting programs in nursing at the baccalaureate and higher levels (AACN, 2005a). In 1998 the CCNE began conducting site accreditation visits, and as of 2005, it accredits approximately 71 percent of baccalaureate programs and 88 percent of master's programs (M. Jackman, personal communication, December 14, 2005). CCNE accreditation focuses on (a) the purposes of accountability in nursing education, (b) evaluating the success of nursing programs based on achievement of their mission and goals, (c) assessing programs based on CCNE accreditation standards, (d) informing the public about accreditation and programs that meet CCNE standards, and (e) fostering improvement in nursing-education programs (AACN, 2005b). The annual fees for CCNE accreditation range from $1,700 to $2,100 depending on baccalaureate- or master's-program accreditation, with additional fees required for evaluation (CCNE, 2004).

In 1996 the AACN also created the Alliance for Nursing Accreditation, of which the CCNE is one of 14 regulatory and credentialing bodies that are dedicated to promoting efficiency in the accreditation process for collegiate and specialized accreditation in nursing (CCNE, 2002). Specialty accreditation agencies in this alliance include nurse practitioner, nurse anesthesia, nurse midwife, and clinical nurse specialist organizations as well as the National Council of State Boards of Nursing and the American Nurses Credentialing Center.

It is easy to see that NLNAC and CCNE accreditation use similar standards to accomplish the primary goal of advancing nursing education. The most obvious difference between the two accrediting bodies is that the NLNAC accredits all nursing programs, from practical programs to doctoral programs, whereas the CCNE focuses only on those programs that educate baccalaureate- and higher-degree nurses. The greatest perceived benefits of accreditation are public recognition of program excellence, professional marketability of programs, and continuous program improvement (Bellack, et al., 1999). It is up to the individual institutions as to which accreditation to seek.

National Council of State Boards of Nursing (NCSBN)

Although the NLNAC and the CCNE are both responsible for accrediting nursing programs, the NCSBN is responsible for nurse licensure testing and nursing practice and regulation, among other endeavors. Nursing regulation is governmental oversight of nursing practice and is provided by 61 boards of nursing (NCSBN, 1998; NCSBN, 2005d).

Governmental regulation of nursing practice is necessary due to the risk of public harm due to incompetence or malfeasance. Each board of nursing is legally authorized to regulate nursing and is granted this power through state legislation that creates Nurse Practice Acts for each state. Boards of nursing develop rules and regulations that are consistent with Nurse Practice Acts to define the scope of nursing practice, license nurses, and discipline nurses for unsafe practice. Boards of nursing were formed early in the twentieth century and include the responsibility of approving nursing programs in each state according to legal standards of nursing education that must remain consistent with Nurse Practice Acts. After organizations such as the NLN and AACN became involved in the accreditation of nursing programs with the purpose of promoting excellence in nurse education according professional standards, a "dual process" of nursing-program evaluation has emerged (NCSBN, 1998).

Currently, boards of nursing fall into three categories: (a) those that grant initial and continuing approval of nursing programs based on a separate review process from accreditation; (b) those that grant initial approval in a separate review and continuing approval based on accreditation by a national organization; and (c) those in which the board is not involved with approval of nursing programs. In Article VIII of the Model Nurse Practice Act, Approval of Nursing Education Programs, approval standards listed concern evaluation, curriculum, students, administration, and faculty, as well as determining compliance with standards and denial and withdrawal of program approval (NCSBN, 2004). A survey conducted by the NCSBN from 1996 to1998 found that the roles identified by state boards of nursing in the regulation of nursing education programs included granting initial approval of basic programs, the monitoring or sanctioning of programs at risk by statutory authority, demonstrating awareness of statewide program needs, and participating in standard setting for basic programs (NCSBN, 1998). As with many processes in today's marketplace, cost is a concern for nursing programs that must meet board-of-nursing approval standards as well as accreditation standards. In fact, in some states, accreditation is a mandatory component of continuing approval for nursing education programs. Thus, nursing education programs are held to the standards of their state board of nursing as well as the voluntary process of accreditation by nongovernmental bodies such as the NLNAC and the CCNE, which help ensure public safety and quality in nursing education.

CASE SCENARIO 9.1

You are the chair of a School of Nursing that contains four nursing education programs: an associate program, a RN to BSN program, a baccalaureate program, and a master's program. The Nurse Practice Act in your state requires that continuing approval for nursing programs be based on either accreditation by a national nursing organization or a separate review by the state board of nursing. The fiscal budget for the School of Nursing is very carefully controlled by the University due to decreases in funding by the state in recent years.

Case Considerations

1. What are the benefits to the School of Nursing in seeking accreditation? What are the drawbacks?

2. What are the options for pursuing accreditation?

3. Should both types of accreditation be sought? Why or why not?

LICENSURE REQUIREMENTS IN NURSING PRACTICE

A formal establishment of professional accountability in nursing was set into motion in 1901 when the **licensure** of nurses was recommended through passage of a worldwide resolution by the International Council of Nurses (ICN). In 1901 at the first meeting of the newly founded ICN, Mrs. Bedford Fenwick of Great Britain addressed the group.

> Whereas at the present time there is no generally accepted term or standard of training nor system of education nor examination for nurses in any country; . . . it is the opinion of this international congress of nurses . . . that it is the duty of the nursing profession of every country to work for suitable legislative enactment regulating the education of nurses and protecting the interests of the public, by securing State examinations and public registration, with the proper penalties for enforcing the same. (Kalisch & Kalisch, 1995, p. 192)

The beginning of the twentieth century was an exciting time for nursing when leaders emerged to change the course of nursing forever and establish nursing as a true profession. Nursing leaders established that nurses would be accountable to the public for their nursing actions. It is interesting to note that during this same time, Florence Nightingale, among others, opposed the regulation of nursing through examination and licensure requirements (McGann, 2004; Palmer, 1984). Nightingale ascertained that the moral character of the nurse and the art of nursing were more important than examinations for licensure, and that nursing was a vocation and not a profession (Palmer, 1984). The character of the nurse, one of Nightingale's primary points of opposition to licensure, became a critical element of licensure and accountability in the profession of nursing. Today the character of the nurse remains an important factor in the health care environment,

wherein drugs screens for chemical dependency or criminal background checks of the nurse are common regulatory methods to protect the public.

In the United States in the early twentieth century the profession of nursing demonstrated a commitment to protect the public through regulation of nursing practice. In 1903 North Carolina, followed by New York, New Jersey, and Virginia, instituted a voluntary licensure that established minimum training standards (NCSBN, 1999). Those states established laws to protect the public by establishing the legal acknowledgement of nursing with title protection, examination, and educational standards (NCSBN, 1999). By 1923 all states had created voluntary licensure with examination, but state requirements and examinations were not standardized as a national effort. With licensure came accountability for the actions and behavior of the nurse: the penalty for unprofessional actions or behavior was removal from the registry (McGann, 2004).

After World War II mandatory licensure was established for registered nurses with the formation of the National Council of State Boards of Nursing (NCSBN). In nursing licensure, it is the regulation of nursing practice through state controls that grant the individual the authority to practice as a registered nurse, licensed practical nurse, or advanced-practice registered nurse (NCSBN, 2004). State legislatures approve the Nurse Practice Act for every state. Each state grants the nurse, who meets licensure requirements, permission to practice within the state. Each state defines and regulates its Nurse Practice Act. The state board of nursing is empowered by the state legislature to regulate nursing and enforce the Nurse Practice Act (NCSBN, 2004). The ultimate goal of the licensure of nurses is to protect the public from harm through methods that establish the competency of the nurse. Nursing is a profession that demands specialized knowledge and skills. It is important that the boundaries of nursing practice be appropriate to the education and experience of the nurse (NCSBN, 1999).

How does a graduate of a BSN, ADN, or diploma program become licensed in a state to practice as a registered nurse? An applicant can obtain a registered-nurse license through the following methods: (a) licensure by exam for a graduate of a board-approved nursing education program; (b) licensure by exam for internationally instructed applicants; (c) licensure by endorsement for a nurse who holds an unencumbered RN license in another state (NCSBN, 2004). In addition, there are other licensure requirements that the nurse must meet, such as conduct requirements by reporting to the board of nursing any related chemical dependency or criminal charges/convictions (NCSBN, 1999; 2004).

In the 1950s a national standardized licensure exam was established (Kalisch & Kalisch, 1995). In the late 1980s the national licensure exam was renamed the National Council Licensure Examination (NCLEX). Graduates of a board-approved nursing-education program are required to pass the National Council Licensure Examination for Registered Nurses (NCLEX-RN) (NCSBN, 2004). The NCLEX-RN provides a measure of "the competencies needed to practice safely and effectively as a newly licensed entry-level RN" (NCSBN, 1999, p. 3). The NCLEX-RN test plan evolved from a job analysis resulting in an exam that "reflects the knowledge, skills and abilities essential for the registered nurse to meet the needs of clients requiring the promotion, maintenance, and restoration of health" (NCSBN, 1999, p. 4). RNs must obtain licensure in each state where they practice. To maintain a license, registered nurses must apply for renewal of the license, pay renewal fees, and meet renewal requirements as specified by their state board of nursing.

How does an advanced-practice registered nurse (APRN) gain licensure to practice within a state? All states require initial licensure as a RN (Bednash, Honig, & Gibbs, 2005). Titling of APRNs varies from state to state (Phillips, 2005). For example, some states use the title advanced-practice nurse or APN instead of APRN. APRNs or APNs may include nurse practitioners, clinical nurse specialists, nurse midwives, and nurse anesthetists (Phillips, 2005). Bednash and colleagues stated that "APNs are licensed, certified, or recognized by state boards of nursing" (2005, p. 263). All states maintain regulatory oversight of APRNs, but licensure

requirements vary from state to state. Eighteen states require a second license to practice as an APRN (Bednash, et al., 2005). States also vary in practice privileges and prescriptive authority for APRNs (Bednash et al., 2005; Phillips, 2005).

Certification and educational preparation requirements also may vary from state to state for APRNs. For example, in California, new legislation affecting APRNs will require a "masters degree in nursing, other masters degree in a clinical field related to nursing or a graduate degree in nursing" for new nurse-practitioner applicants to take effect in 2008 (Phillips, 2005, p. 22). Some states require certification by a national certifying agency for eligibility for licensure for APRNs. Eight professional organizations provide certification for APRNs, such as the American Nurses Credentialing Center and the American Academy of Nurse Practitioners (Bednash, et al., 2005). APRNs should contact their state board of nursing for specific licensure requirements.

MUTUAL RECOGNITION MODEL OF NURSE LICENSURE

In the twenty-first century the rapid changes within nursing through the expanding boundaries of Internet medicine, increasing mobility of the population, and the steadily increasing nursing shortage nationwide have led to the development and implementation of the mutual recognition model of nurse licensure. Prior to 1999 nurses who practiced in more than one state had to acquire separate licenses for each state; this was costly and cumbersome for the nurse. In 1998 the NCSBN developed the **mutual recognition model of nurse licensure,** which led to the Nurse Licensure Compact (NLC), an interstate compact that includes registered nurses (RNs) and licensed practical or vocational nurses (LPN/VNs). The mutual recognition model of nurse licensure is regulatory cooperation between states that gives the nurses the authority to practice in more than one state with one license, provided they meet specific requirements (NLCA, 2004).

Table 9.1 RN and LPN/VN Nurse Licensure Compact States

Compact States	Implementation Date
Arizona	7/1/2002
Arkansas	7/1/2000
Delaware	7/1/2000
Idaho	7/1/2001
Iowa	7/1/2000
Maine	7/1/2001
Maryland	7/1/1999
Mississippi	7/1/2001
Nebraska	1/1/2001
New Mexico	1/1/2004
North Carolina	7/1/2000
North Dakota	1/1/2004
South Dakota	1/1/2004
Tennessee	7/1/2003
Texas	1/1/2000
Utah	1/1/2000
Virginia	1/1/2005
Wisconsin	1/1/2000
Pending Compact States	
New Jersey	Signed by Governor
New Hampshire	Signed by Governor
South Carolina	Pending

NOTE: The table indicates which states have enacted the RN and LPN/VN Nurse Licensure Compact. Note that New Jersey and New Hampshire have enacted the NLC, and these states have not yet implemented the compact (NCSBN, 2005b).

Eighteen states have enacted legislation since 1998 to permit and implement the Nurse Licensure Compact (NCSBN, 2005b). Three additional states have enacted legislation for NLC but have not set an implementation date (NCSBN, 2005b). Through the NLC, nurses gain a multistate licensure privilege that allows them to maintain a license in their state of residence while they practice nursing through physical or electronic means in other compact states (NCSBN, 1998). Under the NLC, registered nurses are required to have an RN license in their home or residence compact state.

The compact agreement facilitates nursing practice among bordering states such as Virginia, North Carolina, and Delaware, whereas nurses may live in Virginia, the residence compact state, but practice nursing in North Carolina, a compact state. If nurses move their primary residence to another state that is in the compact, then a new license must be obtained from the new state of residence (NCSBN, 1998). When nurses relocate from a compact state to a noncompact member state, then they must seek a separate license to practice in the noncompact state.

Which compact state will have the legal authority to regulate nursing practices? Which compact state's Nurse Practice Act will regulate the nursing practice? When nurses are licensed in a compact state, they must consent to the fact that they are legally required to follow the guidelines of the Nurse Practice Act in the compact state where they practice and where the client is located at the time of care (NLCA, 2004). This is an important issue in a world with telemedicine, wherein the client and nurse may be in different locations and even different states. It is the nurse's responsibility to be informed about the Nurse Practice Act in each compact state in which they practice. Both a residence compact state and a nonresidence compact state have the authority to take disciplinary action against a nurse who violates their Nurse Practice Act (NLCA, 2004).

Dorsey (2001) summarizes the advantages of the compact as follows: (a) nurses may practice in multiple states without needing multiple separate licenses, (b) increased interaction between interstate boards of nursing may increase public safety, (c) a mobile workforce, and (d) improved access to nursing care in rural settings. Through the NLC, these advantages could benefit the individual nurse, the public, and health care agencies.

Do APRNs need a licensure compact that would give them multistate privileges to practice? Health care advancements, such as communication

CASE SCENARIO 9.2

Mr. M. has a current and unencumbered registered-nurse license in the state of Virginia, a compact state, where he is a resident. He has worked as an emergency-department registered nurse in a Virginia hospital for 10 years. Recently Mr. M. was offered a job as an emergency-department nurse at a hospital in North Carolina, a compact state. He quit his job in Virginia and accepted the position in North Carolina; however, he plans to continue living in Virginia.

Case Considerations

1. What are the primary issues of nursing practice for Mr. M?

2. In which state must Mr. M. maintain his registered-nurse license?

3. If Mr. M. has an adverse event, such as a medication error, with a client in the hospital in North Carolina, which state's Nurse Practice Act will regulate his practice and why? Which licensing board will investigate the action?

4. Identify whether or not your state is a member of the Nurse Licensure Compact. Discuss with your classmates the advantages and disadvantages of your state's membership or nonmembership in the Nurse Licensure Compact. Give rationale to support your positions on this issue.

technologies, mobility of the APRN, and telemedicine, have led to the development of a separate licensure compact for the advanced-practice registered nurse that was approved in 2002. In 2005 Iowa and Utah approved a mutual recognition of APRN licenses (NCSBN, 2005b; 2005c). The implementation date for this mutual recognition of APRN licenses has not been established. Advantages of a licensure compact that would give the APRN multistate advanced-practice privilege include increased access to health care for the public in underserved areas and promotion of public safety as a result of uniform APRN requirements (NCSBN, 2005a).

Globalization has increased the need for mutual-recognition agreements, which could decrease barriers for professions between countries. The International Council of Nurses [ICN] (2005) reported that several global mutual-recognition agreements in nursing have been implemented or are being negotiated. For example,

- The European Union: Nursing Directives and the emerging Directive on Mutual Recognition of Professional Qualifications

- The Caribbean Community and Common Market: Regional Examination Nurse Registration has enabled the introduction of reciprocity for Registered Nurses among countries of the Region (ICN, 2005).

Global mutual-recognition agreements provide a channel for regulatory cooperation between countries (ICN, 2005).

TRENDS IN MANDATORY CONTINUING EDUCATION IN NURSING

Continuing education (CE) is a voluntary or mandatory method that professional nurses use to maintain competence in nursing practice (Eustace, 2001). In nursing, **mandatory continuing education** is the specific courses or activities that nurses participate in to support their competence to practice nursing (Alabama Board of Nursing,

2004). Either state boards of nursing or certification agencies can require mandatory obligatory continuing education (Smith, 2003). In the 1970s the American Nurses Association created the first validated CE programs (DeSilets & Pinkerton, 2004). In the late 1970s a few states began requiring mandatory continuing education for renewal of the RN license. Some state boards of nursing require mandatory continuing education for reentry into practice and for endorsement of the license from one state to another state (Alabama Board of Nursing, 2004). The American Nurses Association and the National League for Nursing have supported continuing education for the nurse.

Twenty-one states had enacted legislation by 2002 to require mandatory continuing education for the renewal of the license of registered nurses that occurs every 2 to 3 years (Crawford & White, 2002). The nurse must complete the mandated number of CE hours, such as 24 hours per 2-year period, and must follow the specific requirements of licensing boards, such as CE hours being accepted from only approved CE providers. The current standard for measuring a CE is that one contact hour is equal to 50 to 60 minutes of a learning activity (Alabama Board of Nursing, 2004). Some states require specific CE subject content. For example, the Florida Board of Nursing (2005) requires CE credit on the topics of HIV/AIDS, prevention of medication errors, and domestic violence from a Florida-approved provider.

Does mandatory continuing education result in improved competence in nursing practice, improved client outcomes, or improved client safety? There is much discussion in nursing related to MCE. Eustace (2001) discussed the issues of mandatory continuing education from different states. For example, Mississippi endorsed voluntary CE for RNs whereas Colorado repealed the MCE as a requirement for license renewal. Two primary concerns were (a) cost and availability and (b) lack of research supporting the relationship between competence and MCE. Eustace (2001) suggested that nursing should conduct more research in order to study the relationship of CE and client-care outcomes.

Lazarus, Permaloff, and Dickson's (2002) descriptive evaluation study researched mandatory continuing education and the licensee's perceptions of MCE requirements with regard to reasonableness, access, and value. A random sample of 406 RNs and LPNs, residing primarily in Alabama, found that licensees identified CE to be of value and used this knowledge in their nursing practice. The majority of RNs (91 percent) and LPNs (82 percent) reported that the 24 contact hour requirement for renewal of license in Alabama was reasonable.

Table 9.2 States Requiring Mandatory Continuing Education for Renewal of RN License

Alabama

Alaska

Arkansas

California

Delaware

Florida

Iowa

Kansas

Kentucky

Louisiana

Massachusetts

Michigan

Minnesota

Nebraska

Nevada

New Hampshire

New Mexico

Ohio

Texas

West Virginia

Wyoming

Others: Northern Mariana Islands, Puerto Rico, Virgin Islands

SOURCE: Crawford, L. & White, E. (2002). *Profiles of Member Boards*. Chicago: NCSBN.

This study found that the choice of CE was consistent with the type of employment of the majority of nurses choosing CE in their area of nursing practice, clinical technology (including procedures), and specialty practice (Lazarus, et al., 2002). One outcome indicator revealed that reported changes in others' behaviors after attending CE was noted in the improvement or proficiency in technical skills of others in their jobs (34 percent). Researchers concluded that MCE for licensure is an important factor in maintaining nursing-practice competence and safeguarding the public. Lazarus and colleagues (2002) recommended further research to explore MCE and its relatedness to competence in nursing practice.

Other research supports the relationship between CE and competence in nursing practice. Hegge, Powers, Hendricks, and Vinson (2002) studied continuing education, competence, and computers in a random sample of 559 RNs in South Dakota, a state that does not require mandatory CE. Researchers found that most nurses rated themselves as competent. Two-thirds of the RNs reported the belief that nursing competence is linked to CE. Half of the nurses reported the belief that MCE would increase the nurse's competence (Hegge, et al., 2002).

The National Council of State Boards of Nursing (NCSBN) studied the link between MCE and professional competence as well (Smith, 2003). Questionnaires were mailed to a random sample of 2000 RNs and 2000 LPN/VNs with a return rate of 27.7 percent. This study compared nurses from states with mandated CE to nurses from states without mandated CE. Nurses with and without mandatory CE found no differences in the amount of growth in 10 professional ability areas (Smith, 2003).

The American Nurses Credentialing Center Commission on Certification (ANCC, 2005b) requires continuing education and practice as part of the recertification requirements every 5 years. The advanced-practice nurse (nurse practitioners or clinical nurse specialists) must meet the recertification requirements prior to the certification expiration date because there is no grace period. The American Academy of Nurse Practitioners Certification Program (AANPCP) also requires CE and practice for recertification requirements (AANPCP, n.d.). The advanced-practice nurse must have evidence of specific CE and practice experience. Mandatory CE will continue to be an important professional development issue for professional nurses and advanced-practice nurses. Further nursing research is needed in order to explore the questions related to MCE and nursing competence.

CERTIFICATION AND CREDENTIALING REQUIREMENTS IN NURSING

Nursing care in specialty areas and advanced-practice nursing have become increasingly complex. The changing health care environment has increased the demand for highly skilled and knowledgeable nurses. An ANCC (2002) white paper reported an increasing demand for nurses in specialty areas in an era of decreasing numbers of new nurses and an aging nurse workforce. The ANCC white paper presented eight hallmarks or recommendations that "best support professional nursing practice" (p. 5). Nurses of today are working in demanding health care environments. The ANCC white paper reported an increasing demand for nurses in specialty areas in an era of decreasing numbers of new nurses and an aging nurse workforce. These hallmarks apply to all professional nursing-practice sites and are intended to promote the highest level of professional practice for baccalaureate- and higher-degree nurses. ANCC's recommendations included several indicators related to the need for advanced credentialing and specialty certification. These hallmarks of professional nursing practice are excellent guidelines for today's nurses and new graduates.

Professional accountability is essential in the protection of the public from harm. Certification and credentialing are additional regulatory methods that nursing utilizes to advance professional accountability. Certification demonstrates that the nurse has met lengthy practice, testing, and continuing education requirements. The certified nurse has expert knowledge and clinical skills related to the specific area of certification. Through certification, the nurse can develop and maintain the advanced knowledge and skills that are needed in specialty areas of nursing and advanced-practice roles. Certification is awarded by nongovernmental professional organizations. Certification requirements vary according to the professional organizations' established requirements.

The International Council of Nurses Registry on Credentialing (2001) defines certification as "a voluntary and periodic process (recertification) by which an organized professional body confirms that a registered nurse has demonstrated competence in a nursing specialty by having met predetermined standards of that specialty" (para. 3). The International Council of Nurses Registry on Credentialing (2001) defined credentialing as the "processes used to designate that an individual, programme, institution or product have met established standards set by an agent (governmental or non-governmental) recognized as qualified to carry out this task" (para. 4). Credentials inform the public and employers about the level of performance that should be expected from the credentialed nurse or institution.

American Nurses Credentialing Center (ANCC)

Nursing certification began in 1973 through the American Nurses Association (ANA). In 1991 the American Nurses Credentialing Center (ANCC) was developed as a separate corporation for ANA certification programs (ANCC, 2005a). Although there are more than 40 organizations that provide certification for nurses (Yoder-Wise, 2005), the AANC is one of the most widely recognized. The ANCC currently offers certification exams in over 40 specialty areas (including pediatrics, gerontology, home health, medical/surgical, etc.), and has certified more than 151,000 nurses to date (ANCC, 2005c). Nurses may sit for certification on the conditions of an active RN license, appropriate level of education, and experience in the specialty area (ANCC, 2005c).

The credentials that nurses may display after their name reflect the certification requirements level (ANCC, 2005b). For example, associate-degree- and diploma-level- certification nurses use the credentials of RN, C, whereas the baccalaureate-level-certification nurses use the credentials of RN, BC, indicating board certification. Only baccalaureate- and masters-degree-prepared nurses and above may receive "board certified" credentials, which distinguishes between levels of education in nursing (Miller, 2000). The ANCC credentials distinguish the level of certification for the profession and for the consumer (ANCC, 2005b).

Advanced-Practice Certification

For advanced practice, Styles (1998) states that "Certification is a form of credentialing, and credentialing is a form of regulation" (p. 3). Advanced-practice certification may be granted through eight professional organizations, such as ANCC, the American Academy of Nurse Practitioners, or the American Association of Critical-Care Nurses Certification Corporation (Bednash, et al., 2005). In 2001 the ANCC granted reciprocity for advanced-practice certification given by specialty organizations to apply to ANCC certification as well (Anonymous, 2001). Credentials are granted through certification according to educational preparation at the master's degree in nursing level as APRN, BC. However, state boards of nursing regulate the licensure of advanced-practice nurses. Therefore, the legally required credentials may vary from state to state. For example, in Alabama advance-practice roles include (a) certified registered-nurse practitioners (CRNP), (b) certified nurse midwives (CNM), (c) certified registered-nurse anesthetists (CRNA), and (d) clinical nurse specialists (CNS) (Alabama Board of Nursing, 2005). Within each state the Nurse Practice Act will specify the requirements for licensure and the standards of practice as an advance-practice nurse.

Table 9.3 **American Nurses Credentialing Center: Certifications in Nursing Practice, 2005**

Certification Exam	Certification Credential
Advanced Practice Nurses Certification	
Nurse Practitioners	
Acute Care Nurse Practitioner	APRN, BC Advanced Practice Registered Nurse, Board Certified
Adult Nurse Practitioner	APRN, BC
Adult Psychiatric and Mental Health Nurse Practitioner	APRN, BC
Advanced Diabetes Management Nurse Practitioner	APRN, BC
Family Nurse Practitioner	APRN, BC
Family Psychiatric and Mental Health Nurse Practitioner	APRN, BC
Clinical Nurse Specialist	
Clinical Nurse Specialist in Adult Health	APRN, BC
Clinical Nurse Specialist in Adult Psychiatric and Mental Health	APRN, BC
Clinical Nurse Specialist in Advanced Diabetes Management	APRN, BC
Clinical Nurse Specialist in Child/Adolescent Psychiatric and Mental Health	APRN, BC
Clinical Nurse Specialist in Community/Public Health	APRN, BC
Clinical Nurse Specialist in Gerontological	APRN, BC
Clinical Nurse Specialist in Pediatric	APRN, BC
Other Advanced Practice Specialties	
Nursing Administration, Advanced	RN, CNAA, BC Registered Nurse, Certified in Nursing Administration, Advanced, Board Certified
Baccalaureate and Higher Degree	
Cardiac/Vascular Nurse	RN, BC Registered Nurse, Board Certified
Community/Public Health Nurse	RN, BC
Gerontological Nurse	RN, BC
Informatics Nurse: Bachelor's degree in nursing	RN, BC

Table 9.3 (*Continued*)

Certification Exam	Certification Credential
Baccalaureate and Higher Degree (*Continued*)	
Informatics Nurse: Bachelor's degree in other than nursing	RN, BC
Medical/Surgical Nurse	RN, BC
Nursing Administration	RN, CNA, BC
Nursing Professional Development	RN, BC
Pediatric Nurse	RN, BC
Perinatal Nurse	RN, BC
Psychiatric and Mental Health Nurse	RN, BC
Associate Degree or Diploma	
Cardiac/Vascular Nurse	RN, C
	Registered Nurse, Certified
Gerontological Nurse	RN, C
Medical/Surgical Nurse	RN, C
Pediatric Nurse	RN, C
Perinatal Nurse	RN, C
Psychiatric and Mental Health Nurse	RN, C

NOTE: Reprinted with permission from ANCC. (2005d). *ANCC Certification Examinations: General Testing Information*, August 3, 2005. Retrieved October 2, 2005 from, http://www.nursingworld.org/ancc/certification/announce.html.

Accreditation of Certification Programs

The ANCC is also responsible for the accreditation of continuing nursing-education programs for more than 205 organizations around the world (Anonymous, 2002a). ANCC's accreditation program is peer reviewed, international in focus, and uses the ANA's *The Scope and Standards of Practice for Nursing Professional Development* as a foundation for accreditation of CE programs. Additionally, the ANCC created Credentialing International, which provides certification for nurses, accreditation of CE programs, and the Magnet Recognition Program (ANCC, 2005e).

One organization that is devoted solely to the accreditation of nursing certification is the American Board of Nursing Specialties. The ABNS was formed in 1991 to create "uniformity in nursing certification and to increase public awareness of the value of certification" (ABNS, 2005, para 1). The ABNS is peer reviewed and standards based, but it mandates that baccalaureate-level nursing education be required for basic certification (Frank-Stromberg, Berry, Coleman, & Grindel, 1999). Thus, there are only 12 certification boards that are currently recognized by ABNS.

Certification and Outcomes

In 1996 during a conference held by the U.S. Oncology Nursing Certification Corporation to discuss the problems with and future recommendations for nursing certification, 24 representatives of nursing-specialty organizations recommended that the relationship between nursing certification and client outcomes be researched (Frank-Stromberg, et al, 1999.). Questions need to be answered, such as: Does certification result in improved nursing practice and improved client outcomes?

Redd and Alexander (1997) studied the effectiveness of certification with job performance and self-esteem in staff nurses who were certified and noncertified. Work performance was measured by Schwirian's Six Dimension Scale to appraise the participant's and supervisor's work performance. The scale included six subscales of leadership, critical care, teaching/collaboration, planning/evaluation, interpersonal relations/communications, and professional development (Redd & Alexander, 1997). The Rosenberg Self-Esteem Scale was also given to participants to measure self-esteem. Redd and Alexander found that supervisor evaluations of certified nurses were significantly related to higher performance scores in planning/evaluation and teaching/collaboration. Findings also revealed self-esteem scores were significantly higher in certified nurses than in noncertified nurses. Redd and Alexander's study has limited generalizability due to such conditions as small sample size, but this research certainly presents findings that are a valuable contribution to literature related to the importance of certification in nursing practice.

Other studies have not found clear links between certification and job perceptions and client outcomes. Hughes and colleagues (2001) conducted a descriptive correlational study that examined the relationship between certification and job perceptions of 1,217 certified and noncertified oncology nurses. Hughes and colleagues found that certification was weakly correlated with cohesion, commitment, and job satisfaction. Work setting was found to influence differences in job perceptions more than certification. A retroactive study (Frank-Stromberg, et al., 2002) of 20 certified and noncertified nurses and 181 clients examined whether clients cared for by certified oncology nurses experienced superior client outcomes. Contrary to the researchers' hypotheses, client outcomes of symptom management and episodic-care utilization such as admission

to care facilities did not differ between clients cared for by certified nurses and noncertified nurses. The small sample size may have accounted for the findings, however, and the researchers recommended that further study be conducted.

The Joint Commission of Healthcare Organizations (JCAHO) requires that nurses be competent for their assigned responsibility and have the correct credentials for their assignment. In advanced-practice nursing, these requirements include credentialing and privileging. Although the credentialing process in a health care agency will involve verification of education, certification, and experience of the nurse, the privileging process will involve evaluating the nurse's clinical competence, such as written documentation and professional peer judgment, through which the nurse gains within a health care agency the right to perform certain procedures and to care for clients with particular diagnoses (Archibald & Bainbridge, 1994).

Nardini (2000) suggests that certification is critical to employers who should be able to report that their facility employs the most highly qualified nurses to care for their clients. Certification has also been recommended to administrators for the retention and recruitment of the most highly qualified nurses (Woods, 2002). Currently hospitals and many nursing homes have their outcomes published, like report cards for the consumer, in order to provide information about the quality of their health care (Castle & Lowe, 2005). It is important for the public to be reassured that nurses are qualified and competent through accredited education, certification, and licensure, in order to make appropriate clinical judgments related to client care.

ACCREDITING BODIES FOR HEALTH CARE ORGANIZATIONS

Another way in which the public may be assured that nurses and the health care organizations that employ them are qualified and competent is through accreditation of the health care agency.

RESEARCH APPLICATION ARTICLES

Cary, A. H. (2000). Data driven policy: The case for certification research. *Policy, Politics, and Nursing Practice, 1*(3), 165–171.
and
Cary, A. H. (2001). Certified registered nurses: Results of the study of the certified workforce. *American Journal of Nursing, 101*(1), 44–52.

The largest study to date on nursing certification was funded by the American Nurses Credentialing Center and the Nursing Credentialing Research Coalition. This study researched the outcomes of the certification of registered nurses in the United States and Canada and the implications for policy recommendations. The five stages of this study included nurses, clients, and employers in the data collection. Stage 3 included a randomized sample of over 19,000 certified nurse participants. Certified nurses conveyed that several factors were enhanced by certification, such as "more confidence in decision making, ability to detect and initiate early interventions for patient complications . . . fewer adverse incidents in patient care" (Cary, 2000, p. 169). Overall, nurses reported that certification had influenced "personal, professional, and practice outcomes" (Cary, 2000, p. 170). The International Program of Research on the Certified Nurse Workforce study will have implications for nursing policy, practice, and certification with regard to protecting the public and gaining public support for certification.

Other Stage 3 findings included data related to nursing-workforce demographics, practice,

and benefits related to certification. Demographic findings concerning the education levels of certified nurses included (a) 21 percent with a diploma, (b) 16 percent with an associates degree, (c) 35 percent with a bachelors degree, (d) 1 percent with a masters degree, and (e) 1.6 percent with a doctorate (Cary, 2001). The most commonly held credentials included 20 percent with the RN, C (RN, Certified) and 10 percent with the CS (clinical specialist). Other credentials included (a) COHN-S (certified occupational health nurse specialist), (b) CPNP (certified pediatric nurse practitioner), (c) C (certified), (d) ANP (adult nurse practitioner), (e) CCRN-Adult (certified critical care RN, adult), (f) CPAN (certified perianesthesia nurse), (f) CRNH (certified RN, hospice), and (g) CRNA (certified RN, anesthetist) (Cary, 2001). Among nurses who were certified five years or less, the findings revealed that certification enabled (a) 47 percent to feel more confident in their ability to detect early signs and symptoms of complications in clients, (b) 46 percent reported initiating early and prompt interventions for clients experiencing complications, (c) 42 percent reported experiencing more effective communication, (d) 42 percent received higher client satisfaction ratings, and (e) 40 percent experienced fewer adverse incidents (errors) in client care (Cary, 2001, p. 50). This study suggested that certification is related to higher salaries for nurses, higher retention in the field of nursing, and better nursing practice outcomes.

Just as education programs in nursing are accredited by the NLNAC or CCNE, health care organizations are also accredited through agencies such as the Joint Commission on Accreditation of

Healthcare Organizations (JCAHO). JCAHO has been in existence since 1951 and is the oldest and largest accrediting body in existence. JCAHO currently accredits more than 15,000 health care organizations and programs in the United States, including more than 8,200 hospitals and home care organizations, and more than 6,800 other health care organizations that provide long term care, assisted living, behavioral health care, laboratory and ambulatory care services. (JCAHO, 2005, para 1).

Once initial JCAHO accreditation has been achieved, reaccreditation occurs every three years. In 2004 JCAHO revised the reaccreditation process for self-assessment and reporting of compliance with standards for an 18-month period leading up to the 3-year on-site visit.

Although accreditation is a voluntary process, achieving JCAHO accreditation meets the federal conditions that are required for Medicare and Medicaid reimbursement, as well as many insurers (Sandrick, 2004). Accreditation standards include those focused on clients and those focused on organizational and structural functions within the health care organization. Due to the fact that half of all JCAHO standards are focused on client safety during the delivery of care, nursing services are understandably an integral part of JCAHO accreditation. Of particular concern to nursing are standards related to safe staffing levels and workplace environment.

Recognizing that "Nurses are the primary source of care and support for patients at the most vulnerable points in their lives" (JCAHO, 2002, p. 4), JCAHO released a white paper in 2002 entitled "Health Care at the Crossroads: Strategies for Addressing the Evolving Nursing Crisis." This paper addresses the nursing shortage, with recommendations for creating a culture in health care organizations that supports and retains nursing, and for establishing incentives for health care organizations to invest in nursing (Anonymous, 2002b). JCAHO also created the Nursing Advisory Council in 2003, along with other organizations such as the ANA, NLN, and AACN to assist in the implementation of the recommendations in the white paper (Anonymous, 2003). It is clear that JCAHO values and supports professional nursing as an integral component within all health care

organizations and is committed to the future of professional nursing.

Just as voluntary certification is important for the professional development of individual nurses, there is another type of accreditation that is becoming increasingly important to health care organizations. The Magnet Recognition Program, administered by the ANCC, was created in 1994 to recognize (a) excellence in nursing services; (b) adherence to standards for improving client-care services; (c) leadership in nursing administration that supports professional nurse practice and competence; and (d) understanding and respecting cultural and ethnic diversity among all people using health care services (ANCC, 2005f). Unlike JCAHO accreditation, Magnet accreditation focuses on nursing services, and in fact, JCAHO has recommended that health care organizations adopt Magnet characteristics to promote and support nursing within all health care environments (Anonymous, 2002b). As of January 2005, more than 134 health care organizations have been recognized with Magnet status (Schlag, 2005). Magnet accreditation has been associated with higher retention of nurses, higher job satisfaction, and better client outcomes (Bliss-Holtz, Winter, & Scherer, 2004; Schlag, 2005). In today's competitive health care environment, attaining Magnet status is an increasingly desirable achievement.

CHAPTER SUMMARY

Professional accountability in nursing is more important than ever as the profession of nursing refines regulatory processes, such as accreditation, licensure, and certification to protect the public from harm and to protect consumer confidence. Professional accountability continues to guide the profession of nursing to establish measurable standards that improve the quality of nursing practice, nursing education, and the health care environment. These regulatory processes monitor standards of practice, competency, and

WRITING EXERCISE 9.1

The text has discussed certification as it relates to individual nurses, clients, and health care organizations. (1) Identify a specialty certification that would apply to your area of clinical expertise. (2) Identify the benefits of obtaining this certification to your own nursing practice, your clients, and your employer. Or, if you already have a certification, discuss how certification has affected the above three areas. (3) Write your findings and be prepared to discuss them in class or on the discussion board.

quality improvement. Accountability is a multi-leveled concept that may refer to the individual nurse; the institution, such as a school of nursing or health care agency; or the governmental agency, such as a state board of nursing. National, state, and local agencies guide the regulation of the profession of nursing to protect the public's health, safety, and welfare.

> *You are educated. Your certification is in your degree. You may think of it as the ticket to the good life. Let me ask you to think of an alternative. Think of it as your ticket to change the world.*
>
> —Tom Brokaw

REFERENCES

Aiken, L., Clarke, S., Cheung, R., Sloane, D., Sochalski, J., & Silber, J. (2002). Hospital nurse staffing and patient mortality, nurse burnout, and job dissatisfaction. *Journal of the American Medical Association, 288,* 1987–1993.

Aiken, L., Clarke, S., Cheung, R., Sloane, D., & Silber, J. (2003). Educational levels of hospital nurses and surgical patient mortality. *Journal of the American Medical Association, 290,* 1617–1623.

Alabama Board of Nursing. (2004). *Administrative code: Continuing education for license renewal.* Retrieved May 18, 2005, from http://www.abn.state.al.us/main/downloads/admin-code/chapter-610-X-10.html.

American Academy of Nurse Practitioners Certification Program. (nd). *National competency-based certification examinations for adult and family nurse practitioners.* Austin, TX: author.

American Association of Colleges of Nursing. (2005a). *About AACN.* Retrieved on May 31, 2005, from http://www.aacn.nche.edu/ContactUs/about.htm

American Association of Colleges of Nursing. (2005b). *Mission statement and goals: Commission on collegiate nursing education.* Retrieved May 31, 2005, from http://www.aacn.nche.edu/Accreditation/mission.htm.

American Board of Nursing Specialties. (2005). *ABNS: Promoting excellence in nursing certification.* Retrieved June 17, 2005, from http://www.nursingcertification.org/fact_sheet.htm.

American Nurses Association. (1996). *ANA centennial: Voices from the past . . . vision of the future.* Retrieved June 9, 2005, from http://www.nursingworld.org/centenn/cent1990.htm.

American Nurses Association. (2005a). *ANA constituent member associations.* Retrieved November 28, 2005, from http://www.nursingworld.org/cmas/prtcmaaddr.pdf

American Nurses Association. (2005b). *Who we are: ANA's statement of purpose.* Retrieved June 20, 2005, from http://www.nursingworld.org/about/mission.htm.

American Nurses Credentialing Center. (2002). *ANCC white paper: Hallmarks of the professional nursing practice environment.* Washington, DC: author.

American Nurses Credentialing Center. (2005a). *American nurses credentialing center: Certified nursing excellence.* Retrieved June 17, 2005, from: http://nursingworld.org/ancc/inside.html.

American Nurses Credentialing Center. (2005b). *ANCC certification for professional nurses: Certifying excellence in nursing practice.* Retrieved May 19, 2005, from http://nursingworld.org/ancc/inside/about/aboutcert.html.

American Nurses Credentialing Center. (2005c). *American nurses credentialing center: Opening a world of opportunities.* Retrieved June 17, 2005, from http://nursingworld.org/ancc/cert.html.

American Nurses Credentialing Center. (2005d). *ANCC Certification Examinations: General Testing Information,* August 3, 2005. Retrieved October 2, 2005, from http://www.nursingworld.org/ancc/certification/announce.html.

American Nurses Credentialing Center. (2005e). *Credentialing international: Promoting and validating nursing excellence around the world.* Retrieved June 17, 2005, from http://nursingworld.org/ancc/inside/CI/about.html.

American Nurses Credentialing Center. (2005f). *Magnet Recognition Program: Certifying excellence in nursing services.* Retrieved June 17, 2005, from http://nursingworld.org/ancc/inside/about/aboutmagnet.html.

Anonymous. (2001). Nurse practitioner certification reciprocity. *Kansas Nurse, 76*(5), 10.

Anonymous. (2002a). ANCC interview: Accrediting organizations for continuing education in nursing. *The Journal of Continuing education, 33*(4), 152–155.

Anonymous. (2002b). New JCAHO report underscores nursing community concerns. *American Nurse, 34*(5), 1–2.

Anonymous. (2003). JCAHO establishes nursing advisory council. *Nevada RNformation, 12*(3), 12.

Anonymous. (2004). Hallmarks of excellence in nursing education. *Nursing Education Perspectives, 25*(2), 98–102.

Archibald, P., & Bainbridge, D. D. (1994). Capacity and competence: Nurse credentialing and privileging. *Nursing Management, 25*(4), 49–55.

Bellack, J. P., Gelmon, S. B., O'Neil, E. H., & Thomsen, C. L. (1999). Responses in baccalaureate and graduate programs to the emergence of choice in nursing accreditation. *Journal of Nursing Education, 38*(2), 53–62.

Bednash, G., Honig, J., & Gibbs, L. (2005). Formulation and approval of credentialing and clinical privileges. In Joan Stanley (Ed.)., *Advanced Practice Nursing: Emphasizing Common Roles* (2nd ed.), pp. 158–186. Philadelphia: F. A. Davis

Bergman, R. (1981). Accountability—Definition and dimensions. *International Nursing Review, 28*(2), 53–59.

Bliss-Holtz, J., Winter, N., & Scherer, E. M. (2004). An invitation to magnet accreditation. *Nursing Management, 35*(9), 36–43.

Cary, A. H. (2000). Data driven policy: The case for certification research. *Policy, Politics, and Nursing Practice, 1*(3), 165–171.

Cary, A. H. (2001). Certified registered nurses: Results of the study of the certified workforce. *American Journal of Nursing, 101*(1), 44–52.

Castle, N. G., & Lowe, T. J. (2005). Report cards and nursing homes. *The Gerontologist, 45*(1), 48–67.

Commission on Collegiate Nursing Education. (2002). *Annual report 2002.* Retrieved June 17, 2005, from http://www.aacn.nche.edu/Accreditation/PDF/2002AnnualReport.pdf.

Commission on Collegiate Nursing Education. (2004). *Commission on collegiate nursing education: Fee structure.* Retrieved June 15, 2005, from http://www.aacn.nche.edu/Accreditation/pdf/FEESTR06.pdf.

Crawford, L., & White, E. (2002). *Profiles of Member Boards.* Chicago: NCSBN.

DeSilets, L., & Pinkerton, S. (2004). Looking back on 25 years of continuing education. *The Journal of Continuing Education in Nursing, 35*(1), 12.

Dorsey, D. M. (2001). Licensure in nursing: Old vs. new approaches. In Joanne McCloskey Dochterman & Helen Kennedy Grace (Eds.), *Current Issues in Nursing,* (6th ed., pp. 261–266). St Louis, MO: Mosby.

Eustace, L. (2001). Mandatory continuing education: Past, present, and future trends and issues. *The Journal of Continuing Education in Nursing, 32*(3), 133–137.

Florida Board of Nursing. (2005). *Frequently asked questions.* The Florida Department of Health. Retrieved May 16, 2005, from http://www.doh.state.fl.us/mqa/nursing/nur_faq.html#Mandatory.

Frank-Stromberg, M., Berry, D. L., Coleman, E. A., & Grindel, C. G. (1999). Report of a state-of-the-knowledge conference on U.S. nursing certification. Image*: The Journal of Nursing Scholarship, 3*(1), 51–56.

Frank-Stromberg, M., Ward, S., Hughes, L., Brown, K., Coleman, A., Grindel, C. G., & Murphy, C. M. (2002). Does certification status of oncology nurses make a difference in patient outcomes? *Oncology Nursing Forum, 29*(4), 665–678.

Grumet, B. R. (2002). Demystifying accreditation: How NLNAC is making the process relevant for today's educators. *Nursing Education Perspectives, 23*(2), 114–118.

Hegge, M., Powers, P., Hendrickx, L., & Vinson, J. (2002). Competence, continuing education and computers. *The Journal of Continuing Education in Nursing, 33*(1), 24–32.

Hughes, L. C., Ward, S., Grindel, C. G., Coleman, E. A., Berry, D. L., Hinds, P. S., Oleske, D. M., Murphy, C. M., & Frank-Stromberg, M. (2001). Relationships between certification and job perceptions of oncology nurses. *Oncology Nursing Forum, 28*(1), 99–114.

International Council of Nurses. (2005). *Nursing matters: Mutual recognition agreements.* Retrieved May 19, 2005, from https://www.icn.ch/matters_mra.htm.

International Council of Nurses Registry of Credentialing. (2001). *Definitions/Glossary.* Retrieved May 18, 2005, from https://www.icn.ch/rcr/glossary.htm.

Joint Commission on Accreditation of Healthcare Organizations. (2002). *Health care at the crossroads: Strategies for addressing the evolving nursing crisis.* Retrieved June 22, 2005, from http://www.jcaho.org/about+us/public+policy+initiatives/health+care+at+the+crossroads.pdf.

Joint Commission on Accreditation of Healthcare Organizations. (2005). *Frequently asked questions about the joint commission.* Retrieved June 22, 2005, from http://www.jcaho.org/news+room/faqs/index.htm.

Kalisch, P. A., & Kalisch, B. J. (1995). *The advance of American nursing* (3rd ed.). Philadelphia: J. B. Lippincott.

Kohn, L. T., Corrigan, J. M., & Donaldson, M. S. (2000). *To err is human: Building a safer health system.* Washington, DC: National Academy of Sciences.

Laschinger, H., & Wong, C. (1999). Staff nurse empowerment and collective accountability: Effect on perceived productivity and self-rated work effectiveness. *Nursing Economics, 17*(6), 308–317.

Lazarus, J., Permaloff, A., & Dickson, C. (2002). Evaluation of Alabama's mandatory continuing education program for reasonableness, access, and value. *The Journal of Continuing Education in Nursing, 33*(3), 102–111.

Lewis, F. M., & Batey, M. V. (1982). Clarifying autonomy and accountability in nursing service: Part 2. *The Journal of Nursing Administration, 12*(10), 10–15.

McGann, S. (2004). The development of nursing as an accountable profession. In S. Tilley & R. Watson (Eds.), *Accountability in nursing and midwifery* (2nd ed., pp. 38–46). Oxford: Blackwell Science Ltd.

Miller, N. (2000). Certification and advanced practice issues. *Nursing Economics, 18*(4), 211.

Miller, P. J. (2003). Embracing "the 'a' word." *Nursing Management, 34*(5), 10.

Nardini, J. (2000). Certification and credentialing: What does it mean to the patient? *Nephrology Nursing Journal, 27*(5), 457–458.

National Council of State Boards of Nursing. (1998). *Approval of nursing education programs by boards of nursing. National council position paper.* Retrieved May 31, 2005, from http://www.ncsbn.org/resources/complimentary_nscbn_approval.asp.

National Council of State Boards of Nursing. (1999). *Uniform core licensure requirements: A supporting paper.* Retrieved May 12, 2005, from http://ncsbn.org/regulation/nursingpractice_nursing_practice_licensing.asp.

National Council of State Boards of Nursing. (2004). *Model nursing practice act and model nursing administrative rules.* Retrieved May 31, 2005, from http://www.ncsbn.org/pdfs/Chapter8.pdf.

National Council of State Boards of Nursing. (2005a). *Advanced practice registered nurse compact.* Retrieved May 11, 2005, from http://ncsbn.org/nlc/index.asp.

National Council of State Boards of Nursing. (2005b). *Nurse licensure compact.* Retrieved October 6, 2005, from http://ncsbn.org/nlc/index.asp.

National Council of State Boards of Nursing. (2005c). *Nurse licensure compact: APRN compact.* Retrieved May 11, 2005, from http://ncsbn.org/nlc/index.asp.

National Council of State Boards of Nursing. (2005d). *Nursing regulation.* Retrieved November 28, 2005, from http://www.ncsbn.org/regulation/boardsofnursing_ boards_of_nursing_board.asp.

National League for Nursing. (2003). *NLN centers for excellence in nursing education.* Retrieved June 16, 2005, from http://www.nln.org/profdev/excellence.htm.

National League for Nursing Accrediting Commission. (2002). *About NLNAC: Mission.* Retrieved May 31, 2005, from http://www.nlnac.org/About%20NLNAC/AboutNLNAC.htm.

National League for Nursing Accrediting Commission. (2004). *2004 schedule of accreditation fees.* Retrieved June 16, 2005, from http://www.nlnac.org/fees.htm.

Nurse Licensure Compact Administrators. (2004). *Frequently asked questions regarding the national council of state boards of nursing (NCSBN) nurse licensure compact (NLC)*. Retrieved June 8, 2005, from http://ncsbn.org/nlc/index.asp.

Palmer, I. S. (1984) *Nightingale revisited in American Journal of Nursing. Pages from Nursing History* (pp. 4–8). NY: American Journal of Nursing. Reprinted from Nursing Outlook July/August, 1983.

Phillips, S. (2005). A comprehensive look at the legislative issues affecting advanced nursing practice. *The Nurse Practitioner*, 30(1), 14–47.

Redd, M. L., & Alexander, J. W. (1997). Does certification mean better performance? *Nursing Management*, *28*(2), 45–50.

Sandrick, K. (2004). Everything you want to know about the joint commission. *Trustee*, *5*(8), 17–20.

Schlag, M. K. (2005). Education: Key to the magnet culture. *The Journal of Continuing Education in Nursing, 36*(1), 12–13.

Smith, J. (2003). Executive summary: Exploring the value of continuing education mandates. *NCSBN Research Brief*, Volume 6. Chicago: National Council of State Boards of Nursing.

Styles, M. M. (1998). An international perspective: APN credentialing. *Advanced Practice Nursing Quarterly, 4*(3), 105.

Styles, M. M. (2005). Regulation and profession-building: A personal perspective. *International Nursing Review, 52*, 81–82.

Wald, L. (1935). *The house on Henry Street*. New York: Henry Holt. Reprinted in 1915, 1923, 1924, 1927, 1931, 1932.

Watson, R. (2004). Accountability and clinical governance. In S. Tilley & R. Watson (Eds.), *Accountability in nursing and midwifery,* (2nd ed., pp. 38–46). Oxford: Blackwell Science Ltd.

Woods, D. K. (2002). Realizing your marketing influence, part 3: Professional certification as a marketing tool. *The Journal of Nursing Administration, 32*(7/8), 379–386.

Yoder-Wise, P. (2005). State and certifying boards/associations: CE and competency requirements. *The Journal of Continuing Education in Nursing, 36*(1), 3–11.

CHAPTER 10

Health Care Policy Issues

Sharon Guillet

Never doubt that a small group of thoughtful committed citizens can change the world; indeed it's the only thing that ever has.
—Margaret Mead

LEARNING OBJECTIVES

At the completion of the chapter, the learner should be able to do the following:

1. Analyze the different forms of health policy and the contributions each makes to the health of the public.
2. Describe the relationship between health and health policy.
3. Describe the policy process.
4. Analyze the role of politics in the development and implementation of health policy.
5. Discuss U.S. health policy as it relates to health care financing.
6. Develop a policy agenda by applying research findings.
7. Identify contemporary health policy issues.
8. Create a message to a policymaker related to a specific policy issue currently affecting nursing practice.

KEY TERMS

Allocative policy

Health determinants

Health policy

Incrementalism

Medicaid

Medicare

Politics

Regulatory policy

Social policy

INTRODUCTION

The United States is perceived internationally as having the most technologically advanced health care, as well as being the premier provider of high quality medical education in the industrialized world (Kronenfeld, 2002). To outsiders, it would appear that U.S. health care is the best to be found anywhere on the globe. However, those who work within that health care system know that it is in serious trouble (Bailey, 2004). Terms used to describe the American health care system range from "disarray" (Salmon, 2002) to "a shambles" characterized by "high costs and low confidence" (Romano, 2001). Although the system provides advanced care to many, millions of Americans fail to receive even the most basic care services. Some indications of problems with U.S. health care include

- Lack of health insurance resulting in no access to health care for 50 million
- The nursing shortage, which creates a daily struggle to provide basic care to increasingly complex clients
- Case loads that increase as resources to provide care dwindle
- A population that spends more on health care per capita than any industrialized nation in the world and yet has an infant mortality rate that continues to rise (National Coalition on Health Care, 2004)

How health care dollars are spent as well as who receives care and in what settings are all decisions determined by policies, which are established by governments, organizations, and agencies. This chapter will explore how such policies are made, the relationships between health and health policies, and the role that nurses can play in advocating policies that improve the health and well-being of the individuals, families, and communities they serve.

WHAT IS HEALTH POLICY?

A policy is a deliberate course of action developed to deal with a concern (Longest, 2002). Policies provide guidelines for directing behavior. These guidelines reflect the values and beliefs of the people setting the policy. In other words, an institution or organization sets policies that reflect the mission, vision, and values of that entity. People in positions of authority set policy. For example, the dean of a school can determine the policy for readmitting students to the program. Similarly, the Board of Nursing in each state determines the policies related to nursing practice. Such policies belong to the private sector. Business policies that affect health (and therefore may be viewed as health policy) are also made in the private sector. Examples of this include decisions by independent health insurance companies regarding which services and procedures will or will not be covered and automobile insurance companies that offer financial incentives for those who do not smoke or drink alcohol.

Public-sector policies are authoritative decisions (Longest, 2002) made by people within the three branches of government. Such policies reflect the extent to which the government is willing to take action and commit resources to bringing about a desired outcome. When governmental bodies set policy or openly refuse to set policy, their actions are clearly visible. However, sometimes governments take no action at all. It is important to recognize that choosing not to make a decision is in fact a decision (perhaps a deliberate decision) with important consequences.

One type of public policy is **social policy,** which deals with public welfare initiatives, such as mandating that individuals wishing to operate automobiles must be of a certain age and take courses in driver education. Another type of public policy is **health policy.** The goal of any health policy is to improve the health and well-being of the citizenry. Therefore, health policies encompass decisions that are related to how health care is accessed, delivered, and paid for as well as decisions that facilitate the public's ability to pursue and promote healthy behaviors and lifestyles.

Health policies may affect the health of the nation either directly or indirectly. For example, government decisions to mandate immunization of children has a direct effect on health, whereas the decision to offer an insurance benefit to pay for prescription drugs indirectly affects health by making needed drugs more accessible. A policy with an even subtler effect on health is the provision of low-cost student loans to educate more nurses.

TYPES OF HEALTH POLICY

Health policies take many forms, including laws, regulations, judicial interpretations, sanctions, and subsidies. Laws, rules, regulations, and court decisions are referred to as **regulatory policy.** Sanctions and subsidies are called **allocative policy** (Longest 2002). These policies are all directive in nature and have the express purpose of meeting public objectives. Examples of regulatory policies include those related to price setting, licensing, immunizations, the approval of new drugs, and the protection of personal medical information.

Allocative Policies

Allocative policies are made on behalf of specific groups or organizations and generally take the form of subsidies. For example, the government has established several programs to subsidize the health care of vulnerable populations such as the poor, the elderly, and the disabled. Medicare is perhaps the largest federal subsidy for health care, and Medicaid is the largest state subsidy. The federal government also has the power to withdraw its support and uses the threat of financial sanctions to ensure that policies related to special groups are upheld. For example, states send money to hospitals that care for a disproportionately high level of indigent clients. These are referred to as DSH (pronounced dish) dollars. As a part of Medicaid, the federal government reimburses the states between 50 percent and 77 percent of the DSH payment. If the hospital does not have at least 1 percent of its patient days attributed to caring for Medicaid clients, it loses that federal reimbursement. Similarly, under the Emergency Medical Treatment and Active Labor Act (EMTALA), hospitals must treat emergency patients regardless of ability to pay. If a hospital violates EMTALA, there are fines to be paid, but more importantly, there is the potential to lose all government subsidies, a consequence that could force the hospital to close.

Laws

Public health laws are public health policies. According to Gostin (2005), seven of the ten greatest public health achievements of the twentieth century were the result of laws related to vaccinations, safer workplaces, safer and healthier foods, motor-vehicle safety, control of infectious diseases, tobacco control, and fluoridation of drinking water.

Regulations

Regulations are explicit guidelines written by governments that explain how a law is implemented. Federal regulations tend to be very lengthy, sometimes several hundred pages long, depending on the number of agencies involved. For example, the Americans with Disabilities Act (PL101-336), enacted in 1994, is sweeping legislation that affects every aspect of public life. Regulatory policies were developed, which are overseen by nine departments, including the Department of Justice, and the Departments of Transportation, Labor, Lands and Resources, Education, Health and Human Services, Housing, Employment, and Agriculture.

Regulations that address nurse staffing ratios are of practical interest to nursing. Both state and federal governments are proposing or establishing regulations to guide how nurse/patient ratios are established. At the federal level, HR3656 requires Medicare hospitals to regulate the ratios based on patient acuity, whereas the state of California has adopted a fixed minimum-staffing ratio. Policymakers will need to watch the outcomes of these strategies over time in order to make broad policy recommendations (Spetz, 2005).

Court decisions

Court rulings have the potential to change health care policy through the interpretation of the statutes. In recent years the courts have made numerous rulings on end-of-life issues that have created changes in public policies related to termination of life, what measures are considered "extraordinary measures" in preserving life, and who may make end-of-life decisions for another human being.

THE RELATIONSHIP BETWEEN HEALTH AND HEALTH POLICY

The purpose of health policy is to promote health. Therefore, in order to understand what health policies might be developed in a given society, it is important to know how that society defines health. For example, if health is perceived to be the absence of disease, then health policies might address curative approaches to illness rather than preventive approaches. The curative model has long been the approach to health care in the United States. However, over the past decade there has been a shift in societal values to a model of health promotion and disease prevention. Although there are varying definitions of health, U.S. health care providers have universally accepted the World Health Organizations (WHO, 1948) definition of health as being "a state of complete physical, mental, and social well-being and not merely the absence of disease or infirmity."

Generally speaking, attempts to ensure health through the establishment of health policy are made indirectly by addressing those factors that contribute to or interfere with health and its pursuit. (Bell &

Standish, 2005; Kemper, 2003). These factors are referred to as **health determinants** and include biology/genetics, environment (physical, socioeconomic, and cultural), lifestyle choices and behaviors, and the availability of health-related information and services. Policymakers study health determinants to develop strategies that ultimately improve health. For example, the effect of the environment on health is an area about which a great deal of research has been conducted, and much legislation has been enacted especially related to clean air and clean water. As a result, policies made related to asbestos and lead in the environment have reduced the incidence of lead poisoning and lung diseases. Other environmental concerns include violence, homelessness, and more recently, terrorism and poverty. People who live in poverty have poorer health outcomes than the rest of the population. For example, asthma is a major health concern that air-quality policies continue to address. Yet the incidence and prevalence of asthma is disproportionately higher among people of color and people living in low-income communities (Bell & Standish, 2005). Policy analysts and policymakers attempt to understand the relationship between poverty and health and propose policies that are both effective and feasible.

HOW POLICIES ARE MADE

Keller, Strohschein, Lia-Hoagberg, and Schaffer (2003) define policy development as getting an issue on the decision-makers' agenda, making a plan, and determining needed sources. Toofany (2005) describes the policy process as a "simple sequence of thought, action and solution." Although the identification of issues that present health-related problems may not be difficult, getting those issues on the agenda and in front of individuals empowered to make policy is anything but simple. It requires knowledge and diligence and, even though policy and politics are not the same, political savvy is important. Many nurses view **politics** negatively, but it's a neutral term that involves influencing the distribution of resources. More often than not, policies are made through the use of influence and timing. Research is rarely enough to persuade people to take action (Kemper, 2003). An example of this is the fact that evidence linking smoking and lung cancer existed as early as 1950, but significant legislation related to advertising and selling tobacco was not made for several years. Why the delay? Powerful stakeholders such as tobacco companies and farmers would have been adversely affected by antismoking laws and therefore used their political powers to halt action.

Stakeholders are people or groups who will be directly affected by the policy being developed. Nurses are stakeholders in health policy and also serve as advocates for other stakeholders. This advocacy occurs in many forums. It can be part of an organized political process or simply one nurse working for the benefit of one patient. Nurses are uniquely qualified to influence policy and patient outcomes by virtue of their knowledge and hands-on experience. Not only do nurses provide research data, experience, and extensive health care knowledge, they also identify areas of concern and work to bring them to public attention. Nurses are effective because they hold the public trust and are increasingly seen as credible scientists. Nurses are also valuable because they are viewed as being altruistic and as having no particular vested interest other than the good of the public.

There are three general approaches to policy-making: the rational approach, the incrementalist approach, and the stage-sequential approach. The rational approach reflects ideal goals, such as free health care for all; comes up with a plan that weighs the cost/benefit; and tries to bring about a big change all at once. An example of this was the Clinton administration's attempt at sweeping health care reform in the late 1990s. **Incrementalism** is a very political process of making small changes toward the ideal goal. Most policies are made incrementally over time. The advancement of nursing as a profession is an excellent example of incremental shifts in public opinion and subsequent policy. The stage-sequential approach is a systems-based model that treats the development of policy as a

step-by-step process. This is the process used when those in power want to set their own agenda. They start out with the notion that a policy needs to be developed either to maintain or change the status quo. The policy developers then try to find support for their desired position and, if successful, write a policy that guides the development of programs, behaviors, and procedures that will ultimately be evaluated in light of the goals of the policy developed. The steps of this process are generally understood to be

- Problem identification
- Agenda setting
- Policy formulation
- Policy implementation
- Policy evaluation

In reality, policy development is messier than this step-by-step approach might lead you to believe. There is much negotiation before a policy is enacted, and the end result is often not what the designers originally had in mind because of the compromises that are made along the way.

There are a number of models for understanding the policy process. Three of these models, Longest, Kingdon, and Lomas, dominate the research literature and are presented here. The Lomas model (2000), as seen in Figure 10.1, explains the reciprocal relationships between societal values and information and how these relationships influence policy, which in turn alters the relationships. Values are made up of ideas and interests that influence the information made available via knowledge, research, and the media. This information is then used to influence the beliefs that shape values. In the Lomas model, those with persuasion and power have the best opportunity for influencing policy.

According to Kingdon (1995), at any given time, there is a policy stream, a problem stream, and a politics stream flowing in search of an open window of opportunity. The problem stream is a confluence of public problems such as health insurance, the high cost of health care, homelessness, or child care. The policy stream represents the ideas of stakeholders and exists pretty much whether a problem exists or not. For example, if we think nurses should have the

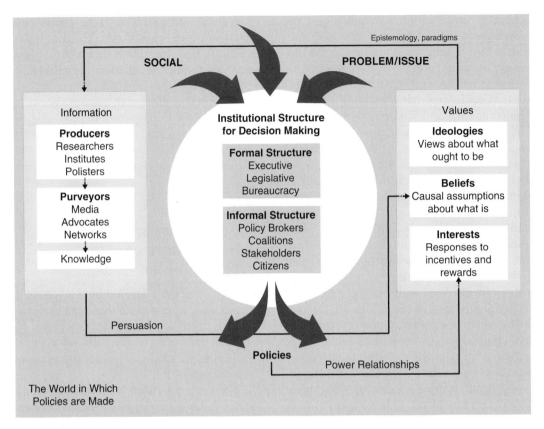

Figure 10.1 **The Lomas Model of the contextual influences on the decision-making process.** Courtesy of Jonathan Lomas.

same prescriptive authority as physicians, that policy notion floats around until a problem arises that allows us to make our case. The political stream is where influence is used to determine what makes it onto the policy agenda. It may be a tragedy in the world, a change in elected officials, or something that happens to a public figure; one example is the Brady Law. James S. Brady was President Reagan's press secretary, who was wounded in the assassination attempt on the president in 1981. Mr. Brady was shot in the head, and the event was recorded and played on television across the country. This event helped the passage of legislation that requires a seven-day waiting period for purchasing handguns, even though the National Rifle Association (with a very strong political lobby) was opposed.

Political processes and the media are very important in advancing problems and solutions to the point that they receive local or national attention. If two streams come together, it can open a window of opportunity, or world events may create an opening (like the terrorist attacks of Sept. 11, 2001), but policy change can happen only if the window is open. Once the opportunity passes, the potential policies go back into the stream of problems that need solving.

The Longest Model (2002), as seen in Figure 10.2, incorporates the Kingdon model into a more complete, dynamic, systems-based conceptualization of the policy process. This model includes the implementation and evaluation phases of the policy process and demonstrates how that information is linked back to the streams of problems, policy, and politics. The key

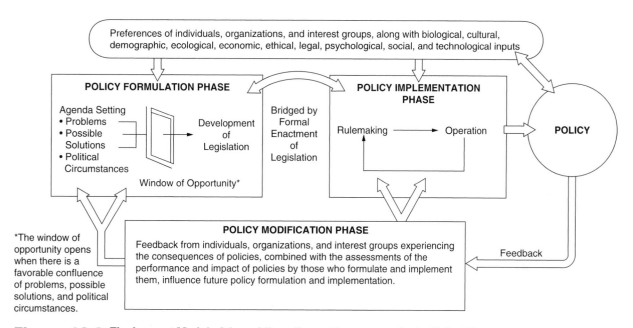

Figure 10.2 **The Longest Model of the public policymaking process in the United States.** Courtesy of Beaufort B. Longest.

feature of this model is its cyclical nature, allowing for changes to be made anywhere along the process. This model supports the incremental approach to policymaking.

HEALTH POLICY AND HEALTH CARE FINANCE

Health care spending currently accounts for 15 percent of the U.S. gross domestic product (GDP), and the Center for Medicare and Medicaid Services (CMS, 2005) projects that by 2014 this will increase to 18.7 percent. This spending reflects payments for services as well as durable medical equipment, technology, and prescription drugs. How is this care paid for? In the United States, health care is financed through numerous public- and private-sector programs. The predominant system for financing health care in both sectors is managed care, with over 165 million enrollees in private plans and over

59 million in federally operated Medicaid-managed care plans (CMS, 2005). See Chapter 7 for a more thorough discussion of managed care.

Public-Sector Financing

Public-sector programs exist at federal, state, and local levels and include Medicare, Medicaid, children's health-insurance program (SCHIP), military programs, veterans programs, federal-employee health-benefits programs (FEHBP), the native American program, and the maternal-child block-grant program. Another federal program that has a significant impact on health is the Social Security program, although it is not a health care financing mechanism per se.

Medicare

Medicare is national health insurance for Americans over the age of 65, the disabled, and people with end-stage renal disease. It was established in 1965 in an effort to reduce the financial burden of

RESEARCH APPLICATION ARTICLE

Deschaine, J. E. & Schaffer, M. A. (2003) Strengthening the role of public health nurse leaders in policy development. *Policy, Politics & Nursing Practice, 4*(4), 266–74.

Using the Longest model of policymaking, Deschaine and Schaffer (2003) interviewed eight leaders in public-health nursing in order to identify and analyze factors that interfered with the ability of public-health nurses to influence public policy. Several barriers were identified, including gender bias; lack of resources (fiscal and human); lack of political skill and power; varying levels of leadership competency; lack of academic preparation, especially in the area of policy development; and lack of public understanding. The authors recommended strengthening the academic preparation of nurses in the area of policy and politics and creating support for ongoing development of leadership, research, and political skill.

It is interesting to note that the nurses interviewed identified the same barriers to policy development regardless of their settings—rural, urban, or suburban. Because the study used qualitative methods, the findings were not generalizable beyond those specific nurses. However, the research supports earlier studies that identified similar barriers (Cramer, 2002; Gebbie, Wakefield, & Kerfoot, 2001). The role of gender that was identified in this study is a new finding and warrants further investigation.

health care on the elderly. In the 40 years of its existence, it has been administered by a variety of federal agencies and currently is under the Centers for Medicaid and Medicare (CMS, 2005). Medicare has two parts: Part A pays for hospitalization and is funded by payroll deductions, and Part B pays for medical expenses such as health care provider visits and is funded by member premiums. Most Medicare recipients are happy with their services, but there are concerns about the gap between health care costs and Medicare reimbursement rates because Medicare pays only a percentage of the actual costs and for a limited time. For example, Medicare pays for only the first 60 days of hospitalization.

WRITING EXERCISE 10.1

Policy analysts look at problems and either propose policy or look at proposed policies and offer opinions about outcomes. This is usually done via a policy-issue paper that (1) identifies the problem, (2) explains why the problem is important (economically, ethically, socially, etc.), (3) asks a policy question about the problem, (4) identifies the stakeholders, and (5) proposes a list of solutions to the problem.

For example, an issue brief on the nursing shortage would identify the lack of RNs in hospitals as the problem and ask the question, how can the nursing shortage be ameliorated? Or it may ask, how can patient safety be maintained in the face of the shortage? Select a policy issue of interest and develop a policy brief on the issue. Be sure to include the components enumerated above.

Average beneficiaries pay about 22 percent of their income for out-of-pocket expenses (Longest, 2002). The original Medicare program was a fee-for-service program that allowed individuals to go to any physician or hospital they chose that participated in Medicare. In 2003 the Medicare Modernization Act (MMA, P.L. 108-173) was passed, which allows beneficiaries to participate in a wide array of HMOs and PPOs and, for the first time, provides a prescription drug benefit. A number of demonstration projects were also mandated as part of MMA. These projects include feasibility studies related to rural hospitals, expanding chiropractic services, and improving quality of care for people with chronic illnesses, to name a few (CMS, 2005). Policymakers find themselves on the horns of a dilemma with Medicare because, although it is a valued program, it is very costly, and future reforms are likely to add to the federal government's financial burden. Who will pay for the program and how it is best administered are questions that policymakers continue to struggle with.

Medicaid

Medicaid is a program jointly funded by federal and state governments to provide health-related services to special groups of people such as the blind, disabled, the aged, women who are pregnant, and children and teenagers who meet eligibility requirements related to income and resources. Medicaid is the largest source of health services funding for people with low incomes and limited resources. Eligibility rules are federally mandated, but states have flexibility in the way that resources are counted, so there is considerable variation from state to state in who is eligible for Medicaid. Unlike Medicare, Medicaid funds can be used to pay for long-term care. However, recipients must "spend down" their resources to be eligible for reimbursement of long-term care. The amount an individual is allowed to keep varies from state to state but is somewhere in the neighborhood of $1500. Individuals may have a separate savings account in which money is earmarked for burial expenses, but that money cannot be used for anything else. Because long-term care is so expensive, many people started shifting

assets or transferring funds to family members in order to be eligible for Medicaid. This behavior became so widespread that a policy change was made as part of the Health Insurance Portability and Accountability Act of 1996 (HIPAA), making it a federal crime to intentionally transfer or hide funds within three years of applying for Medicaid services. This policy applies to individuals as well as their attorneys and estate planners, if they knowingly try to cheat or "game" the system.

State Children's Health Insurance Plan (SCHIP)

SCHIP, like Medicaid, is a jointly administered program. It was instituted in 1997 as part of the Balanced Budget Act. Forty million dollars was made available to states with the goal of expanding health insurance to children whose families earn too much money to be eligible for Medicaid, but not enough money to purchase private insurance.

SCHIP is designed to provide coverage to "targeted low-income children." A "targeted low-income child" is one who resides in a family with income below 200 percent of the Federal Poverty Level (FPL) or whose family has an income 50 percent higher than the state's Medicaid eligibility threshold (CMS, 2005). Like Medicaid, states have a lot of flexibility in how they administer the SCHIP program. Some states expand eligibility beyond the 200 percent FPL limit, and others cover entire families and not just children. States can use their SCHIP funds to expand Medicaid coverage, set up their own insurance plan, or develop a hybrid with elements of each. Whatever the design, the state plan must be approved by the federal government.

Military Insurance

The Department of Defense (DOD) provides health care coverage for active-duty servicemen and women and their dependent families. The insurance plan sounds and operates much like civilian health plans. Active-duty servicemen and women must enroll in TRICARE Prime, which operates like an HMO. Individuals who are not active duty automatically belong to TRICARE Standard, which functions like a PPO, with yearly deductibles and increased out-of-pocket expenses. There is an added benefit called TRICARE Extra, which offers a discount to nonactive-duty members who use in-plan (HMO-like) providers.

Veterans are covered through the Department of Veterans Affairs. The Veterans Health Administration (VHA) oversees more than 1100 facilities within 21 integrated health care networks, which include clinics, hospice centers, long-term care facilities, and over 160 hospitals across the nation.

Social Security

The Social Security Act (SSA) was passed in 1935 in order to secure the economic future of older Americans. In 2005 more than 48 million people were receiving Social Security benefits at a cost of more than $500 billion. Social Security is the major source of income for over 66 percent of America's senior citizens and the only source of income for another 22 percent (Social Security Administration, 2005). In addition to retirement income, the SSA also provides survivor and disability benefits to a large number of Americans who have not reached retirement age. Money for Social Security benefits comes from payroll contributions that are matched by employers. There is widespread concern that because people are living well after retirement age, Social Security funds will be depleted by the middle of this century, and workers who are contributing today will not reap the benefits of the money that was taken from them. This presents a policy crisis for the federal government, and the political platform that most successfully addresses the issue is likely to find its candidate as the leader of the nation.

Private-Sector Financing

Private-sector financing is made up of all nongovernmental agencies, providers, and commercial enterprises. It is the largest sector because private companies or corporations provide the majority of health care services. Along with pharmaceutical, technology, and information systems, the health insurance industry is part of the private sector. Approximately 60 percent of Americans are covered by employer-based insurance, 9 percent are covered by direct-pay insurance, and an estimated 15 percent

are either uninsured or underinsured (Denavas, Walt, Proctor, & Mills, 2004). Lack of insurance has a documented negative affect on health because the uninsured receive less preventive care, are diagnosed at more advanced disease stages, and once diagnosed, tend to receive less therapeutic care and have higher mortality rates than the insured. Insurance companies provide a variety of benefits and set their own policies regarding coverage and eligibility. In an effort to protect the public from the vagaries of the health insurance industry, the Health Insurance Portability and Accountability Act (P.L. 104-191) was passed in 1997 and implemented in 2000. This act prevents insurance companies from denying coverage on the basis of preexisting conditions and provides for continuous coverage when individuals change jobs. Unfortunately HIPAA has no power to control costs or maintain quality. The National Committee for Quality Assurance (NCQA) has standards for health insurance plans and collects data to demonstrate whether a health plan meets those standards. However, participation in data collection is voluntary. In 2004, with almost 600 health plans reporting, NCQA data indicated that there was a tremendous disparity in health plans with the majority of Americans receiving "less than optimal care" (NCQA, 2005). Dissatisfaction with private- sector health plans and negative outcomes are creating public pressure for policy reform.

HEALTH POLICY ISSUES— THE BIG THREE: COST, QUALITY, AND ACCESS

The discussion thus far illustrates that the current health care system in the United States has three major interwoven problems: it is expensive, large segments of the population have either limited or no access to services, and there is significant disparity in the quality of care provided (NCHC, 2004). Issues related to cost, quality, and access have dominated policy discussions for the last decade and will continue to be front and center for the foreseeable future.

Cost

The United States spends more on health care than any other country in the world. In 2003 total spending on health care was $1.7 trillion, accounting for more than 15 percent of the U.S. gross domestic product, and this is expected to reach $2.6 trillion by 2010 (NCHC, 2004). In spite of this, as many as many 59 million Americans are periodically uninsured in any given year and between 20 and 30 million are without health insurance for the entire year. (Congressional Budget Office, 2004). Consequently, those with insurance bear an increased burden as costs go up to compensate for the financial shortfalls that health care agencies experience. A Kaiser Commission report to the Urban Institute (2003b) estimated that each year uninsured Americans receive about $34.5 billion in uncompensated health care while paying $26.4 billion out of their own pockets. According to the Institute of Medicine (2001), the United States loses between $65 billion and $130 billion annually as a result of poor health and early death due to lack of insurance. An area of particular concern is the cost of prescription drugs. Medicare, Medicaid, and TRICARE are continually assessing policies related to drug coverage and have mandated the use of generics, removed drugs from the approved drug list, and limited the amounts available at any given time in an effort to control expenditures in this arena. A prescription drug benefit is being added to Medicare.

The National Governors Association (2005) has adopted the following policy position related to prescription drugs: "A number of policy changes must be enacted that will help decrease costs and improve quality and efficiency of care. The goal of reducing both state and federal expenditures will require policy changes that impact all segments of the pharmaceutical marketplace, including (but not limited to) increased rebates from manufacturers, reforms to the Average Wholesale Price (AWP), and tiered, enforceable co-pays for beneficiaries. States must have additional tools to properly manage this complicated and critical benefit."

Quality

The Institute of Medicine began evaluating the quality of health care in the United States in 1996 and has published numerous reports on the topic. The report *To Err is Human* (Kohn, Corrigan, & Donaldson, 2000) estimated that between 44,000 and 98,000 Americans die each year from preventable medical errors in hospitals. Those figures do not include the 88,000 deaths that occur because of nosocomial infections or the 300,000 deaths that occur due to preventable medical errors (NCHC, 2004). To put that number in perspective, it is about nine times the number of deaths attributed to highway accidents each year. In *Crossing the Quality Chasm* (2001), the IOM identifies 10 rules for improving the quality of the health care system (see Table 10.1).

Access

In the United States, health insurance is the gateway to services. Individuals without insurance are forced to access the system via "safety net" facilities such as free clinics, health department clinics, and increasingly, emergency rooms. According to a report by the Kaiser Family Foundation (2003a), 27 million workers were uninsured in 2003 because many employers do not offer health benefits, and many employees cannot afford to pay the premiums. Increasing numbers of individuals are likely to be without health insurance due to the rising costs of providing such insurance. According to the NCHC (2004), several studies predict that premiums will continue to increase at double-digit rates over the next several years, with premium rates (approximately $14,545) for employer-sponsored family health coverage in 2006 more than doubling those of 2001.

Healthy People 2010

Health policy in the United States focuses on achieving the goals of Healthy People 2010, a document developed under the Department of Health and Human Services (DHHS, 2000) by scientists with public input, which establishes the national health agenda for the current decade. Two overarching goals have been identified: eliminating health disparities

Table 10.1 **Simple Rules for the 21st Century Health System**

Current Approach	New Rule
Care is based on primary visits	Care is based on continuous healing relationships
Professional autonomy drives variability	Care is customized according to patient needs and values
Professional is in control	The patient is the source of control
Information is a record	Knowledge is shared and information flows freely
Decision making is based on training and experience	Decision making is evidence based
Do no harm is an individual responsibility	Safety is a system property
Secrecy is necessary	Transparency is necessary
The system reacts to needs	Needs are anticipated
Cost reduction is sought	Waste is continually decreased
Preference is given to professional roles over the system	Cooperation among clinicians is a priority

SOURCE: *Crossing the quality chasm: A new health system for the 21st century.* IOM, 2001.

Table 10.2 **Healthy People 2010 Focus Areas**

1. Access to Quality Health Services	15. Injury and Violence Prevention
2. Arthritis, Osteoporosis, and Chronic Back Conditions	16. Maternal, Infant, and Child Health
3. Cancer	17. Medical Product Safety
4. Chronic Kidney Disease	18. Mental Health and Mental Disorders
5. Diabetes	19. Nutrition and Overweight
6. Disability and Secondary Conditions	20. Occupational Safety and Health
7. Educational and Community-Based Programs	21. Oral Health
8. Environmental Health	22. Physical Activity and Fitness
9. Family Planning	23. Public Health Infrastructure
10. Food Safety	24. Respiratory Diseases
11. Health Communication	25. Sexually Transmitted Diseases
12. Heart Disease and Stroke	26. Substance Abuse
13. HIV	27. Tobacco Use
14. Immunization and Infectious Diseases	28. Vision and Hearing

A Systematic Approach to Health Improvement

```
                          ┌─────────────────────────────────┐
                          │              Goals              │
                          └─────────────────────────────────┘
                          ┌─────────────────────────────────┐
                          │           Objectives            │
                          └─────────────────────────────────┘

         ┌───────────────────────────────────────────────────────────┐
         │                   Determinants of health                  │
         │        ┌──────────────────────────────────────┐           │
         │        │       Policies and interventions      │          │
         │        └──────────────────────────────────────┘           │
         │   ┌───────────────────────────────────────────────┐       │
         │   │                   Behavior                    │       │
         │   │   Physical           Individual        Social │       │
         │   │   environment                      environment│       │
         │   │                   Biology                     │       │
         │   └───────────────────────────────────────────────┘       │
         │        ┌──────────────────────────────────────┐           │
         │        │      Access to quality health care     │          │
         │        └──────────────────────────────────────┘           │
         └───────────────────────────────────────────────────────────┘
                          ┌─────────────────────────────────┐
                          │          Health status          │
                          └─────────────────────────────────┘
```

Figure 10.3 **Healthy People 2010. Retrieved March 24, 2006 from http://www.health.gov/healthypeople/document/pdf/uih/2010uih.pdf.**

and increasing the number and quality of healthy life years. Twenty-eight focus areas have been established to accomplish these goals, and each focus area has a number of objectives to support it (see Table 10.2). The Healthy People objectives allow agencies and communities to work together to improve the health of the individuals they serve. The objectives also provide a mechanism for measuring success. Policymakers are much more likely to be successful in advancing their positions and garnering support for their initiatives when they address or are aligned with these objectives. The Healthy People objectives have been specified by Congress as the measure for assessing

the progress of the Indian Health Care Improvement Act, the Maternal and Child Health Block Grant, and the Preventive Health and Health Services Block Grant. (DHHS, 2000).

The goals of Healthy People 2010 were developed after identifying the 10 leading health indicators that reflected the major national health concerns at the beginning of the century (see Table 10.3). They were chosen on the basis of their ability to motivate action, the availability of data to measure outcomes, and their importance to the health of the public. Figure 10.3 illustrates a systematic approach to health improvement.

Table 10.3 **Leading Health Indicators for the United States**

- Physical Activity
- Overweight and Obesity
- Tobacco Use
- Substance Abuse
- Responsible Sexual Behavior
- Mental Health
- Injury and Violence
- Environmental Quality
- Immunization
- Access to Health Care

Another significant policy-focused event that incorporates input from scientists, experts, and the lay public is the White House Conference on Aging. This event takes place once a decade. The purpose of the event is to develop policies that support the Older Americans Act (PL). The 2005 Conference focused on financing and planning for long-term care, reemployment, flexible work settings, housing and transportation, opportunities for lifelong learning, and social engagement through volunteering and leisure activities.

Policy Issues Confronting the Health Professions

There are numerous policy issues confronting the health professions. These issues fall into four major categories: global issues, government issues, community issues, and workplace issues.

Global Issues

Global issues within this context refer to issues relevant to society at large, as opposed to issues of international importance, although the two are not mutually exclusive. Issues of hunger, abuse, violence, and war certainly represent major concerns to all people around the globe. The amount of attention

given to these issues by policymakers waxes and wanes based on how relevant they are to their constituents at the time. For example, terrorism has been an international issue for decades, but only recently has become a policy concern for Americans. Following the attack on the World Trade Center in 2001, policies have been implemented at federal, state, and local levels to prepare for future disasters, and schools of nursing now include disaster preparedness and bioterrorism in their curricula.

Two related issues with global implications are the aging of society and the matter of long-term care (LTC). While Reinhardt (2003) maintains that the aging of the population is "too gradual a process to be the major cost driver in health care, it is still an important issue for policymakers and health care providers." Healthy aging and reducing frailty are at the forefront of concerns of baby boomers who are reaching the age of 65. To address these concerns, the Robert Wood Johnson Foundation, as part of the Aging Partnership, has established the National Blueprint for healthy aging, which includes policy initiatives that will increase the ability of senior citizens to engage in physical activity, which has been shown to decrease disability and improve quality of life. The blueprint can be found at www.agingblueprint.org.

Long-term care (LTC) refers to a broad range of supportive medical, personal, and social services needed by people who are unable to meet their basic living needs for an extended period of time. Contrary to popular belief, the majority of long-term care is received at home and in community facilities, not in nursing homes. As many as one-fourth of all American households are directly or indirectly involved in caregiving. Although this is an issue that will escalate as the baby boomers age, it is also a concern for the under-65 age group because 43 percent of people receiving LTC fall into this age group. LTC is expensive. The cost of a nursing home ranges from $30,000 to $80,000 per year, and home and community care ranges from $12,000 to $50,000 per year (Day, 2006). But cost is not the only problem; quality has been a concern for decades. The IOM report (2001) on LTC identified "serious problems . . . including

CASE SCENARIO 10.1

Mrs. G is an 83-year-old woman who until about 6 months ago worked part time for a county agency as a home health aide. The county disbanded the program due to lack of funding, and Mrs. G decided to take a well-earned retirement. One month ago she called her son, who is living in another state, saying she had had a heart attack, and she couldn't remember how to get home. She was agitated and tearful. When the son went to see her, he found that she in fact had not sustained a heart attack but had experienced some angina for which she was taking NTG gr 1/150 sublingually prn. More distressing was the fact that she weighed only 89 pounds, was shaky on her feet, and was having significant problems with her short-term memory. He brought her back to his home to try to get her well and have her evaluated by a gerontologist. She began to gain weight and had no episodes of chest pain, but her memory was so impaired she was no longer able to live alone safely. The son suspected that the reason for her weight loss may be that she forgot to eat.

The problem was what to do with her. Nursing homes cost about $1000 per week, and she was not eligible for Medicaid. She still had a home and some land holdings in her home state, and she wanted to return home. Her son wanted her to move in with him, but he could not stay home with her because he had to work to support his family of four.

Case Considerations

1. What are some options for this family to consider when planning LTC for Mrs. G?

2. What federal and state level resources are available for this family?

3. What type of LTC policy would you recommend to help families who are facing these types of circumstances?

4. What policies related to Healthy People 2010 or the National Blueprint would be helpful in this situation?

---

pain management, pressure sores, incontinence and malnutrition." Kayser-Jones (2003) has done a number of studies on the quality of care in nursing homes and found that patients frequently suffer from dehydration, malnutrition, and pressure ulcers (2002a) and die without appropriate end of life care (2002b). Her findings indicate that these negative outcomes are related to inadequate staffing (Kayser-Jones et al., 2003). Kemper (2003) identified seven policy issues related to LTC that need more research: eligibility systems, payment systems, societal values related to LTC (i.e., what constitutes quality of life in this setting), the performance of LTC insurance/fiscal preparedness, the affect of technology on LTC, the effects of community environment on the quality of the LTC experience, and LTC delivery systems.

Another global issue related to health involves genetic engineering. According to Ojha and Thertulien (2005), there are four issues related to genetics that have universal policy implications: genetic privacy, regulation and standardization of genetic testing, gene patenting, and education. Education is important for both health providers and individuals undergoing genetic testing.

Government Issues

It is critically important for health professionals to be aware of attempts to change language in any of the rules and regulations that relate to their scope of practice. For example, in an era of cost constraints, agencies such as the Centers for Medicare and Medicaid are tempted to change regulations stipulating the number or level of essential personnel in specific health care environments. For example, a proposal to change regulatory language related to operating room personnel was successfully quashed at the federal level, and the Association of Operating Room Nurses (AORN) is working at the state level to ensure that all states require the presence of a licensed RN or physician in the circulating role in the OR (Franko, 2004).

Other government issues are related to funding workforce development. Title VIII of the Public Health Service Act was expanded by the Nurse Reinvestment Act (PL 107-205) to provide grants for advanced education, workforce diversity programs, faculty loan programs, geriatric education programs, and nurse loan-repayment programs. Money to sustain these grants must be appropriated annually by the federal government. It is important for nurses to be aware of the funding cycle (typically June and July) and contact legislators reminding them of the importance of continuing to invest in the nursing workforce.

Nursing organizations such as the American Nurses Association (ANA), American Organization of Nurse Executives (AONE), Emergency Nurses Association (ENA), Oncology Nurses Association (ONA), and others work to accomplish global objectives related to nursing and health. Unfortunately, to date these organizations have not succeeded in mobilizing the more than 2 million nurses in the United States in any united fashion. Imagine the changes that could be accomplished if nursing could speak with one voice on an issue. The American Medical Association (AMA) continues to exert a strong influence on policy by virtue of its unified stand on the issues.

At the state level, nurses must be aware of the State Board regulations related to licensure and any changes made to the scope of their practice.

Community Issues

Policies that affect community health are similar to those that affect national health. The difference is that they reflect the values of the people involved more directly. A continuing problem that the majority of communities face is affordable quality childcare. This is especially true in rural areas. In addition to the problem of finding quality care is the problem of transporting children to and from care. The need for childcare in off hours is of particular concern to nurses and other providers who work evening and night shifts.

Other community concerns generally involve schools and community services such as fire, safety, and acute and emergency health care.

Workplace Issues

Factors related to the nursing work environment affect the health of nurses as well as patients. In addition to nurse/patient ratios, policymakers are looking at the research related to workplace issues, such as the number of hours worked in a shift, the days worked in a week, and mandatory overtime. The educational preparation of RNs is also an important issue, as illustrated in a study by Aiken (2003), which demonstrated that clients cared for in hospitals with higher percentages of nurses prepared at the BSN level had better outcomes. The American Nurses Association (ANA) listed the following issues as priorities for the 109th Congress to address: the nursing shortage, appropriate staffing, fair labor standards, workplace safety/ergonomics, and whistle blowing. Another growing concern is related to immigration policies and the use of foreign nurses to ease the nursing shortage. The ANA, in collaboration with other nursing organizations, developed a document entitled Nursing's Agenda for the Future, which identifies a strategic plan for addressing these issues. The plan can be obtained from the Web site http://www.NursingWorld.org/naf.

CHAPTER SUMMARY

The health of any nation is significantly affected by the policies established by that nation. These policies may have a direct impact on health, such as bans on tobacco smoking, or, as is the case more often than not, they might affect health indirectly through mechanisms that regulate the economy and the environment. Nurses are uniquely positioned to affect health policy by virtue of their knowledge,

CASE SCENARIO 10.2

A number of nurses from your organization are planning to attend the State Board hearing on the educational preparation of nurses. The American Nurses Association established the BSN as the entry level for practice over 30 years ago. Traditionally, the majority of hospitals and other health care organizations have treated associate-degree nurses and baccalaureate nurses the same regarding pay and assignment. This practice is shifting as more evidence points to better patient outcomes with BSN-prepared nurses. The American Association of Community Colleges argues that the ADN is sufficient and points to the fact that both groups of nurses take the same licensing exam and therefore are "just as qualified." The State Board is considering a regulation that would give ADNs a provisional license and require them to get the BSN within 10 years or the license would expire. You are preparing to offer your views on the subject to the board.

Case Considerations

1. What data would you gather to help you formulate an opinion?

2. What role, if any, should experience play in shaping the debate?

3. Should entry-level requirements be different for students who have a previous bachelor's degree in another field?

4. Some authors have argued that the focus should be on exit level rather than entry level. What are your thoughts about that?

their expertise, and their ethical obligations to the individuals, families, and communities they serve. Research indicates that nurses frequently encounter barriers to policy development. How can nurses overcome these barriers? According to a survey of nurse leaders who have been successful in the policy arena, it requires expertise, networking, collective action, influence, the ability to take the broad view, and perseverance (Warner, 2003). Nurses must become informed about the issues and get involved in the policy process in order to ensure healthy working environments for themselves, and secure the safety, health, and quality of life of the patients they currently treat and those they have yet to meet.

Whatever we allow to happen . . . will happen.
                    —Leslie Neal, PhD, RN, FNP-C

REFERENCES

Aiken, L. (2003). Educational levels of hospital nurses and surgical patient mortality. *JAMA, 290*(12), 1617–23.

Bailey, R. (2004). Mandatory health insurance now. *Reason, 36*(6), 38–39.

Bell, J., & Standish, M. (2005). Communities and health policy: A pathway for change. *Health Affairs, 24*(2), 339–43.

Centers for Medicare and Medicaid (2005). CMS Demonstration projects under the Medicare Modernization Act (MMA). Retrieved on July 2, 2005, from http://www.cms.hhs.gov/researchers/demos/MMAdemolist.asp.

Clarke, S. P. (2005). The policy implications of staffing-outcomes research. *JONA, 35*(1), 17–19.

Cramer, M. E. (2002). Factors influencing organized political participation in nursing. *Policy, Politics, & Nursing Practice, 3*(2), 97–107.

Congressional Budget Office (2004). The uninsured and rising health insurance premiums. Report before the Subcommittee on Health. Committee on Ways and

Means. U.S. House of Representatives. Retrieved on July 8, 2005, from http://www.cbo.gov/showdoc.cfm?index=5152&sequence=0.

Cummings, G., & McLennan, M. (2005). Advanced practice nursing: Leadership to effect policy change. *JONA, 35*(2), 61–66.

Day, T. (2006). Retrieved on September 1, 2006, from http://www. Longtermcarelink.net/about_nursing_homes.html.

DeNavas-Walt, C., Proctor, B. D., & Mills, J. (2004). Income, poverty, and health insurance coverage in the United States: 2003. *Current Population Reports*. U.S. Census Bureau P60-226. Washington, DC: U.S. Government Printing Office.

Deschaine, J. E., & Schaffer, M. A. (2003). Strengthening the role of public health nurse leaders in policy development. *Policy, Politics, & Nursing Practice, 4*(4), 266–74.

Franko, F. (2004). The RN in the circulator role—A proactive approach. *AORN Journal, 79*, 3.

Gebbie, K. M., Wakefield, M., & Kerfoot, K. (2000). Nursing and health policy. *Journal of Nursing Scholarship, 32*(3), 307–315.

Gostin, L. (2005). Law and the public's health. *Issues in Science and Technology, 21*(3), 71–78.

Institute of Medicine (2001). *Crossing the quality chasm: A new health system for the 21st century.* Washington, DC: National Academies Press.

Kaiser Family Foundation (2003a). *The uninsured and their access to healthcare.* Fact sheet 1420-05. Kaiser Commission on Medicaid and the Uninsured.

Kaiser Family Foundation (2003b). *The uninsured: A primer.* Kaiser Commission on Medicaid and the Uninsured. Retrieved on July 5, 2003, from www.kff.org/uninsured/7216.cfm.

Kayser-Jones, J. (2002a). Malnutrition, dehydration, and starvation in the midst of plenty: The political impact of qualitative inquiry. *Qualitative Health Research, 12*(10), 1391–1405.

Kayser-Jones, J. (2002b). The experience of dying: An ethnographic nursing home study. *The Gerontologist, 42*, 11–19.

Kayser-Jones, J. (2003). Continuing to conduct research in nursing homes despite controversial findings. *Qualitative Health Research, 13*, 114–118.

Kayser-Jones, J., Schell, E., Lyons, W., Kris, A. E., Chan, J., & Beard, R. L. (2003). Factors that influence end-of-life care in nursing homes: The physical environment, inadequate staffing, and lack of supervision. *The Gerontologist, 43, Spec. No. 2,* 76–84.

Keller, L., Strohschein, S., Lia-Hoagberg, B., & Schaffer, M. (2003). *Population-based public health nursing interventions: Practice-based and evidence-supported.* Manuscript submitted for publication, Minnesota Department of Health.

Kemper, P. (2003). Long term care research and policy. *The Gerontologist, 43*(4), 436.

Kingdon, J. (1995). *Agendas, alternatives, and public policies.* (2nd cd.). New York: Harper Collins.

Kohn, L. T., Corrigan, J. M., & Donaldson, M. S. (2000). *To err is human: Building a safer health system.* Institute of Medicine Report. Washington, DC: National Academies Press.

Kronenfield, J. (2002). *Healthcare policy issues and trends.* Westport, CT: Praeger.

Lomas, J. (2000). Connecting research and policy. *ISUMA, 1*(1), 140–44.

Longest, B. (2002). *Healthpolicy making in the United States.* (3rd ed., pp. 9–35). Chicago: Health Administration Press.

Mason, D. Leavitt, J., & Chaffee, M. (2002). Policy and politics: A framework for action. In D. Mason, J. Leavitt, & M. Chaffee (Eds.), Policy and Politics in Nursing and Health Care (4th ed., p. 9). Saunders.

National Coalition on Health Care (2004). *Building a better health care system: Specifications for reform.* Retrieved on July 2, 2005, from http://www.nchc.org/materials/studies/reform.pdf.

National Commission for Quality Assurance (2005). *The state of health care (2004).* Retrieved on July 2, 2005, from http://www.ncqa.org/communications/SOMC/SOHC2004.pdf.

National Governors Association (2005). *Medicaid improvement: A preliminary report.* Retrieved on July 2, 2005, from http://www.nga.org/cda/files/0506medicaid.pdf.

Ojha, R., & Thertulien, R. (2005). Health care policy issues as a result of the genetic revolution: Implications for public health. *American Journal of Public Health, 95*(3), 385–389.

Reinhardt, U. E. (2003). Does the aging of the population really drive demand for health care? *Health Affairs, 22*(6), 27–39.

Romano, M. (2001). Woe is us: Stinging reports criticize health industry, detail a widespread dissatisfaction. *Modern Healthcare, 31*, 4–5.

Salmon, M. (2002). Foreword. In D. Mason, J. Leavitt, & M. Chaffee (Eds.) *Policy and Politics in Nursing and Health Care* by (4th ed., p. XXV). Saunders.

Social Security Administration (2005). *The future of social security*. SSA Publication No. 05-10055. Retrieved on July 8, 2005, from http://www.ssa.gov/pubs/10055.html.

Spetz, J. (2005). Public policy and nurse staffing: What approach is best? *JONA, 35*(1), 14–16.

Sudano, J., & Baker, D. (2003). Intermittent lack of health insurance coverage and use of preventive services. *American Journal of Public Health, 98*(1), 130–137.

Toofany, S. (2005). Nurses and health policy. *Nursing Management, 2*(3), 26–31.

U.S. Department of Health and Human Services (November, 2000). *Healthy people 2010: Understanding & improving health.* (2nd ed.). Washington DC: U.S. Government Printing Office.

World Health Organization (1948). Preamble to the Constitution of the World Health Organization as adopted by the International Health Conference, New York, 19–22 June, 1946; signed on 22 July 1946 by the representatives of 61 States (Official Records of the World Health Organization, no. 2, p. 100) and entered into force on 7 April 1948. Retrieved on June 20, 2005, from http://www.who.int/about/definition/en/.

Warner, J. R. (2003). A phenomenological approach to political competence: Stories of nurse activists. *Policy, Politics, & Nursing Practice, 4*(2), 135–143.

Wunderlich, G. S., & Kohler, P. (2000). *Improving the quality of long term insurance*. Institute of Medicine Report. Washington, DC: National Academies Press.

CHAPTER 11

Diversity

Karin A. Polifko

We have become not a melting pot but a beautiful mosaic. Different people, different beliefs, different yearnings, different hopes, different dreams.
—Jimmy Carter

LEARNING OBJECTIVES

At the completion of the chapter, the learner should be able to do the following:

1. Identify significant employment trends in the health care industry.
2. Describe current diversity issues.
3. Apply specific cultural nursing theories to patient-care delivery.
4. Analyze the intertwining issues of race, nursing, and society.
5. Discuss specific gender issues within the nursing profession.
6. Synthesize the impact of the aging nursing workforce on health care delivery.
7. Identify concerns regarding sexual orientation in the nursing profession.
8. Describe methods for supervising patient-care delivery in a diverse environment.

KEY TERMS

Acculturation

Cultural Heritage Model

Diversity

Gender issues

Role strain

Transcultural Assessment Model

Transcultural nursing

One of the greatest challenges facing health care employers in this current decade is the hiring and retention of a labor force composed of diverse, professional employees. The United States was built on diversity—diversity of religious beliefs; diversity of race, ethnicity, and cultures; diversity of thoughts. Diversity also includes factors of socioeconomic class, physical abilities, and sexual orientation. The face of the United States in general, and subsequently reflected within the health care environment, is rapidly changing. In several parts of the county, some minority races are quickly replacing the previously majority races, especially in California, Texas, and Florida. Health care professionals are not keeping pace racially or culturally with reflecting those populations served. Our continuously aging nursing workforce, with its increasingly anticipated retirements and fewer young nurses entering the field, is an accelerating challenge. Additionally, nursing is yet to become a profession of choice for many males, with the exception of a few specialty areas.

SIGNIFICANT EMPLOYMENT TRENDS

The 1990s became a turning point for the nursing profession for many reasons. The continued effect of the prospective payment system directly touched the bottom line of the many health care systems, which in cost-cutting efforts dramatically decreased the number of registered nurses, substituting instead unlicensed assistive personnel (UAP) to care for clients. Nurse educators, often seen by health care administrators as nonessential, were eliminated, as were numerous education departments. Along with their education departments, the clinical nurse specialists (CNS) were often eliminated as well, with administrators believing that the CNS was oftentimes an expensive staff nurse. Computer and biomedical advances enhanced patient care through improved diagnostics, yet challenged the system and personnel who had to learn, apply, and troubleshoot the new technologies. Paper charting systems are still transitioning to computerized systems in many health care facilities, with the goal of eliminating as much of the handwritten orders and reports as possible in an effort not only to decrease medical errors, but also to allow for electronic transfer of information. The net result of all these advances was a dramatic decrease in the number of direct nurse caregivers and nurses in support positions throughout the health care system.

A significant result in the late 1990s and early 2000s was the renewed focus on patient outcomes that directly related to the level and amount of nursing care provided. Aiken, Clark, Sloan, Cheung, & Silber (2003) directly linked educational preparation to the outcomes of surgical patients. The Institute of Medicine (2001) produced a seminal work linking the patient error rate to the numbers and types of health care workers, including nurses, resulting in hospitals changing how they review their mistakes and to whom and how quickly these mistakes are reported. Hospitals and health care systems soon began to realize that the dramatic cuts in the professional nursing staff in the late 1990s resulted in fewer interested prospective nurse applicants, higher dissatisfaction among those employed, and higher turnover (Buiser, 2000).

The changing demographics of the United States is altering health care usage. The population continues to age, demanding more physician and nurse time, while increasing the need for more personnel. Similarly, the provider population is aging at the same speed, with retirement expected for many at the same time that there will be an increased need by the patient population. The numbers of young workers in the United States aged 18 to 30 are declining, resulting in a lower number who could potentially be attracted to the health care fields in sufficient enough numbers to replace the retired workers. Conversely, the age cohort of those 60 years and older is growing in America; it is projected by the U.S. Census (2001a) that this group's size will continue to increase over the next few decades.

The cost of health care continues to rise, especially among the elderly population, who will require more services from insurers, including Medicare and Medicaid. Further, the racial and cultural make-up of the United States is constantly evolving, with each group viewing health care differently and with varying expectations of the health care providers, who increasingly do not look like they do. Access to adequate health care has been an issue for years, with the gaps growing as minority populations swell.

The National Center for Health Workforce Analysis (2003), in its report entitled *Changing Demographics: Implications for Physicians, Nurses and Other Health Workers,* detailed the impact for the registered-nurse workforce. As in prior studies, it is projected that the need for registered nurses will continue to grow from 2 million in year 2000 to 2.8 million in year 2020 (p. V). Similarly, the need for licensed practical nurses and nurse aides will continue to increase. The hospital setting will persist in experiencing slower growth with the outpatient setting seeing a more robust growth. Acute hospital settings will continue to expand technology and care into outpatient settings, as patient days continue to decline. Additionally, as the population continues to age, so does the registered-nurse workforce. One of the greatest concerns in health care today is that as the demand for services increases due to an aging population, the actual number of registered nurses able to provide care will decrease due to retirements or simply inability to perform direct patient-care services any longer. Direct patient care is physically challenging, and the aging workforce does not have the stamina or the physical strength to perform many of the functions consistently during a 12-hour shift, such as lifting patients or putting them in their beds, resulting in a greater number of occupational injuries.

DEFINING DIVERSITY

Diversity is often viewed as existing in a state of difference, with heterogeneity among common elements. The United States has always embraced and encouraged people from different cultures, backgrounds, races, and ethnicities, and it is a country that values diversity. According to the 2000 Census, 17.9 percent of the U.S. population, almost 50 million people, speak a language other than English in their home, with Spanish being the predominant language after English.

A person's culture, race, and ethnicity influence everyday decisions and actions and often guide relationships in the work, social, and home environments. Culture is based upon belief sets, values, norms, and folkways of a specific group; we grow up within a certain culture in our community, where particular behaviors are either valued or discouraged. Culture may be expressed in the form of particular clothing, foods, celebrations, and social expectations. Values are concepts that are taught as right or wrong, moral or immoral, ethical or unethical (Yukle, 1994). With the majority of one's values developed by age seven, it is critical for parents to understand a child's moral development, and to appreciate the influence that they, the family, the school system, and the larger community have on a child at such a young age. Values are strongly driven by culture; what may be acceptable for one culture is not acceptable for another. One example of a culturally driven value is that of a woman's place in society. In a strongly patriarchal society, such as China, women are not as valued as men and do not hold an equal place in society as they do in a less patriarchal society, such as Denmark.

People who have similar biological variations, such as skin tone, facial features, and bone structure are said to belong to a specific race. Ethiopians have a much different biological make-up than the Danish: hence, two divergent races.

Whom you identify with is a component of ethnicity; it is marked by perceptions of who someone is and to what group you feel you belong. Ethnicity is socially driven, allowing the group members a self-identification and sense of belonging. The belief that any given culture or ethnic group is superior to another is considered to be ethnocentric thinking. Figure 11.1 illustrates the many ways in which people differ.

Acculturation is the process by which new behaviors are adopted as part of the immediate culture, resulting in new values, knowledge, or belief sets that are shared by all members. Assimilation is often used interchangeably with the word acculturation and can mean that someone of a different background may be absorbed into the larger community of people of another culture. On the other hand, someone may choose to actively assimilate to

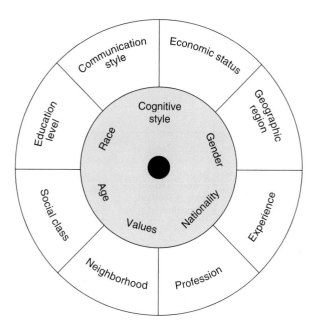

Figure 11.1 Ways in which people differ.

the larger culture in an effort to decrease the perceived differences. Choosing western-style dress, eating American foods, or using some of the colloquial phrases in speech are examples of active cultural assimilation.

SELECTED CULTURAL NURSING THEORIES

Anthropologist Madeline Leininger developed the Transcultural Nursing Theory (Leininger, 1997). She began her studies of **transcultural nursing** in the 1960s, studying the world's different cultures and how various cultures responded to nursing care, and specifically, caring behaviors practiced by nurses. In addition, Leininger also studied the relationships between nursing care and health/illness values, beliefs, and patterns of behavior. She began the Transcultural Nursing Society in 1974 as a subspecialty of nursing, combining both of her loves—nursing and

anthropology. The goal of transcultural nursing is to provide care that is consistent with a patient's expectations and cultural belief set. Everyone has been raised in a society that has certain values, beliefs, and norms, with clear guidelines for what behaviors are both accepted and not accepted by others. Leininger goes on to say (1978, p. 8) that the application of transcultural nursing is the "comparative study of and analysis of different cultures and subcultures in the work with respect to their caring behavior, nursing care and health-illness values, beliefs and patterns of behavior with the goal of developing a scientific and humanistic body of knowledge to provide culture-specific and culture-universal nursing care practices."

There are several assumptions in understanding Leininger's Transcultural Nursing Theory, which has three primary precepts. The first is that of caring: all cultures have a defined concept of caring and how caring behaviors are exhibited to others. The second notion is that of the provision of "good" care: each culture has an accepted standard for what is expected by a care provider. The third concept defines the care provided to a client or client system as based upon an awareness of the culture's self-identification in terms of symbols, communications, and in shared meanings between members of the group.

The bulk of patient-care records used by registered nurses to document care do not provide the opportunity to document cultural assessment results. Giger and Davidhizar's **Transcultural Assessment Model** (1999) offers nurses a culturally sensitive instrument with which to perform patient assessment and evaluate the various meanings of cultural responses. In order to provide a cultural assessment for a patient, Giger and Davidhizar recommend a review of six concepts as described in the Transcultural Assessment Model (see Figure 11.2). These concepts are communication, space, social organization, time, environmental control, and biological variations. Each culture has its own perceptions of these six concepts and oftentimes the variance between different cultures can be quite significant.

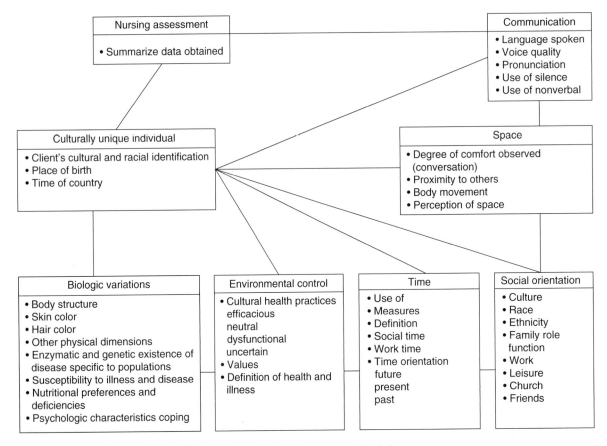

Figure 11.2 **Giger and Davidhizar's Transcultural Assessment Model.**

SOURCE: From Giger, J. N. & Davidhizar, R. E. (1995). *Transcultural nursing: Assessment and intervention*, St. Louis: Mosby-Yearbook. Reprinted with permission.

In applying the Transcultural Assessment Model to patient assessment, the nurse is afforded the opportunity to take into account numerous factors when ascertaining why certain behaviors occur or why particular outcomes are sought that may not be consistent with the nurse's goals and objectives. For example, the American culture is very cognizant of time, expecting appointments to begin and end as scheduled, versus the Filipino culture in which it is a more accepted behavior to be late. Other cultures have unspoken rules about personal space and touching unfamiliar people; the Hispanic culture has much smaller personal space than the Japanese culture, which is much more reserved and needs a more expansive space for a person to feel comfortable. All six concepts take into account an individual's unique characteristics as the nurse plans for culturally sensitive care.

Some minority cultures aspire to assimilate to the majority culture, often changing their expectations and notions of what is right and wrong based upon the fit of the majority culture. One can see this assimilation in newly arrived immigrants

WRITING EXERCISE 10-1

The text has presented three popular transcultural theories: Leininger's Transcultural Nursing Theory, Giger and Davidhizar's Transcultural Assessment Model, and Spector's Cultural Heritage Model. (1) Identify one client from your clinical practice that is from a culture/ethnic background that is different from yours. (2) Using one of the above three theoretical models illustrated, perform a cultural assessment of your client. (3) Write up your assessment and be prepared to discuss in class.

who want to dress like, sound like, and be viewed as Americans. On the other hand, there are some cultures that remain segregated from the mainstream culture by their language, dress, and behaviors, which are clearly those of their primary culture; they may even be physically isolated in a different section of town, such as Chinatown in San Francisco, California.

Spector's (2000) **Cultural Heritage Model** examines a client through his culture, religion, and ethnicity. Additionally, Spector adapts concepts from Giger and Davidhizer's Transcultural Assessment Model to provide a well-rounded client assessment. The six categories from the Transcultural Assessment Model include environmental control, social organization, biological variations, space, time and communication and are part of the Spector's Cultural Assessment Model.

One facet of Spector's model is the inclusion of the patient as well as primary and extended family members, with the belief that all contribute to the socialization of an individual, who in turn becomes part of the larger society. Spector's model assumes that people maintain their traditional folkways, beliefs, and values, resulting in a consistent heritage. A heritage becomes inconsistent when the person develops acculturation features, wanting to assimilate to the primary culture. Often acculturation occurs more quickly when the host culture is friendly and embracing versus alienating and forbidding. Figure 11.3 offers an example of a cultural assessment interview guide.

RACE, NURSING, AND SOCIETY

The predominant race in the United States continues to be white, non-Hispanic, approximately 69 percent of the population (U.S. Census, 2001b). The percentage of white, non-Hispanic Americans has continued to decrease throughout the years, with the Hispanic population quickly becoming the largest minority group in 2002 at 13.5 percent of the total population, increased from 4.5 percent in 1970, which was the first year that Hispanics were separately identified in a census. Likewise, the African American population maintains about 13 percent of the overall U.S. population, with Asian/Pacific Islanders at 4 percent. Native Americans and Alaskan Indians remain at approximately 1 percent of the total population. Interestingly, 2002 was the first year that people were able to claim membership in more than one race; 2.4 percent of the U.S. populations did so in 2002. Those with dual-race identities were younger (42 percent were under 18), and lived predominately in the West.

One intriguing point about the Hispanic culture is that while Hispanic share the same ethnicity, they may be of different races. Hispanics are composed of peoples from Cuba, Puerto Rico, and Central and South America, races that have markedly different physical features. However, in the United States the

Cultural Assessment Interview Guide

Name: _____

Nickname or other names or special meaning attributed to your name: _____

Primary language:

    When speaking _____

    When writing _____

Date of birth: _____

Place of birth: _____

Educational level or specialized training: _____

To which ethnic group do you belong? _____

To what extent do you identify with your cultural group? _____

Who is the spokesperson for your family? _____

Describe some of the customs or beliefs that you have about the following:

    Health _____

    Life _____

    Illness _____

    Death _____

How do you learn information best?

    ☐ Reading

    ☐ Having someone explain verbally

    ☐ Having someone demonstrate

Describe some of your family's dietary habits and your personal food preferences. _____

_____

Are there any foods forbidden from your diet for religious or cultural reasons? _____

_____

Describe your religious affiliation. _____

What role do your religious beliefs and practices play in your life during times of good health and bad health? _____

_____

On whom do you rely on for health care services or healing and what type of cultural health practices
have you been exposed to? _____

_____

Are there any sanctions or restrictions in your culture that the person taking care of you should know? _____

_____

Describe your current living arrangements: _____

How do members of your family communicate with each other? _____

Describe your strengths: _____

Who/what is your primary source of information about your health? _____

Is there anything else that is important about your cultural beliefs that you want to tell me? _____

Figure 11.3 Cultural Assessment Interview Guide.

SOURCE: From DeLaune, S.C. & Ladner, P. K. (1998) *Fundamentals of nursing: Standards and practice*. Clifton Park, NY: Delmar. Reprinted with permission.

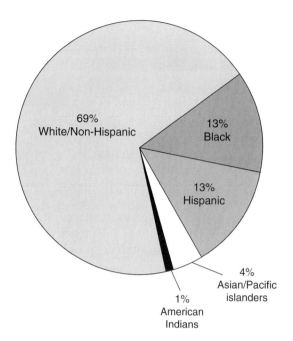

Figure 11.4 **2002 Racial and ethnic demographics in US.**

half of the U.S. Asian population lives in the western part of the country, primarily in California and Hawaii. New York has the highest Asian population of states in the east.

Like the previously mentioned groups, the Native American and Alaskan Indian groups are increasing in number faster than the general white, non-Hispanic group in the states. There are over 562 tribes that have federal identification. The Native American population has grown tremendously from the early 1920s (350,000) to almost 4 million today. Of this 4 million, only 2.5 million reported that they were of a single Native American race. Over 79 percent of those who identify as Native Americans state a specific tribe, with the 6 largest tribes being Cherokee, Navajo, Latin American Indian, Choctaw, Sioux, and Chippewa. Eskimo is the largest identified subgroup of Alaskan Indian. Figure 11.4 contains the 2002 racial and ethnic demographics of the U.S.

NURSING DIVERSITY

How does the nursing profession compare to the general population in terms of racial and ethnic diversity? Many nursing groups hold the belief that the profession should reflect the communities in which they live and serve, and value diverse backgrounds in race, gender, age, religious beliefs, sexual affiliations, and physical abilities. When interpreting information from previous studies from the National Sample Survey of Registered Nurses, it is important to keep in mind the manner in which the data were collected, because it reflected more closely how the U.S. Census Bureau collected racial and ethnic data. Respondents to the 2000 Survey were able to choose more than one category, yielding a new category that included non-Hispanic nurses in two or more races.

The number of nurses who identified themselves as minorities grew from 1996 to 2000. In 2000 approximately 86.6 percent of all nurses stated that they were white, non-Hispanic—almost 12 percent of all registered nurses viewed themselves as a member of one or more minority groups, up from 7 percent in 1980. The breakdown of the self-reported groups

vast majority (over 60 percent) of those who self-identify as Hispanic are Mexican, followed by Puerto Rican, and then Cuban. In several large cities in the United States, Hispanics are the majority population, such as in Los Angeles, El Paso, and Miami. In fact, over half of the U.S. Hispanic population resides in just two states: California and Texas.

Although many Hispanics live in the states on the border of Mexico and the United States, the African American population lives predominately in the southern states, with over 54 percent choosing to live there in 2000. Like the Hispanic population, the African American population is growing faster than the white, non-Hispanic population, at a rate of over 21 percent between 1990 and 2000. It is projected by the U.S. Census Bureau that by the year 2050, almost 25 percent of the total population of the United States will be Hispanic (U.S. Census Bureau, 2004).

Asian and Pacific Islander populations are the fastest growing minority segment of the United States, with an increase of over 72 percent in the last decade. The predominant Asian subgroup is Chinese, followed by Filipinos and Indians. Over

RESEARCH APPLICATION ARTICLE

Anderson, L. M, Scrimshaw, S. C., Fullilove, M. T., Fielding, J. E., Normand, J. & the Taskforce on Community Preventative Services (2003). *Culturally competent healthcare systems: A systematic review.* American Journal of Preventive Medicine, 24(3S), 68–79.

As the population continues to evolve, creating a more multicultural environment, health care systems, with their inherent diversity issues and concerns, are challenged to provide services that meet the needs of these populations. A multidisciplinary team (Anderson et al., 2003) evaluated the current literature and published studies in the health care literature that addressed the effectiveness of specific interventions to increase the cultural competency and sensitivity of health care systems and their personnel. Although there are numerous interventions that have the potential to reduce health disparities based upon cultural, racial, ethnic, and socioeconomic variables, there have been few focused studies with measurable results proving the effectiveness of the intervention. If there is an underlying lack of trust, respect, understanding, or even ability to successfully communicate, then the health care quality diminishes.

The team reviewed five programs that focused on establishing cultural competence: recruitment and retention programs of minority members; interpreter services/bilingual providers; cultural competency and sensitivity training for health care providers; the use of health education materials that were culturally sensitive, including language appropriateness; and evaluation of the specific health care settings for a culturally cognizant environment. The interesting results of the literature review showed that even though numerous institutions have many of these programs intact and working, the literature could not illustrate the outcomes of these five categorical interventions.

is 4.9 percent African American, non-Hispanic; 3.7 percent Asian/Pacific Islander; 2 percent Hispanic; 0.5 percent Native American/Alaskan Native; and 1.2 percent self-identified as two or more races. When compared with the overall U.S. population, the most underrepresented group among nurses is Hispanics. Not only is 13.5 percent of the general U.S. population Hispanic, but this is also the fastest growing minority group in the United States, clearly reflecting the extraordinary need to develop concentrated recruiting efforts into the profession.

Why is it an issue that there is a disparity between minority health care providers and those they treat? There are several reasons, but one of the most compelling is that oftentimes members of a minority group may have different health care practices and patterns of health care usage than a nonminority group member. There may be issues of trust, respect, and even basic communication. Barriers to care access, whether physical or monetary, are other issues that may lead to a poor initiation of services and subsequently inadequate follow-through by the client. Additionally, access to medical insurance can be a barrier to affordable medical services; the U.S. Census Bureau (1999) reported that 89 percent of non-Hispanic whites had medical insurance, whereas 79 percent of African Americans and only 67 percent of Hispanics carried insurance. Clearly there is a correlation between access to care and the resultant health status of the individual. It is well known that limited access to health care services results in less preventative care and more complicated comorbities when care is finally achieved.

One of the directives from the 1998 Pew Health Professions Commission was to "ensure that the

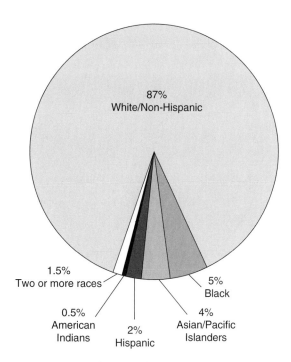

Figure 11.5 **2000 Racial and ethnic diversity within the registered nurse population.**

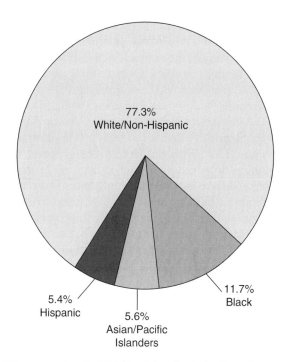

Figure 11.6 **2000 Racial and ethnic diversity within the student registered nurse population.**

health profession workforce reflects the diversity of the nation's population" (Pew Commission, 1998, p. iv). It is particularly obvious that in the nursing profession, just as in medicine, minority populations are not well represented, which can dramatically affect the delivery of health care to specific populations. Figure 11.5 demonstrates the 2000 RN population in terms of racial and ethnic diversity proportion. It is a long-held observation that those professionals of a minority background will better understand the cultural beliefs, values and, folkways than those not of the minority group and therefore will be able to communicate and provide care in a culturally competent manner.

The number of racial and ethnic minority nursing students has shown recent improvement; from 1996 to 2000 the number has grown from 10.3 percent to 13.4 percent. The largest minority group of enrolled undergraduate students nationally is African Americans (11.7 percent), followed by Asians,

Native Hawaiians or other Pacific Islanders (5.6 percent), and Hispanics or Latinos (5.4 percent), as seen in Figure 11.5. Florida's statistics for enrolled baccalaureate nursing students ranks African Americans (19.5 percent) first, followed by Hispanics or Latinos (13.5 percent), Asians (4.0 percent), and self-identified as Other (3.3 percent) (SREB, 2002).

Some possible reasons why there are so few minority nurses are family and a culture's perceptions of the role of nurses (for many it is subservient and submissive); the current images of nurses as seen in the media are not always positive and competent, but physicians usually are; and the strong need to have positive role models with whom potential students can identify and confide. The first role models that many nursing students encounter are their nursing faculty, who can especially encourage those students who may not see themselves reflected in their peer group.

With few role models in the academic ranks, the number of minority nursing faculty is not increasing,

(Staiger, Auerbach, & Buerhaus, 2001). According to the latest available AACN data, there has been no significant increase in the numbers of full-time, minority nursing faculty members. Overall, 89.9 percent are white, 5.3 percent are African American, 1.9 percent are Hispanic, 1.7 percent are Asian/Pacific Islander, and 0.4 percent are Native American/Alaskan Native (Berlin, Stennett & Bednash, 2004, p. 69), illustrated in Figure 11.7. With the United States just at the beginning of yet another intense nursing shortage, having adequate numbers of faculty to teach is just as important as finding the potential students. There is an increasing scarcity of not only frontline nurses but also nurses prepared at the master's and doctoral levels, who can teach the next generation of nurses, which unfortunately results in many well-qualified applicants being turned away from nursing programs. There are several factors that contribute to this continuing faculty shortage, including the increasing age of nurse faculty, the increasing retirement projections, and a decline in younger faculty who work in colleges or universities. With the average age of a nurse faculty member at 53.3 for doctoral faculty, and 48.8 for master's-prepared faculty, the aging trend continues to increase (Berlin, Stennett & Bednash, 2003). In addition to the aging and retirement issues and the lack of faculty of diverse backgrounds, another problem is that many potential nursing students who could have been recruited to the profession are often turned away just as the need for skilled BSN nurses is intensifying.

GENDER ISSUES IN THE PROFESSION

Historically, nursing has been thought of as a profession for women, a career that allows someone to enter and exit when family demands increase or decrease, a career that one "can always find a job in," and a career that, for at least entry level, offers a reasonable salary. However, nursing often is not thought of as a career of choice for men, with **gender issues**

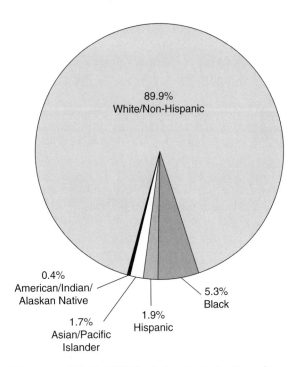

Figure 11.7 **2004 Racial and ethnic diversity within the nursing faculty population (AACN, 2004).**

and perceptions being deciding factors against joining this profession. Other previously male-dominated professions have made significant concerted efforts to attract and maintain females, yet nursing has made little effort over the years to attempt to rebalance its predominately female ranks.

According to the 2000 Registered Nurse Population study funded by the U.S. Department of Health and Human Services (Spratley, Johnson, Sochalski, Fritz, & Spencer, 2001), there are currently 146,902 male registered nurses of the total 2,694,540 registered nurses in the United States, representing 5.4 percent of the total registered nurse population. Of those 2,311,000 employed in nursing during 2002, 7.1 percent were men (U.S. Department of Labor, 2004). Many more male-dominated professions, such as medicine, engineering, and business, have made better inroads by increasing the numbers of women in the workforce, yet nursing continues to struggle to achieve an improved representation from males.

CASE SCENARIO 11.1

In your community there is a great interest in RN to BSN education by associate-degree nurses; however, the size of each new incoming class at nearby Prestigious University has not increased in several years, even though there are many qualified nurses who have applied. Many of the registered nurses working at Good Faith Hospital have expressed their frustration to the Vice President for Patient Services. Although there may be several educational options for you and your colleagues to earn a BSN, including attending one of several local colleges, or even earning a degree through an online college, the majority want the opportunity to attend Prestigious University and enroll in the College of Nursing.

Case Considerations

1. What is the primary issue at hand in this scenario? Why is it an issue?

2. From the University's perspective, identify some of the reasons behind limiting the size of the new RN to BSN class. Why can't the College of Nursing just admit all those who are qualified?

3. Discuss several options for you and your classmates at this point. Which ones are attractive options and why?

4. Who may be able to advocate to the Dean of the College of Nursing on behalf of you and your colleagues? Devise at least three solutions that this person(s) may be able to negotiate with the Dean of the College of Nursing.

Since the beginning of the first documented monastic nursing care in the fourth and fifth centuries, men have provided care to members of religious orders (Evans, 2004). There are documented stories throughout medieval times of orders of knights who provided care to the sick and infirm; however, this care was considered to be best performed by someone of low position, with nursing care often delegated to women, who were considered of lower status than men.

Florence Nightingale changed the gender of nursing with her strongly espoused belief set that every woman was essentially a nurse (Nightingale, 1969, first published in 1860). Nightingale also proposed the notion that nursing was women's work, and that men were generally not needed in nursing "except where physical strength was needed" (Kalisch & Kalisch, 1986, p. 166). The majority of men who pursued nursing as a career during this time went to work in the asylums and psychiatric wards, where they were valued because of their brute strength and ability to restrain combative patients, rather than being valued because of their nursing knowledge (Evans, 2004).

With the advent of World War I men were barred from enlisting in the Army Nurse Corps, and this ban continued through World War II, even though there was still a significant nursing shortage in the services. National laws were put into place that prohibited male nurses from 1901 to 1955, which had detrimental effects on the long-term perceptions of men's work versus women's work (Mericle, 1983). In fact, men were not even granted commissioned-officer status in the armed services until 1955 (Kelly, 1969).

Male nurses continue to choose certain specialty areas, most notably psychiatric care, anesthesia, emergency and critical-care services, and nursing administration. Even as recently as 1960 a full year of psychiatric nursing was required of first-year students enrolled in the Pennsylvania Hospital School for Men; and most men in nursing schools were banned from even registering for obstetrics courses, both theory and clinical (Villeneuve, 1994). According to Larsen and George (1992), only 15 percent of American nursing schools even took applications from prospective male students, with some schools refusing to admit male students as recently as the 1980s. As late as 1982 a landmark decision from the U.S. Supreme Court required Mississippi University for Women to cease excluding males from enrollment in nursing classes; males had been allowed to audit nursing courses but not to actually enroll, progress, and graduate from the nursing school (Villeneuve, 1994).

What are some of the possible reasons for such a low percentage of males engaged in the nursing profession? There are similar threads throughout the literature, one of which is **role strain**, which occurs when there is tension between the expectations and the actualities of the role.

Many of the desired characteristics in a nurse are thought to be strongly feminine in nature—caring, nurturing, gentleness, and self-sacrifice—which are not initially perceived as male characteristics. Gaze (1987) speaks of a misperception of assumed homosexuality among male nurses, which creates a destructive yet powerful stereotype that can lead prospective male nursing students to choose alternative health care careers. Many interested teenage males are afraid that they are not choosing a "masculine" career when compared with their schoolmates who are focusing on the more macho fields of premedicine, allied health technologies, or even health care administration. In addition, due to the low percentage of male nurses in the field, both prospective and working male nurses have limited access to successful role models, both in their college coursework and in the work setting. There is much to be said for mentoring a new nurse as he progresses, especially during the critical first year when first impressions regarding the role and its expectations are established.

These issues, along with perceptions and negative stereotyping of men who choose a nursing career, continue to be problematic for the profession. Another significant barrier to increasing the percentage of male nurses is that of the image, or the portrayal of today's nurse. Nurses have evolved from the image of the handmaiden, to Nurse Ratchet, to the sex symbol, and in some more recent scenarios, a valued team member providing nuturing and competent care. Recently there have been print advertisements sponsored by Johnson & Johnson, audiovisual and television media, of a racially and ethnically diverse group of male and female nursing professionals in a variety of settings.

THE AGING NURSING WORKFORCE

As the massive baby-boomer population (born between 1946 and 1964) ages, so does the entire workforce in the United States, including the nursing profession. With this aging population comes numerous implications for those needing health care services; among them are increasingly complicated chronic disease processes with a subsequent rise in comorbidities, dwindling financial resources, loss of family members, and in many cases, social isolation. According to the U.S. Census Bureau (2000), 35 million people (12.4 percent) in the U.S. population are over 65 years of age. The fastest growing group of elders is also the oldest: in the year 2000, almost 12.1 percent of older Americans were at least 85 years of age.

Interestingly, as the population ages, it becomes more imbalanced in terms of gender. For the age group 55 to 64, there were almost 92 men for every 100 women, but that number becomes more skewed as age increases. For those over 65, there were 70 men for every 100 women; and by 85 and older, there were only 41 men per every 100 women (see Figure 11.8). Further, the majority of elderly live either in the West (20 percent) or the South (16 percent) according to the 2000 census.

With the aging of the U.S. population, many more registered nurses are coming closer to retirement than in previous decades. Much has been written on the state of the registered nurse shortage (Aiken, Clark, Cheung, Sloan, & Silber, 2002; Buerhaus, Staiger, & Auerbach, 2000) in the last five years, with predictions that the profession will continue to lose nurses as they age, retire, or simply

CASE SCENARIO 11.2

Your nurse manager has recently assigned you to a new committee consisting of six staff nurses from a variety of patient-care units, two nurse managers, and one nursing faculty member from the local college, which has clinicals in your hospital. The goal of the committee is to increase diversity within the nursing-services division, including the recruitment of more men, because there are only 2 out of 848 registered nurses employed. You and one manager are to focus on male nurse recruitment; other committee members will focus on the recruitment of more diverse nursing candidates.

Case Considerations

1. How would you begin to research some of the reasons that there are few male and racially/ethnically diverse nurses at your facility? Of whom would you ask questions and why did you choose these specific people?

2. Identify five questions that you would want to ask those people.

3. What do you assume are some of the reasons that more male nurses are not choosing this particular facility? Reasons for the racially/ethnically diverse nurses not choosing this facility?

4. Are there any special recruiting methods to employ?

5. Several nurses whom you have spoken to about your committee assignment are curious why Nursing Administration even wants to recruit more male nurses; after all, they feel that nurses should be women. What do you say to them?

6. Identify at least three recruitment strategies for nursing education to increase male and racially/ethnically diverse enrollment in nursing schools. Are there any perceived barriers to these nonmajority students being successful in nursing school?

choose other careers. With over 2,696,540 licensed registered nurses, almost 500,000 are not employed in nursing (Sprately, Johnson, Sochalski, Fritz, & Spencer, 2001). In 2000 only 31.7 percent of the

2,694,540 registered nurses in the United States were under 40, as compared with 52.9 percent in 1980. The largest decline in the last two decades occurred among the under-30 group of registered nurses, with the total numbers dropping from 25.1 percent (1980) to only 9.1 percent (2000). The U.S. Bureau of Labor Statistics predicted in its Monthly Labor Review (November, 2001) that by the year 2010, one million new nurses will be needed in the United States health care workforce (Fullerton, 2001).

The aging of the registered nurse workforce can be directly attributed to the declining number of new students entering into nursing, coupled with the higher age of the entering students. Enrollment in baccalaureate nursing programs declined in the latter part of the 1990s, with only a recent small improvement (American Association of Colleges of Nursing, 2003), which unfortunately does not

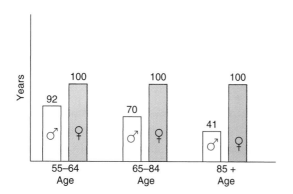

Figure 11.8 **Proportion of men to women by age.**

significantly affect the overall shortage. In 2003 the vast majority of nursing programs turned away many well-qualified applicants who met the admission requirements. There are numerous justifications for turning away prospective nursing students, but the most frequently cited is the lack of resources, both in faculty and clinical sites. Nursing education is in a strange situation at this point, with more applicants than available facilities to serve them.

Currently, the average age of a registered nurse in the United States is 45.2 years, gaining almost a year in age from the 1996 survey (Spratley et al., 2001). The primary concern of employers and consumers alike is that a large group of registered nurses is seeking to retire at about the same time as health care services are expected to increase for those 65 and older. Technological, pharmacological, and biomedical advances continue to improve life expectancy. Coupled with the significant decrease in younger nurses entering the workforce, a huge gap exists in the health care profession's ability to offer quality nursing services to those who need them the most. We would be losing not only a significant human resource upon these aging nurses' retirements, but many years of wisdom and knowledge in a variety of clinical areas. In a study performed by Letvak (2002), hospital administrators were surveyed regarding their perceptions of the aging registered nurse workforce. Although many of these administrators were well aware of their aging workforce and possessed a strong desire to retain them in the workplace, virtually none of the facilities had any specific recommendations or policies in place for the retention of this highly desirable group of men and women.

SEXUAL ORIENTATION

Most world societies have some history of identified homosexual activity. Based upon a society's attitudes toward nonheterosexual behaviors, sexual orientation has not always been clearly recognized,

which leads many individuals to hide or deny their sexual orientation.

Sexual orientation is a term that refers to "an individual's pattern of physical and emotional arousal toward other persons" (Frankowski, 2004, p. 1827). The three primary identifiers are heterosexual, bisexual, and homosexual. Heterosexual people are attracted to those of the opposite gender, whereas bisexuals are attracted equally to both males and females. Homosexual males, often labeled "gay," are attracted to other men, while homosexual females, referred to as "lesbians," are solely attracted to other women. There are two additional categories that often present confusion: transgendered individuals and transvestites. Transgendered people do not identify with their given anatomical or chromosomal gender, with some opting for radical reconstructive surgery and medical treatments. Transvestites dress and act in the manner of the opposite gender: for example, a male who gets gratification from dressing in women's clothing. Transgendered people and transvestites can be heterosexual, homosexual, or bisexual.

It is difficult to ascertain with any precision the number of Americans who self-identify as heterosexual, homosexual, or bisexual. Unfortunately, there is still a significant stigma to professing homosexuality or bisexuality, and therefore, like in many other countries around the world, exact numbers are hard to obtain in these particular categories. In his landmark text, *Sexual Behavior in the Human Male*, Alfred Kinsey (1948) stated, "Ten per cent of all the males are more or less exclusively homosexual for at least three years between the ages of 16 and 55. This is one male in ten in the white male population" (p. 651). For years this percentage has been quoted as accurate; however, today there is much scrutiny over the methods by which Kinsey obtained his subjects (many were prisoners and sex offenders; all were volunteers). With suspicions that the actual number is much lower, no one knows just what the statistics are. In one review, even the homosexual advocacy group, the National Gay and Lesbian Task Force (NGLTF), did not specify statistics of those who self-identify as gay or lesbian.

Additionally, there have been few population-based studies undertaken to date; information from such studies would greatly enhance our understanding of the prevalence of homosexuality in the United States. One later study completed by Seidmand and Rieder (1994) estimated that approximately 2 percent of men were homosexual and 3 percent were bisexual, with another source estimating the total population of gay, lesbian, bisexual, and transgendered individuals to stand between 11 million and 23 million Americans (Nayyar, 2001). Regardless of the actual number, it is important to note that the standard figure that stood for several decades has just recently been challenged for its accuracy.

MANAGING A DIVERSE TEAM

One of the greatest challenges that those of us in health care settings face is the changing diversity of our environment, including those with whom we work directly. Supervising those who are of a different background, race, ethnicity, or even gender than us can be a challenge. There are several instruments available to assist nurses in assessing the culturally diverse patient; but these tools do not necessarily provide additional assistance for the management of a culturally diverse health care team.

Work habits are as varied as types of people. Not everyone values intangible actions such as promptness, task completion, or eagerness to learn in the same way. There are cultures, for example, wherein it is acceptable to be late for an appointment, or missing a deadline may be more tolerated in some cultures than others. Likewise, people learn from their families and social environments various coping mechanisms for dealing with stress, tension, change, and conflict, with these values transcending the workplace. People don't switch their values on and off at work, or how they deal with certain situations, and it is these scenarios that are a challenge for even the most experienced manager.

Communication (or the lack thereof) is probably the one area that lends itself to more issues than any other. Communications can be verbal, nonverbal, or written, and all can be misinterpreted on some level. People bring their various experiences to work, including how they deal with change, conflict, anxiety, authority, and even members of the opposite sex. Not everyone responds in the same manner, or would respond as you would, so keep in mind that there are many ways to view and react to any given situation.

Nonverbal communication is an area that is subject to more misunderstanding than most. For example, in one country it may be a sign of forthrightness to look at someone directly in the eyes when speaking with them, yet in another country, this can be taken for dishonesty or insincerity. The use of touch (or the absence of) can also be an area of broad differences in that some cultures may be very demonstrative, and others are distinctly hands-off. How one approaches the opposite gender is also a consideration; in some countries males and females are viewed equally, whereas in other areas there is clearly a subordination of gender, most frequently female, that needs careful attention from the health care provider. In some cultures, it is the male who is the decision maker; in others it is the female. The point of this discussion is not that one culture is better than another or has superior values, but that all are to be recognized for their differences; and varied approaches must be taken, especially if groups of people are to work effectively together.

What methods can a leader employ to make a multicultural team effective? They are many and varied, but all can assist the group in achieving success.

- Avoid making judgments and decisions without evaluating as much of the environment as possible. By being nonjudgmental and reviewing the details of a situation, the leader will have the opportunity to make the best decision with as much data as possible. It's very easy to jump to conclusions when framing the situation in your own comfort zone, but an effective leader will take into account all the variables that affect the circumstances, including diversity issues, previous experiences, and the personalities involved.

■ Value the differences of others. This is a great first step in understanding and helping team members evaluate situations that may be problematic. It goes a long way toward bridging gaps and achieving successful relationships.

■ Model behaviors that you would like to see demonstrated by others on your team, behaviors that are conducive to team building, not team destruction. Respect others on your team and listen to what they have to say. If there is a misunderstanding due to cultural differences, prejudice, bias, or any reason, seek to clarify the situation in a respectful and considerate manner rather than to merely assume that the others are wrong and you are correct.

■ It is better to appreciate the value that diversity brings to a team rather than become irritated at the nuances of difference.

■ Do not assume that everyone from a specific group has the same values, that they think and act alike regardless of circumstance. Not all Americans have the same value for being on time, not all Mexicans love spicy foods, and not all Filipinos avoid eye contact.

■ Assist those in a minority group to be heard and respected as equally as those in the majority. Sometimes this is difficult, but in order for the group to meet with success, all members must participate equally in achieving outcomes.

■ When developing a team from the bottom up, remember that diversity of viewpoint and background is a rich and fertile ground from which to reap the richest outcomes. Through a multiplicity of talents, you have the potential to achieve far more than you might normally expect.

CHAPTER SUMMARY

The United States is becoming a more racially, ethnically, and culturally diverse nation than ever before, with minorities becoming the majority population in various locations of the country. Although it has maintained approximately the same gender ratios and diversity statistics for years, significant change is occurring within the nursing profession. Not only are fewer young people entering the nursing field, but current nurses are approaching and reaching retirement age, portending a crisis in the field of nursing just when the aging U.S. population will have the most need for health care services. As the profession continues to evolve, bold new ideas will be required in order to continue to attract new entrants into nursing, perhaps looking beyond those whom we traditionally think of as "nurse"

One day our descendants will think it incredible that we paid so much attention to things like the amount of melanin in our skin or the shape of our eyes or our gender instead of the unique identities of each of us as complex human beings.

—Gloria Steinem

REFERENCES

Aiken, L. H., Clark, S. P., Cheung, R. B., Sloan, D. M., & Silber, J. H. (2003). Educational levels of hospital nurses and surgical patient mortality. *Journal of the American Medical Association, 290,* 1617–1623.

Anderson, L. M., Scrimshaw, S. C., Fullilove, M. T., Fielding, J. E., Normand, J., & the Taskforce on Community Preventative Services (2003). Culturally competent healthcare systems: A systematic review. *American Journal of Preventive Medicine,* 24(3S), 68–79.

Berlin, L. E., Stennett, J., & Bednash, G. D. (2003a). *2002–2003 enrollment and graduations in baccalaureate and graduate programs in nursing.* Washington, DC: American Association of Colleges of Nursing.

Berlin, L. E., Stennett, J., & Bednash, G. D. (2003b). *2002–2003 salaries of instructional and administrative nursing faculty in baccalaureate and graduate programs in nursing.* Washington, DC: American Association of Colleges of Nursing.

Buerhaus, P. I., Staiger, D. O., & Auerbach, D. I. (2000). Implications of an aging registered nurse workforce. *Journal of the American Medical Association, 283*, 2948–2954.

Buiser, M. (2000). Surviving managed care: The effect on job satisfaction in hospital-based nursing. *MEDSURG Nursing, 9*(3), 129–135.

Evans, J. (2004). Men nurses: A historical and feminist perspective. *Journal of Advanced Nursing, 47*(3), 321–328.

Frankowski, B. (2004). Sexual orientation and adolescents. *Pediatrics, 113*(6), 1827–1832.

Fullerton, H. (2001). Labor force projections to 2010: Steady growth and changing composition. *Monthly Labor Review Online, 124*(11), 21–38. Retrieved November 12, 2004, from http://www.bls.gov/opub/mlr/2001/11/art2full.pdf.

Gaze, H. (1987). Man appeal. *Nursing Times, 83*(20), 24–27.

Giger, J. N., & Davidhizer, R. E. (2004). *Transcultural nursing: Assessment and intervention.* (4th ed.). St. Louis: Mosby.

Haden, T. (2004). After decades of discrimination, poverty and despair, American Indians can finally look toward a better future. Retrieved October 9, 2004, from http://www.usnews.com/usnews/issue/041004/misc/4native.htm.

Institute of Medicine, Committee on Quality of Health Care in America (2001). *Crossing the quality chasm: A new health system for the 21st century.* Washington, DC: National Academy Press.

Kalisch, P., & Kalisch, B. (1986). *The advance of American nursing* (2nd ed.). Boston: Little, Brown.

Kelly, K. (1969). Men nurses are there in the military services. *American Journal of Nursing, 69*(2), 310–315.

Kinsey, A. C., Pomeroy, W. B., & Martin, C. E. (1948). *Sexual behavior in the human male.* Philadelphia: W. B. Saunders.

Larsen, J., & George T. (1992). Nursing: A culture in transition in A. Baumgalt & J. Larsen (Eds.). Canadian nursing faces the future (2nd ed.). (pp. 71–94). St. Louis: Mosby.

Leininger, M. (1997). Transcultural nursing research to transform nursing education and practice: 40 years. *Image, 29*(4), 341–347.

Leininger, M. (1998). *Transcultural nursing: Concepts, theories and practices.* New York: Wiley.

Letvak, S. (2002). Retaining the older nurse. *Journal of Nursing Administration, 32*(7–8), 387–392.

Mericle, B. (1983). The male as psychiatric nurse. *Journal of Psychosocial Nursing and Mental Health Services, 21*(1), 28–34.

Nayyar, S. (2001). The missed market. *American Demographics, 23*(11), 6.

Nightingale, F. (1969). *Notes on nursing: What it is and what it is not.* Dover: NY.

Pew Health Professions Commission (1998). Recreating Health Professional Practice for a New Century: The Fourth Report of the Pew Health Professions Commission. San Francisco: The Center for the Health Professions, University of California. Retrieved November 10, 2004, from http://www.futurehealth.ucsf.edu/pdf_files/recreate.pdf.

Seidman, S. N., & Rieder, R. O. (1994). A review of sexual behavior in the United States. *American Journal of Psychiatry, 151*(3), 330–341.

Southern Regional Education Board: Racial/Ethnic and Gender Diversity in Nursing Education. (2002). Retrieved November 16, 2004, from http://www.sreb.org/programs/nursing/publications/Diversity_In_Nursing.

Spector, R. (2000). *Cultural diversity in health and illness.* Norwalk, CT: Appleton & Lange.

Spratley, E., Johnson, A., Sochalski, J., Fritz, M., & Spencer, W. (2001). The registered nurse population March 2000: Findings from the National Sample Survey of Registered Nurses. Rockville, MD: Division of Nursing, Bureau of Health Professions, Health Resources and Services Administration, U.S.A.

Staiger, D. O., Auerbach, D. I., & Buerhaus, P. I. (2001). Minority enrollments up, but not minority faculty. Retrieved August 18, 2004, from http://minoritynurse.com/features/faculty/07-09-01c.html.

U.S. Bureau of Labor Statistics (2001, November). Monthly Labor Review.

U.S. Census Bureau (1999). Washington, DC: U.S. Department of Commerce. Retrieved August 12, 2004, from http://www.census.gov/hhes/hlthins/hlthins99/hi99tc.html.

U.S. Census Bureau Quick Tables DP-1 Profile of General Demographic Characteristics: 2000. Retrieved November 10, 2004, from http://factfinder.census.gov/servlet/QTTable?_bm=n&_lang=en&qr_name=DEC_2000_SF1_U_DP1&ds_name=DEC_2000_SF1_U&geo_id=04000US12.

U.S. Census Bureau (2001a). International database. Washington, DC: U.S. Department of Commerce. Retrieved August 11, 2004, from http://www.census.gov/ipc/www/idbnew.html.

U.S. Census Bureau (2001b). Hispanic population in the United States. Washington, DC: U.S. Department of Commerce. Retrieved August 18, 2004, from http://www.census.gov/prod/cen2000.

U.S. Department of Health and Human Services, The National Center for Health Workforce Analysis (2003). Changing demographics: Implications for physicians, nurses and other health workers. Washington, DC: Author.

U.S. Department of Labor (2004, February). Retrieved July 2, 2004, from http://bls.gov/cps/wlf-databook.htm.

Villeneuve, M. J. (1994). Recruiting and retaining men in nursing: A review of the literature. *Journal of Professional Nursing, 10*(4), 217–227.

Yukle, G. (1994). *Leadership in organizations* (3rd ed.). Englewood Cliffs, NJ: Prentice Hall.

CHAPTER 12

Legal Accountabilities in the Health Care Environment

Mary Ann Brown

The law is reason, free from passion.
—Aristotle

LEARNING OBJECTIVES

At the completion of this chapter, the learner should be able to do the following:

1. Identify emerging trends restricting mandatory overtime.
2. Define the four elements of negligence.
3. Describe current trends contributing to the nursing shortage.
4. Analyze the nurse's role in the informed-consent process.
5. Identify nursing practices that can reduce the risk of a lawsuit.
6. Describe the purpose of the Health Insurance Portability and Accountability Act.
7. Describe key provisions in a Nurse Practice Act.

KEY TERMS

Advance directive	Mandatory overtime	Nurse Practice Act
Informed consent	Negligence	Power of Attorney

The clinical practice environment for today's nurses is vastly different from the previous two decades. Today, nurses are faced with myriad challenges in their daily practice: short staffing, mandatory overtime, threats of dismissal and accusations of insubordination when mandatory overtime cannot be worked, higher patient acuity, greater professional accountability, shorter patient hospitalization stays, greater patient and family discharge teaching needs, maintenance of patient confidentiality, and increasing litigation claims. Given this working environment, it is incumbent upon nurses to know and understand the legal implications of their practice. This involves an understanding of nurses' clinical accountability, their rights regarding their practice, and their professional limitations. Armed with this knowledge and a calm, professional demeanor, nurses can go a long way toward enhancing their profession and protecting themselves against lawsuits.

EMPLOYMENT ISSUES

During the past decade health care organizations have been under tremendous pressure to reduce costs. As a result many facilities have chosen to reduce nursing positions, their largest expense. Unfortunately, the reduction in nursing staffing has occurred at the same time that patient acuity, decreased length of stay, and sophisticated technology is on the rise. The aggregate result of these factors has been an inability to provide safe, quality patient care.

Recent studies draw a direct correlation between staffing and patient outcome. The Institute of Medicine published a report that shocked both the health care workforce and the general public (Kohn et al., 1999). It showed that as many as 98,000 hospital patients died each year from preventable errors.

A study published in the *Journal of the American Medical Association* (Aiken, et al., 2002) found a high correlation between staffing ratios and patient deaths, as well as job burnout and job dissatisfaction. The study reported that whenever a nurse was assigned more than four surgical patients, the increased risk of death rose seven percent for each additional patient. Hospitals having the lowest nurse staffing levels, which was defined as eight patients per nurse, showed that patients had a 31 percent greater risk of dying than those in hospitals that assigned four patients per nurse.

A study conducted by the American Nurses Association in 2001 (Houle, 2001) revealed that 75 percent of nurses felt the quality of nursing care had declined over the past two years. More than 54 percent of those surveyed said they would not recommend a nursing career to their children or friends. Of the 7,299 respondents to the survey, 5,067 cited inadequate staffing as the main reason for a decline in the quality of care. This was followed by a decrease in nurse satisfaction and delays in providing basic care. When asked to describe what they were experiencing in the workplace, many nurses said they were "skipping meals and breaks to care for patients"; feeling "an increased pressure to accomplish work"; and "are pressured to work voluntary overtime" (Houle, 2001). As a result, many nurses reported feeling discouraged and exhausted when leaving work, regretting what they could not provide to their patients.

One of the tools employed by nursing management as a solution to inadequate nurse staffing has been **mandatory overtime.** Nurses who refuse to work mandatory overtime are threatened with dismissal, accused of patient abandonment, and reported to appropriate licensing boards. A study commissioned by the Agency for Health Care Research and Quality (Rodgers et al., 2004) found that nurses were three times more likely to make errors when the working shift lasted longer than 12.5 hours. That study noted that nurse participants reported not being able to leave work at the end of the scheduled shift 80 percent of the time. Nurses worked at least 12.5 consecutive hours on 40 percent of the shifts studied.

In 2003 the U. S. Department of Health and Human Services Agency for Health Care Research and Quality charged the Institute of Medicine to identify environmental work factors for nurses that have an impact on patient safety, and to identify improvements that would increase patient safety. In the report (Page, 2003), the Institute of Medicine identified three areas that created an environment that threatened patient safety.

The first was the loss of trust in hospital administration that nurses experienced based on the perception that initiatives in patient care and nursing work redesign placed emphasis on efficiency rather than patient safety. The second area of concern was a reduction of nursing leadership at different levels throughout an institution. The loss of separate departments of nursing, a decrease in the number of nurse managers, failure to fill vacant chief nursing officers' positions, and increasing the nurse managers' responsibilities for more than one clinical unit all had the effect of reducing direct managerial support to the clinical staff who provided direct patient care. Nurses also perceived a loss of power and authority among chief nursing executives and directors as compared with other top hospital officials. This loss of support served as an impediment to nurses' ability to solve problems in their work setting that threatened patient safety.

The third finding that posed the most serious threat to patient safety was the long hours worked by nurses. One study reviewed by the Institute of Medicine found that 3.5 percent of scheduled shifts exceeded 12 hours, and some of those shifts were 22.5 hours long. Another area of concern was the reduction in continuing education and sufficient orientation due to budgetary constraints. The Institute of Medicine recommended that nurses not be allowed to work any combination of shifts, be they voluntary or mandatory, in excess of 12 hours in a 24-hour period, or more than 60 hours in a 7-day period. The report noted that the more hours worked, the greater the risk of medical error. The report concluded that eliminating mandatory overtime was essential for patient safety.

Nurses are of the opinion that reliance by administration on mandatory overtime "alleviates a sense of urgency or necessity to proactively find safer and more appropriate staffing." (Nursing World, 2001). However, initiatives pending at the federal level to severely limit mandatory overtime will hopefully force health care facilities to increase staffing rather than force nurses into the untenable situation of mandatory overtime. The American Nurses Association (2001) adopted the position that mandatory overtime should not be utilized as a staffing tool, and that elimination of this practice is critical to improving working conditions for nurses.

Although several states have enacted legislation to prohibit mandatory overtime for nurses, this issue has now reached the national level. Representative Pete Stark (D-CA) and Representative Steven LaTourette (R-OH) have introduced the Safe Nursing and Patient Care Act of 2005 (H.R. 791/S.351). If passed, this legislation would place limits on the use of mandatory overtime. The Act would first prohibit federally funded health care facilities from requiring a registered nurse or licensed practical nurse from working hours beyond an established scheduled shift. In no instance could a nurse be required to work more than 12 hours in a 24-hour period or more than 80 hours in a two-week period. Second, nurses who refuse to work overtime would have nondiscrimination protection. Third, funding would be provided to the Department of Health and Human Services to conduct a study on the maximum number of hours that may be worked by a nurse without compromising patient care. Fourth, an exception would be included for mandatory overtime in the event of an emergency situation in response to a disaster. This important legislation would stop the dangerous practice that has contributed to a decline in safe, quality patient care, and an exodus of nurses from the nation's hospitals.

THE RIGHT TO REJECT AN ASSIGNMENT

The registered nurse's primary responsibility is to the patient; the nurse is accountable for judgments made and actions taken in the course of providing patient care. Management tactics of threatening nurses with charges of patient abandonment for refusal of mandatory overtime places the nurse in a precarious position. The Standards of Clinical Nursing Practice delineate the clinical responsibilities of the profession of nursing. The standards set a level of competence for nursing care and professional performance that is common to all nurses. A review of these guidelines makes it clear that the nurse will be ultimately accountable for the nursing decisions that are made and the care that is given. Therefore, the American Nurses Association believes that nurses should decline any assignment that places either the patient or themselves in serious jeopardy (Nursing World, 1997).

Some state nursing associations have developed operating principles within the framework of their individual Nurse Practice Acts on this issue. For instance, the North Carolina State Nurses Association has established and published Guidelines for the Registered Nurse in Giving, Accepting, or Rejecting a Work Assignment. The New York State Nurses Association developed an Assignment Despite Objection (ADO) form that nurses can sign when they feel they have an assignment that places them or their patients in a compromising position.

In March of 2005 Congress introduced an amendment to the Public Health Act that would address the nursing shortage and staffing issue. The bill mandates required staffing ratios for direct nurse-to-patient care for certain health care facilities (Minimum Direct Care Registered Nurse Staffing Requirements, H.R. 1222, 2005). This legislation was in response to recent studies showing that patient outcomes directly correlate to staffing levels. One of the purposes of the legislation is to address the shortage of registered nurses in the United States by aiding in the recruitment of new nurses, and improve retention of experienced nurses who are considering leaving direct patient care due to the demands created by inadequate staffing.

The bill lists specific factors to be evaluated by a health care facility in determining staffing ratios. These factors include (1) the number and acuity of patients; (2) anticipated admissions and discharges per shift; (3) specialized experience needed by the nurse; (4) staffing levels of ancillary personnel; and (5) the familiarity of agency registered nurses to the hospital practices, policies, and procedures.

Under the bill, a hospital is required to annually evaluate its staffing plan for each unit with relation to actual patient-care requirements and the accuracy of the acuity system. In addition, the staffing plan must be developed based on the input of nurses who provide direct patient care. The hospital is required to submit its staffing plan to the Secretary of Health and Human Services, with annual updates. The bill also requires hospitals to post, in a visible spot that is accessible to staff, patients, and the public, the requirements of the bill and the direct-care nurse-to-patient ratios during each shift.

The bill allows for nurses to refuse an assignment if "the nurse is not prepared by education, training, or experience to fulfill the assignment without compromising the safety of any patient or jeopardizing the license of the nurse." The bill forbids a hospital to discharge, retaliate, or discriminate against a nurse based on the nurse's refusal to accept a particular assignment. The bill further prohibits a hospital from filing a complaint or a report against a nurse with the appropriate state professional disciplinary agency because of the nurse's refusal to accept a work assignment.

If action has been taken by the hospital against the nurse in violation of the act, the nurse may bring a lawsuit to the U.S. District Court. The nurse may also file a complaint with the Secretary of Health and Human Services, who will investigate the complaint. A notice will be posted in each hospital explaining

WRITING EXERCISE 12.1

Using the information described above, identify one instance wherein you were required to work overtime or received an unreasonably heavy patient assignment. Identify the factors that may have placed you or your patient(s) in jeopardy. Describe the steps you would take, after reading this material, if you were placed in the same position today. Write down your responses, and be prepared to discuss them in class.

the right of nurses under the Act, including a statement that a nurse may file a complaint with the Secretary for violation of the Act, and providing instructions for how to file a complaint.

DISCRIMINATION

There are many federal statutes that relate to employment discrimination, including discrimination based on race, color, religion, gender, sexual harassment, pregnancy, age discrimination, and disability. Employees who believe they are the target of an employer's discrimination may file a claim with the Equal Employment Opportunity Commission (EEOC). Employees are required to present evidence that they were treated differently from other employees and that such treatment was based on a discriminatory motive. In order to successfully defend a charge of discrimination, employers must be able to demonstrate legitimate, nondiscriminatory reasons for their decisions. If the EEOC finds that the employee was a victim of discrimination, the employee is entitled to back pay, front pay (if applicable), and punitive damages.

Employees may bring a sexual harassment suit if they are the target of unwelcome verbal or physical conduct of a sexual nature that is made as a condition of employment in return for sexual favors. The employee can also bring an action if the unwelcome conduct unreasonably interferes with the employee's ability to perform job functions.

The Americans with Disabilities Act (ADA), 42 USC § 12101 et seq., protects qualified individuals with a recognized disability from discrimination. The ADA defines a qualified individual as "an individual with a disability who, with or without reasonable accommodation, can perform the essential functions of the employment position that such individual holds or desires." Under the ADA, an employer is required to make reasonable accommodations to permit the qualified disabled individual to meet the essential job functions. These accommodations may include modifying facility accessibility, changing work schedules, or reassigning employees. The employer is not, however, required to make modifications that would prove to be an undue hardship, which would include any modification that requires significant expense or difficulty.

An area that may pose particular problems in the workplace is that of employees with a dependency on alcohol or drugs. Such individuals will eventually exhibit a pattern of signs and symptoms that will become obvious to others, necessitating an intervention. Some of the physical symptoms can include tremors, dilated pupils, runny nose, diaphoresis, and an increasing lack of personal grooming. The individual will also exhibit behavioral changes such as mood swings, frequent absenteeism or tardiness, frequent trips to the bathroom immediately after accessing the narcotic cabinet, strong interest in medicating patients for pain, isolation from staff, and a decrease in work performance. Drug diversion should be suspected if there are frequent incorrect narcotic counts, an increase in patient complaints regarding ineffective pain management, or an unusually large number of narcotics needed on a unit. Once an individual is suspected of having an alcohol problem or diverting narcotics from the workplace, a confidential investigation needs to take place. The focus of the investigation should be in the following areas:

1. Documented evidence of decreased performance.
2. Documented observations of behavior patterns and psychosocial behavior consistent with chemical dependency.
3. Documented discrepancies between oral and written reports given by the nurse in question.
4. Errors in charting and record keeping.
5. Errors in recording usage of control drugs.
6. Poor personal hygiene, odor of alcohol, or tremors.
7. Absenteeism.
8. Reference for assignments linked with drugs available.
9. Health history/physical signs and symptoms.

If the investigation reveals a suspected chemical dependency problem, the appropriate nursing administration personnel should review the evidence to determine if is conclusive. If the information is sufficient, the intervention process will follow in accordance with facility guidelines. An intervention usually includes a professional counselor or nursing colleagues who are in recovery. The nurse is confronted with the problems that have been observed, unprofessional conduct, and possible drug-related behavior. The nurse should be given information about treatment options, and arrangements should be made for an evaluation with a professional counselor.

The intervention, although conducted in a caring manner, must make clear to the nurse the different options for treatment and the consequences of rejection of the treatment. If treatment is accepted, the nurse should be accompanied to the treatment center, and the intervention should be documented.

Under the ADA, drug-dependent individuals are considered handicapped and cannot be discriminated against. However, illegal use of drugs is not protected by the ADA. The ADA also allows employers to hold individuals with alcoholism to the same performance standards as other employees, including policies that prohibit drinking on the job. This being said, the employer may have to accommodate individuals with alcoholism by adjusting their work schedule so they can attend support meetings or allowing them personal phone calls to an AA sponsor. Employers are permitted to establish polices that govern the use of drugs and alcohol in the workplace and may establish a drug-testing program.

The Age Discrimination in Employment Act (ADEA), 29 U.S.C. § 621 et seq., protects those employees over 40 years of age from discrimination based on age with regard to hiring, discharge, and compensation, as well as other employment issues. Employers are prohibited from publishing any advertisement or notice that expresses any age limitations or preferences. An employee who proves a claim of age discrimination is entitled to attorney's fees, back pay, and reinstatement or front pay.

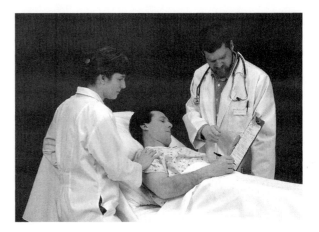

Figure 12.1 **Witnessing the signature of a consent form after the physician has fully informed the client about the proposed treatment is often a nurse's responsibility.**

LEGAL INSTRUMENTS

No one likes to think about what would happen if they became incapacitated and could not make their own health care decisions. However, recent events portrayed in the media such as the Terry Schiavo case show how planning for an incapacitating event can keep these important personal decisions out of the courtroom and in the hands of individuals who can be trusted to carry out financial and health care wishes.

Power of Attorney

A **Power of Attorney** (POA) is a legal instrument whereby the person who signs it, called the principal, delegates legal authority to another individual, called the agent or agent-in-fact, to make legal, financial, and property decisions on the principal's behalf. A "nondurable" POA remains in effect until the principal becomes mentally incompetent, dies, or revokes the instrument. Normally a non-durable POA is used in limited transactions, such as closing on a real estate transaction when the individual cannot be present to sign the documents.

Durable Power of Attorney

A durable POA (see Figure 12.2) allows the agent to act on the principal's behalf even after the principal becomes mentally incompetent or is physically unable to make decisions. The durable POA is revoked at the time of the principal's death or upon revocation by the principal. Regardless of whether the POA is durable or not, it grants sweeping authority to the agent. The POA gives the agent the power to (1) buy or sell real estate, (2) handle tax matters, (3) conduct all banking transactions, (4) engage in litigation, and (5) manage the principal's property. In light of the broad authority granted by a POA, an individual should choose an agent carefully: a trusted family member, a professional with a stellar reputation for honesty, or a good friend. The POA must be signed in the presence of a Notary Public.

Advance Directive

Depending on the state, an **advance directive** is known by different names, including Living Will, directive to physicians, medical power of attorney, and health care directive (see Figure 12.3). An advance directive allows individuals to write down what extended medical treatment should be provided or withheld should they become unable to communicate their wishes. This document in essence creates a contract with an individual's attending physician, who is obligated to honor its instructions. In *Cruzan v. Director, Mo. Dep't of Health*, 497 U.S. 261 (1990), the Supreme Court held that not only do individuals have a constitutional right to control their medical treatment, but medical personnel also must follow "clear and convincing evidence" of a person's medical treatment wishes, even if they do not share those wishes. If physicians cannot honor the document, they must transfer the care to another provider who can honor it. An advanced directive is used not only to instruct physicians to withhold extraordinary measures, such as the use of artificial breathing or

cardiac apparatus, but also to reinforce the treatment the individual wishes to receive, even if that includes all medical treatment available. In some states individuals can state their preference for the administration of food and water.

A durable power of attorney for health care, also called a health care proxy in some states, is a legal document wherein individuals may grant another person authority to make medical decisions on their behalf if they can no longer make them. This person, called an agent or attorney-in-fact, can access medical records, speak to the treating physicians, and seek intervention by the court, if necessary, on the individual's behalf.

It is important that several factors are taken into consideration when choosing a health care agent. First, it is important the person be assertive and strong-willed. An agent may have to engage in a protracted fight against family members who have different values and beliefs, as well as an obstinate medical establishment. The agent needs to have the fortitude to see the person's wishes through to the end, which can sometimes be an arduous journey.

Second, geographical proximity may become a crucial factor if the individual has a long illness. Therefore, whereas agents don't have to live in the same city or state, it is important to keep in mind that they may have to remain close by for weeks, or even months, at a time depending on the nature of the illness, in order to ensure the individual's wishes are being carried out.

Third, while it is never recommended that the health care provider be the named agent, it is usually a good idea to have the financial agent and health care agent be the same person. If the health care agent is different from the durable power of attorney who oversees the financial affairs, the possibility exists that these two individuals could become at odds with each other, allowing the financial agent to interfere with the health care agent's wishes by withholding payment (Shae, 2005).

If an individual does not feel comfortable naming someone as a health care agent, the individual will have the advance directive that health care personnel are required to follow.

Part I. Durable Power of Attorney for Health Care

• If you do NOT wish to name an agent to make health care decisions for you, write your initials in the box

[Initials]

This form has been prepared to comply with the "Durable Power of Attorney for Health Care Act" of Missouri.

1. Selection of agent. I appoint:
Name:_____
Address:_____

It is suggested that only one Agent be named. However, if more than one Agent is named, anyone may act individually unless you specify otherwise.

Telephone:_____
as my Agent.

2. Alternate Agents. Only an Agent named by me may act under this Durable Power of Attorney. If my Agent resigns or is not able or available to make health care decisions for me, or if an Agent named by me is divorced from me or is my spouse and legally separated from me, I appoint the person(s) named below (in the order named if more than one):

First Alternate Agent

Name:_____

Address:_____

_____

Telephone:_____

Second Alternate Agent

Name:_____

Address:_____

_____

Telephone:_____

This is a Durable Power of Attorney, and the authority of my Agent shall not terminate if I become disabled or incapacitated.

Part I. Durable Power of Attorney for Health Care (Continued)

3. Effective date and durability. This Durable Power of Attorney is effective when two physicians decide and certify that I am incapacitated and unable to make and communicate a health care decision.

• If you want ONE physician, instead of TWO, to decide whether you are incapacitated, write your initials in the box to the right.

[Initials]

4. Agent's powers. I grant to my Agent full authority to:

[Initials]

A. Give consent to, prohibit, or withdraw any type of health care, medical care, treatment, or procedure, even if my death may result;

• If you wish to AUTHORIZE your Agent to direct a health care provider to withhold or withdraw artificially supplied nutrition and hydration (including tube feeding of food and water), write your initials in the box to the right.

[Initials]

• If you DO NOT WISH TO AUTHORIZE your Agent to direct a health care provider to withhold or withdraw artificially supplied nutrition and hydration (including tube feeding of food and water), write your initials in the box to the right.

[Initials]

B. Make all necessary arrangements for health care services on my behalf, and to hire and fire medical personnel responsible for my care;

C. Move me into or out of any health care facility (even if against medical advice) to obtain compliance with the decisions of my Agent; and

D. Take any other action necessary to do what I authorize here, including (but not limited to) granting any waiver or release from liability required by any health care provider, and taking any legal action at the expense of my estate to enforce this Durable Power of Attorney.

5. Agent's Financial Liability and Compensation. My Agent acting under this Durable Power of Attorney will incur no personal financial liability. My Agent shall not be entitled to compensation for services performed under this Durable Power of Attorney, but my Agent shall be entitled to reimbursement for all reasonable expenses incurred as a result of carrying out any provision hereof.

Part II. Health Care Directive

• If you DO NOT WISH to make a health care directive, write your initials in the box to the right, and go to Part III.

[Initials]

I make this HEALTH CARE DIRECTIVE ("Directive") to exercise my right to determine the course of my health care and to provide clear and convincing proof of my wishes and instructions about my treatment.

If I am persistently unconscious or there is no reasonable expectation of my recovery from a seriously incapacitating or terminal illness or condition, I direct that all of the life-prolonging procedures which I have initialed below be withheld or withdrawn.

I want the following life-prolonging procedures to be withheld or withdrawn:

• artificially supplied nutrition and hydration (including tube feeding of food and water) . . . . [Initials]

• surgery or other invasive procedures. [Initials]

• heart-lung resuscitation (CPR) . . . . [Initials]

• antibiotic. . . . . [Initials]

• dialysis. . . . . [Initials]

• mechanical ventilator (respirator). . . . . [Initials]

• chemotherapy. . . . . [Initials]

• radiation therapy. . . . . [Initials]

• all other "life-prolonging" medical or surgical procedures that are merely intended to keep me alive without reasonable hope of improving my condition or curing my illness or injury. . . . . [Initials]

However, if my physician believes that any life-prolonging procedure may lead to significant recovery, I direct my physician to try the treatment for a reasonable period of time. If it does not improve my condition, I direct the treatment be withdrawn even if it shortens my life. I also direct that I be given medical treatment to relieve pain or to provide comfort, even if such treatment might shorten my life, suppress my appetite or my breathing, or be habit forming.

IF I HAVE NOT DESIGNATED AN AGENT IN THE DURABLE POWER OF ATTORNEY, THIS DOCUMENT IS MEANT TO BE IN FULL FORCE AND EFFECT AS MY HEALTH CARE DIRECTIVE.

Part III. General Provisions Included in the Directive and Durable Power of Attorney

YOU MUST SIGN THIS DOCUMENT IN THE PRESENCE OF TWO WITNESSES. IN WITNESS WHEREOF, I have executed this document this_____day of _____, year____.

_____
Signature

Print name _____
Address _____

The person who signed this document is of sound mind and voluntarily signed this document in our presence. Each of the undersigned witnesses is at least eighteen years of age.

Signature_____   Signature_____

Print name _____   Print name _____

Address _____   Address _____

ONLY REQUIRED FOR PART I — DURABLE POWER OF ATTORNEY

STATE OF MISSOURI   )
) as
_____OF _____   )

On this_____day of _____, year_____, before me personally appeared to me known to be the person described in and who executed the foregoing instrument and acknowledged that he/she executed the same as his/her free act and deed.

IN WITNESS WHEREOF, I have hereunto set my hand and affixed my official seal in the County of _____, State of Missouri, the day and year first above written.

_____
Notary Public

My Commision Expires:

Figure 12.2 Durable power of attorney for health care and health care directive.

SOURCE: Reprinted with permission of the Missouri Bar.

Sample Living Will

Declaration made this _____ day of _____, year_____.

I, _____, willfully and voluntarily make known my desire that my dying not be artificially prolonged under the circumstances set forth below, and I do hereby declare:

If at any time I have a terminal condition and if my attending or treating physician and another consulting physician have determined that there is no medical probability of my recovery from such condition, I direct that life-prolonging procedures be withheld or withdrawn when the application of such procedures would serve only to prolong artificially the process of dying, and that I be permitted to die naturally with only the administration of medication or the performance of any medical procedure deemed necessary to provide me with comfort care or to alleviate pain.

It is my intention that this declaration be honored by my family and physician as the final expression of my legal right to refuse medical or surgical treatment and to accept the consequences for such refusal.

In the event that I have been determined to be unable to provide express and informed consent regarding the withholding, withdrawal, or continuation of life-prolonging procedures, I wish to designate, as my surrogate to carry out the provisions of this declaration:

Name: _____
Address: _____
_____ Zip Code: _____
Phone: _____

I wish to designate the following person as my alternate surrogate, to carry out the provisions of this declaration should my surrogate be unwilling or unable to act on my behalf:

Name: _____
Address: _____
_____ Zip Code: _____
Phone: _____

Additional instructions (optional):

I understand the full importance of this declaration, and I am emotionally and mentally competent to make this declaration.
Signed: _____

Witness 1:
     Signed: _____
     Address: _____

Witness 2:
     Signed: _____
     Address: _____

Figure 12.3 Sample living will.

SOURCE: Reprinted by permission of Choice in Dying, 200 Varick Street, New York, NY 10014

THE HEALTH INSURANCE PORTABILITY AND ACCOUNTABILITY ACT OF 1996

The Health Insurance Portability and Accountability Act (HIPAA) was enacted by Congress to reduce administrative costs by standardizing the format of certain electronic health care transactions and to encourage the electronic transmission for these transactions. The privacy provisions of HIPAA protect health care consumers against the "unauthorized use of disclosure" of individually identifiable medical information. The Privacy Rule delineates rights for individuals regarding their health information. (45 C.F.R. Parts 160–164). Facilities are required to provide patients with a Notice of Privacy Practices. This notice informs patients of their rights (1) to receive confidential communications about their protected health information, (2) to inspect and obtain a copy of their record, (3) to request corrections or amendments to the record, (4) to request restrictions on the disclosure of the protected information, and (5) to receive an accounting of disclosures.

Individuals may inspect and copy their own protected health information provided the information is maintained in a "designated record set," which is a group of records including medical and billing records, maintained by the entity. An entity may require the individual to submit a written request. The entity has a set time frame in which to respond, depending on the location of the health information. Although individuals have the right to inspect or copy their own protected health information, they do not have the right to protected health information (PHI) relating to psychotherapy notes, information compiled in anticipation of litigation, PHI created or obtained by a health care provider in the course of a clinical study, or PHI that could endanger the safety of an individual.

In certain circumstances, covered entities are required to obtain a written authorization from individuals (or the individual's personal representative) to use or disclose their PHI. If a signed authorization is required, it must contain the following elements:

1. A description of the information to be used or disclosed

2. Identification of the person(s) to whom disclosure will be made

3. A description of each purpose of the disclosure

4. Identification of the person(s) who will make the disclosure

5. An expiration date

6. The individual's signature and date

7. If signed by the individual's personal representative, a description of the representative's authority to sign

8. The patient's right to revoke the authorization in writing

9. A statement that the covered entity may not condition payment, treatment, or enrollment based on whether the individual provides a signature

10. The possibility that the information disclosed may be further disclosed by the recipient receiving the information

11. Specific provisions are spelled out in the authorization regarding psychotherapy notes, research, and marketing.

The Privacy Rule provides for disclosure of PHI without an individual's authorization for public health activities, reports of abuse, neglect and domestic violence, disclosures for judicial proceedings, worker's compensation, disclosures for law enforcement, government-related disclosures, and donors.

Entities under HIPAA are required to adopt policies and procedures to ensure that protected health information is managed properly. Each entity must appoint a privacy officer to develop and implement policies and procedures, as well as conduct in-house training of employees. At the direct patient-care level, staff must follow the facility's policies and procedures to ensure that protected health information is not accessible or visible to other patients or visitors. Nurses and other physicians should use care when speaking to patients in multibed wards. If a patient has visitors, the patient must be asked if the visitor has permission to hear the medical information that is about to be disclosed. Facilities often post reminder notices for staff in elevators, hallways, and the cafeteria to observe patient confidentiality. These small but important measures can minimize the risk of disclosure of a patient's protected health information.

NEGLIGENCE

Negligence is defined as "conduct which falls below the standard established by law for the protection of others against unreasonable risk of harm," Restatement (Second) of Torts §282 (1965). In medical malpractice litigation, negligence is the predominant theory of liability. In order to establish a malpractice case, a patient must prove four requisite elements.

First the patient must show that the nurse owed the individual a duty of care. This is the most straightforward element to prove in a malpractice case. Normally this is shown by reliance on hospital records that document the nurse's involvement with the patient. Once nurses accept an assignment, they have agreed to treat patients with the degree of skill, care, and diligence possessed or exercised by competent and careful nurses.

Second, the patient must prove that the nurse breached the standard of care. The standard of care is defined as the care a reasonable, prudent, or careful health care practitioner would provide in similar circumstances. Nurse Practice Acts, state boards of nursing, hospitals, and nursing departments all have established policies and procedures that give guidance to nurses and ancillary staff for different patient-care situations.

Third, the patients must show that a breach of the standard of care resulted in their injury, and that if the standard of care had been followed, the injury would not have occurred. If there is more than one method of care, a nurse will normally not be found negligent if one of the approved methods was followed, even if it is later discovered that it was the wrong choice.

Fourth, the patient must show that the injury caused actual damage. Injuries caused by a breach in the standard of care that satisfy the damages element include death, disability, severe or prolonged pain, additional surgery or hospitalization to correct an error, or deformity. A key doctrine in the law of agency, known as *respondeat superior* (Latin for "let the master answer"), provides that a principal (employer) is responsible for the actions of its agent (employee) during the course of employment. Therefore, a hospital is vicariously liable for the negligence of its nurses. This liability allows a patient to bring a lawsuit against the nurse, the hospital, or both. Two conditions must exist in order for the hospital to be vicariously liable. First, an employer/employee relationship must exist between the hospital and nurse; and second, the injury has to occur within the scope of the employment. The imposition of vicarious liability assures injured patients that they will "deep pocket" to seek redress, and allows the party who bears the loss to spread the loss through higher charges for services and goods.

INFORMED CONSENT

Informed consent encompasses an individual's granting consent, whether expressed or implied, as well as exercising the right to refuse treatment, Gray 697 F. Supp. 580 (D.R.I. 1985). Although the informed consent doctrine serves several functions, the central premise is that patients are the ones to decide what shall be done with their body.

It is the responsibility of the health care provider who is going to perform the proposed treatment to obtain informed consent from the patient. There are several required elements that must be disclosed in order to make sure that the consent is informed. These elements include

1. Disclosure of the nature and reason for the treatment

2. A discussion of the risks, benefits, and alternatives to the treatment

Table 12.1 Actions to Decrease the Risk of Liability

Communicate with your clients by keeping them informed and listening to what they say.

Acknowledge unfortunate incidents, and express concern about these events without either taking the blame, blaming others, or reacting defensively.

Chart and time your observations immediately, while facts are still fresh in your mind.

Take appropriate actions to meet the client's nursing needs.

Follow the facility's policies and procedures for administering care and reporting incidents.

Acknowledge and document the reason for any omission or deviation from agency policy, procedure, or standard.

Maintain clinical competency, and acknowledge your limitations. If you do not know how to do something, ask for help.

Promptly report any concern regarding the quality of care, including the lack of resources with which to provide care, to a nursing administration representative.

Use appropriate standards of care.

Document the time of changes in conditions requiring notification of the physician, and include the response of the physician.

Delegate client care based on the documented skills of licensed and unlicensed personnel.

Treat all clients and their families with kindness and respect.

RESEARCH APPLICATION ARTICLE

Croke, E. M (2003). Nurses, negligence, and malpractice. *American Journal of Nursing, 103*(9), 54.

Croke (2003) reviewed 250 case summaries wherein nurses were sued for malpractice. The criteria for these cases was that the nurse was engaged in the practice of nursing as defined in the Nurse Practice Act of the involved state, the nurse was a named as a defendant in a civil lawsuit, and all trials were held between 1995 and 2001. Croke identified six categories of negligence: failure to follow standards of care, failure to document, failure to assess and monitor, failure to use equipment responsibly, failure to communicate, and failure to serve as a patient advocate.

Croke identified thirteen specialty-practice areas of nursing involved in the malpractice cases. Seven specialties were identified within the acute-care setting. The greatest frequency of reported cases of negligence occurred in the medical/surgical unit, followed by obstetrics. The areas of nursing with the least litigation activity were the coronary and intensive care units, operating rooms, and pediatrics, followed by recovery room and emergency room.

Croke also identified several steps to help nurses reduce the potential for being named in a lawsuit. First, maintain open, respectful communication with patients and families. It is a well-known fact that patients are less likely to sue if they perceive a nurse to be caring and professional. Second, maintain competence in the specialty area. Third, incorporate legal principals into daily practice. Fourth, know your strengths and weaknesses. Nurses should accept only those assignments that they feel competent to handle and should allow more experienced nurses to handle specialized duties. Fifth, all nursing care should be documented factually, accurately, completely, and timely. If care is not documented, it will be assumed that it was not rendered. It is difficult to prove something was done when there is no supporting documentation in the record.

The risk of nurses being named in a lawsuit is on the rise. The best weapons nurses have in their arsenal is to utilize good judgment, critical thinking, discretion when reviewing an assignment, good documentation, and kindness toward the patient and family. All of these methods, employed together, can help avoid being named a defendant in a lawsuit.

3. A discussion of the risks and benefits of foregoing the treatment

4. A discussion of alternative treatments

5. The consent is given voluntarily and free of coercion.

The discussion regarding consent must be in language the patient understands. Medical terminology should not be used because most patients can't understand it. The extent or degree of disclosure is a matter of legal difference of views. The majority opinion applies the patient-need standard, which requires disclosure of significant information that a reasonable person in a same or similar position as the patient would want to know. The minority view is based on what the medical community thinks the patient should know.

There is an assumption in law that people should have the required mental capacity to make a decision regarding their treatment. If a court declares a person legally incompetent, it will appoint a guardian to make health care decisions on behalf of

CASE SCENARIO 12.1

A 45-year-old female is admitted for a diagnostic hysteroscopy. Part of the surgery involves the use of a hystercope, an optical device connected to a pump. The purpose of the pump is to continuously fill the uterus with fluid to enhance the view of the interior. The pump contains four tubes: one is an irrigation tube through which fluid flows into the uterus, one is for suction to draw fluid out of the uterus, a third is connected to compressed nitrogen, and the fourth is an exhaust tube. One of the tubes was connected improperly, causing nitrogen to be pumped into the patient's uterus. As a result, she suffered an air embolism to the coronary arteries resulting in death. At trial, evidence showed that neither nurse in the operating room had training or experience operating the hystercope; the charge nurse who assigned the nurses to the case was unaware of the fact (Chin v. St. Barnabas Medical Center, 160 NJ 454 App. Div. 1999).

Case Considerations

1. What is the main issue in this case?

2. What action, if any, should the nurses have taken prior to accepting the assignment?

3. Three nurses were assigned to this case: an experienced circulating nurse, an inexperienced circulating nurse, and an experienced scrub nurse. Which nurses do you think were found liable? Why?

4. What procedures would you implement to avoid this scenario from happening in the future?

the patient. When the decision-making ability of the patient is questioned, often a psychiatric exam will be requested. A mental health diagnosis or condition should not, in and of itself, preclude a patient from having the ability to make a decision, unless it is determined that the patient is incapable of making an informed decision. In order to evaluate the patient's knowledge base, the use of open-ended questions made in a nonthreatening way can be useful in soliciting what the patient understands. For instance, health care providers can ask patients what their understanding is of their condition, what treatment was recommended, what they think will happen if they do or do not receive the recommended treatment, and what their decision is. Going through this process with the patient will help the health care provider assess whether additional information or clarification of information is necessary.

If language barriers exist, it is the nurse's responsibility to make sure that patients understand what they are signing when the nurse witnesses the patient's signature on the permit. The nurse should follow hospital policy for obtaining a translator.

Informed consent requires that the patient voluntarily agree to the procedure and does not sign under emotional duress. The nurse can observe both verbal and nonverbal cues to determine if the consent is voluntarily. This point is important for several reasons. Normally, practitioners do not want to go ahead with a procedure to which the patient has not completely consented. In addition, a patient who is hesitant about a procedure may be more likely to find fault with the outcome, even if it is one of the possible complications about which the patient was forewarned. Make sure that patients are aware of their rights, including the right to change their mind.

The law recognizes several exceptions to a valid informed consent, among them the emergency exception and therapeutic privilege. Under the emergency exception, informed consent is not necessary if the patient presents with a life-threatening injury that requires immediate attention, the patient is unable to communicate, or there is no time to obtain consent from another authorized individual due to the nature of the injury.

The therapeutic exception is one in which full disclosure is not required if such disclosure would cause the patient significant psychological harm. To use this exception, an expert in psychiatry who is not otherwise involved with the client's care should perform an assessment.

Absent an emergency, if the patient is a minor, consent must be obtained from the minor's parent or guardian before treatment. However, some statutes provide that "emancipated" or married minors can give consent. Although the legal definition of emancipation varies from state to state, it often requires that minors be married or living independently from their parents and financially independent. A number of states allow for a minor's consent for sexually transmitted disease, alcohol or drug treatment, and treatment of the minor's children.

Litigation surrounding informed-consent issues used to be based on battery, which is an intentional tort involving unauthorized treatment. Actual proof of harm did not need to be established for a patient to bring a successful claim of battery. Although battery is now the minority opinion, the majority of consent litigation is based on a negligence theory, sometimes requiring expert testimony. While the health care provider is expected to disclose a risk to the patient, the provider is expected to disclose only those risks that a similarly situated practitioner would be expected to know.

Although emphasis has been placed on disclosures of risk for a proposed treatment, the California case of *Truman v. Thomas*, 27 Cal.3d 285, 165 Cal.Rptr. 308, 611 P.2d 902, 905 (1980), places a duty on physicians to disclose the risks of refusing medical treatment to their patients. In *Truman*, the physician informed the patient that she should have a Pap smear even though he never told her the risks of not having the test done. The patient refused, citing cost as an issue. She subsequently died of cervical cancer, and her children brought the lawsuit. The court held that a physician owes a duty to inform a patient of any material risks, not only of an accepted procedure, but also of a refused procedure. The court defined material information as that "which the physician knows or should know would be

CASE SCENARIO 12.2

You work in the outpatient surgery unit and are preparing a patient for surgery. The patient arrives alone because her husband is overseas on business. The patient is a 42-year-old female admitted for a hysterectomy for dysfunctional uterine bleeding. She tells you that she has been trying unsuccessfully for years to conceive. She says that although she knows she will feel better after the surgery, she does not really want it. She admits to being sexually active and thinks her last menstrual period was "about two months ago." You have barely started your patient assessment when the charge nurse tells you the operating room is coming for the patient in 15 minutes.

Case Considerations

1. What are the issues with this patient?

2. How would you handle the preoperative preparation of this patient at this point?

3. What interventions, if any, do you need to take to protect the patient before sending her to the operating room?

4. Would you consult with your charge nurse? Why or why not?

regarded as significant by a reasonable person in the patient's position when deciding to accept or reject the recommended medical procedure" (Id. at 905).

THE NURSE PRACTICE ACT

The purpose of the **Nurse Practice Act** is to protect the public from unsafe practitioners and to ensure quality nursing practice rendered by qualified practitioners. Nurse Practice Acts define for each state what nursing is and the standards of nursing practice, and they provide guidance to individual state Boards of Nursing to impose disciplinary measures for violations of the Nurse Practice Act.

The National Council of State Boards of Nursing (NCSBN) enacted the first Model Nurse Practice Act in 1983, in response to NCSBN member boards recognizing the need for a regulatory body. The model serves as a guide to state boards for new ideas and to allow boards to examine their existing regulatory language when considering Nurse Practice Act revisions in light of state laws and rules. Models also allow for a degree of uniformity among states regarding the practice of nursing.

Nurse Practice Acts grant boards authority to discipline a licensee or applicant for various violations, including failure to meet requirements, licensing examination violations, unethical conduct, criminal convictions, unsafe practice, drug diversion, and failure to comply with alternative program requirements. The board has the authority to refuse to issue or renew a license; limit, restrict, suspend, or revoke a license; place a license on probation or place conditions on a license; reprimand a licensee; and impose civil penalties. The board can also recover the costs of any proceeding resulting in the revocation, suspension, or restriction of a nursing license. The costs can include those paid by the board to the office of administrative hearings, the office of the attorney general, any investigative or legal services, board staff expenses including time and travel, and any other costs associated with the proceedings.

In most states, health regulatory boards, such as nursing boards, come under the jurisdiction of the Department of Health Professions (DHP). The DPH is responsible for administering regulations and laws that pertain to health care practitioners. For example, in Virginia, complaints or allegations are first made to the Virginia DPH Complaint Intake Unit. The information received by the DPH must pertain to a violation of law in order to warrant an investigation. If the complaint is not a violation of law, it does not warrant an investigation. Sources of complaints include health care practitioners, law enforcement agencies, employers, or concerned citizens.

If a complaint justifies an investigation, the case is opened, given a priority rating, assigned an investigator, and entered into a computer tracking system. The assigned investigator interviews witnesses, accumulates evidence, and obtains relevant documents. Persons who are involved in the case can communicate directly with the investigator, and the investigator can periodically advise the sources of the information on the status of the case. Once the investigation is complete, the investigator submits a comprehensive report, along with all records and evidence, to the appropriate regulatory board for further action.

When the Board of Nursing receives an investigative report, a review of the case is conducted to determine if sufficient evidence exists to warrant further investigation. If the board determines sufficient evidence does exist, then an informal conference is held wherein a committee meets with the licensee. The source of the information is also allowed to attend the conference. The informal conference committee can recommend one of three actions: (1) close the case, (2) have the licensee consent to board action pursuant to a board order, or (3) send the case to the full board for full review.

A formal board hearing is required if the licensee requests it, if the proposed sanction is suspension or revocation of the license, or the informal conference committee recommends the hearing. A formal hearing involves the parties calling witnesses and the introduction of evidence. The hearing is presided over by an administrative law judge, who makes a recommendation to the board whether the burden of proof has been met showing that one or more violations by the licensee has occurred, thereby establishing grounds for disciplinary action. The board reviews the record from the hearing and is responsible for making a final decision. Disciplinary actions can be any of the following:

- Remedial or corrective action
- Reprimand or censure
- Suspension of license either indefinitely or for a specific period of time
- Monetary penalty
- Probation
- Limitations on the licensee's practice privileges
- Revocation of license.

The board communicates disciplinary action as required by law to federal databanks, the National Council of State Boards of Nursing centralized licensing and discipline databank (Nursys), as well as other entities.

For nurses with chemical dependency, the board can establish rules for an Alternative to Discipline Monitoring Program. Program objectives include early identification of and treatment for a nurse with chemical dependency; monitoring when the nurse returns to work to assure the safety of the public; and monitoring to assure the nurse's compliance with treatment, recovery, and work practice. The program is a nonpunitive and nonpublic process designed to monitor the participant's recovery and his/her ability to provide safe nursing care. The program has specific criteria for entry, and admission can be denied for a number of reasons. Nurses who qualify must meet all the requirements set forth in the program and agree to inform any and all employers of their participation in the program. Participants complete the program once they have complied with all the terms and conditions of the program. Failure to comply with the provisions of the program, inability to practice according to acceptable standards of care, or receipt of a felony conviction are some of the grounds for termination from the program.

All board notices and final orders are public documents and available upon request. They are also placed in the licensee's official record. Copies of final orders may be mailed to the original source of the complaint. Other aspects of a disciplinary case are considered confidential and are not available to the public.

GOOD SAMARITAN STATUTES

The Good Samaritan Doctrine comes from a New Testament parable in which a Samaritan is the only passerby to help a man beaten by thieves. Although this parable suggests that one may have a moral obligation to come to the aid of another, traditional common law imposes no duty on individuals to help another in distress. Whereas the "no duty to rescue" doctrine applies, once a person renders assistance, common law imposes a duty to do so in a reasonable manner. The intent of the Good Samaritan legislation is to encourage providers to render "good faith" medical treatment to those who otherwise would not receive it. California was the first state to pass such legislation, with the remaining states following suit.

Good Samaritan statutes are laws enacted by various states that serve as a shield form tort liability for injury and damages that may result when a health care worker or other rescuer provides emergency assistance when not legally obligated to do so. Most state Good Samaritan statutes follow this basic principal: "[a]ny person who in good faith, renders emergency care or assistance, without compensation, to any ill or injured person at the scene of an accident, fire, or any life-threatening emergency, or enroute therefrom to any hospital, medical clinic or doctor's office, shall not be liable for any civil damages for acts or omissions resulting from the rendering of such care or assistance" (Medi Smart, Nursing Education Resources, 2006). However, acts or omissions of gross negligence or willful or wanton misconduct will not receive the protection from suit under the statute.

In order to receive the protection under the statute, the act must be volunteer in nature, the person receiving the help must not object to being helped, and the rescuer must be acting in good faith.

The Virginia statute contains a substantial number of defined classes of Good Samaritans protected from civil liability rendering assistance in a variety of emergency situations. Pursuant to Va. Code Ann. § 8.01-225 (as amended 2000), immunity is granted in the following medical situations provided that the individual giving assistance is not compensated by the victim and acts in good faith: assisting a female in labor; assisting as an emergency technician or attendant; assisting in an accident involving hazardous waste or material, liquefied petroleum gas, liquid natural gas; rendering emergency resuscitative treatments, including the use of an automatic external defibrillator; and administering epinephrine to a person to whom an insect sting treatment kit has been prescribed and having the belief that the individual receiving the injection is suffering or about to suffer a life-threatening anaphylactic reaction.

In addition, immunity is granted to volunteers certified to render emergency care by the National Ski Patrol System, Inc.; employees of a school board authorized and trained to administer insulin and glucagons to a student diagnosed with diabetes; a licensed physician serving as the operational medical director for a licensed emergency medical services agency without compensation; licensed or professional engineers participating in rescue or relief assistance; and any volunteer engaging in rescue work at a mine.

Individuals who render emergency services receive immunity from civil liability for the death or injury to any persons or damage to property sustained as a result of the rendering of emergency assistance (Va. Code § 44–146.23). Hospice volunteers, veterinarians, and sports-team physicians rendering emergency assistance all have civil liability immunity from any damages resulting from the treatment. The services must be provided free of charge, rendered in good faith, and fall within the limits of physician's license.

Health care professionals also receive protection from Good Samaritan statutes provided that the medical care professional has no preexisting duty to care for the victim, and there is no expectation of compensation. In *Boccasile v. Cajun Music Ltd.*, 694 A.2d 686 (S Ct. RI, 1997), a family brought a wrongful death suit against a nurse and physician who, as volunteers at a music festival, assisted a man in anaphylactic shock from eating seafood. The nurse and physician were the only two volunteers in the first-aid tent at an outdoor music festival. Both were unpaid volunteers. Upon receiving word that a male patron was in distress, the physician went to his aid. Recognizing the man was in anaphylactic shock, the physician instructed others to call paramedics and administered epinephrine to the man.

After being relieved in the first-aid tent, the nurse also went to the man's aid and stayed with him while waiting for the paramedics' arrival. The man went into respiratory distress and despite CPR by the physician and nurse, the man died en route to the hospital. The Rhode Island Supreme Court used the Good Samaritan statute to throw out the wrongful death suit filed by the family against the nurse and physician. The court found that the nurse and physician were volunteers rendering gratuitous services in an emergency situation, and there was no proof they were guilty of "gross, willful, or wanton misconduct."

Although issues of negligence are a matter for individual court interpretation, it appears that the Good Samaritan statute will protect health care professionals who voluntarily render assistance in an emergency.

CHAPTER SUMMARY

The focus of health care has changed dramatically from "the physician knows best" to patient self-determination. The Internet has enabled health care consumers to become educated about their health and act as a partner, rather than a recipient, regarding their health care. The publication of hospital studies and surveys have pulled back the covers on health care and exposed the frightening inner challenges nurses face every day in their working environment. Legislation can improve the work environment for nurses and provide patient safety. However, only nurses can protect themselves, most of all through education about patient rights, establishment of appropriate professional boundaries regarding patient care, and personal fulfillment. Attainment of these goals will result in nurses feeling secure in their working environment, which will ultimately translate into satisfied, healthier patients.

If we desire respect for the law, we must first make the law respectable.
—Louise D. Brandeis

REFERENCES

Age Discrimination in Employment Act of 1967, 29 U.S.C. § 621 et seq.

Aiken, L. H., Clarke, S. P., Sloane, D. M., Sochalski, J., & Silber, J. H. (2002). Hospital nurse staffing and patient mortality, nurse burnout, and job dissatisfaction. *Journal of the American Medical Association, 288*: 1987–1993.

American Nurses Association, Opposition to Mandatory Overtime (2001, October 17). Retrieved June 27, 2005, from www.nursingworld.org/readroom/position/workplac/revmot2.htm.

Americans with Disabilities Act, 42 U.S.C. § 12010 et seq.

Carroll, R. (2004). *Risk Management Handbook*. Jossey-Bass, Inc.

Chin v. St. Barnabas Medical Center, 160 NJ 454 (App. Div. 1999).

Croke, E. M. (2003). Nurses, negligence, and malpractice. *American Journal of Nursing, 103*(9), 54. Retrieved June 28, 2005, from www.nursingcenter.com/library/journalarticleprint.asp?Article_ID=423284.

Cruzan v. Director, MO. Dep't of Health, 497 U.S. 261 (1990).

Giordano, K. (2003). Examining nursing malpractice: A defense attorney's perspective. Retrieved July 19, 2005, from www.findarticle.com/p/articles/mi_monuc/is_2_23/ai_100543074.

Health Insurance Portability and Accountability Act of 1996, Pub.L.No.104–191 (1996).

Houle, J. (2001). Health and Safety Survey. *Nursing World.* Retrieved July 8, 2005, from http://www.nursingworld.org/surveys/hssurvey.pdf.

King, J. (1986). *The law of medical malpractice.* St. Paul, MN: West.

Kohn, L. T., Corrigan, J. M., & Donaldson, M. S., Eds. (1999). *To err is human: Building a safer health system.* Washington, DC, National Academy Press.

Medi Smart, Nursing Education Resources, What is a good Samaritan statute? Retrieved September 7, 2006, from http://medi-smart.com/gslaw.htm.

Minimum Direct Care Registered Nurse Staffing Requirements: H. R. 1222, 109th Cong. (2005).

National Council of State Boards of Nursing, Nursing Regulation, Model Nurse Practice Act and Rules. Retrieved December 16, 2005, from www.ncsbn.org/regulation/nursingpractice_nursing_practice_model_act_and_rules.asp.

Nursing World (1997). The right to accept or reject an assignment. Nursing World Position Statement. Retrieved June 27, 2005, from www.nursingworld.org/readroom/position/workplac/wkassign.htm.

Nursing World (2001). Opposition to mandatory overtime. Nursing World Position Statement. Retrieved June 27, 2005, from www.nursingworld.org/readroom/position/workplac/revmot2.htm.

Page, A. (2003). Keeping patients safe: Transforming the work environment of nurses. Committee on the Work Environment for Nurses and Patient Safety. Institute of Medicine of the National Academies. National Academy Press. Retrieved July 1, 2005, from http://books.nap.edu/catalog/10851.html.

Rodgers, A. E., Wei-Ting, H., Scott, L. D., Aiken, L. H., & Dinger, D. F. (2004). The working hours of hospital staff nurses and patient safety. *Health Affairs, 23*: 202–212.

Safe Nursing and Patient Care Act of 2005: H. R. 791, 109th Cong. (2005).

Shae, I., J. D. (2005). Choosing your health care agent. Retrieved June 24, 2005, from http://print.estate.findlaw.com/estateplanning/living-will/choosing-health-care-agent.html.

Truman v. Thomas, 27 Cal.3d 285, 165 Cal.Rptr.308, 611 P.2d 902 (1980).

Virginia Department of Health Professions. The disciplinary process for licensed health professional. Retrieved December 16, 2005, from http://www.dph.state.va.us/Enforcement/enf_DisciplineProcess.htm.

CHAPTER 13

Ethical Considerations in the Health Care Environment

Linda M. Sigsby

Everywhere, the ethical predicament of our time imposes itself with an urgency which suggests that even the question "Have we anything to eat?" will be answered not in material but in ethical terms.

—Hugo Ball (1886–1927)

LEARNING OBJECTIVES

After completing this chapter, the learner should be able to:

1. Discriminate among terms that are often confused and used inappropriately in ethics debates.
2. Identify how law, ethics, and culture interrelate.
3. Discuss selected ethics theories used in health care.
4. Describe how a health care issue becomes an ethical dilemma.
5. Analyze an ethical dilemma to determine rationale and justifications for positions.
6. Discuss specific applications of ethics in health care in the United States today.

KEY TERMS

Autonomy	Justice	Religion
Beliefs	Moral behavior	Values
Beneficence	Morals	
Ethics	Nonmaleficence	

Many young women and men enter the nursing profession each year with a desire to help people. They want to care for sick people and help make them better. Nurses want to do the right thing in helping patients make good health care decisions. These value-laden ideas and concerns about the public are important elements in ethics. They show respect for others and an interest in the population's well-being.

For these reasons, it is imperative that terms are used appropriately and with specific meaning.

SIMILARITIES AND DIFFERENTIATION OF TERMS

Basic to any discussion about ethics is the need to clearly understand the use of terms that are often used interchangeably, but have different meanings. Some of these are listed in the Key Terms for this chapter and include values, morals, ethics, beliefs, and religion. **Ethics** is the study of morals and of moral choices. When a person or issue is considered **moral,** the reference is usually used to describe a decision that is good versus evil or right versus wrong. **Moral behavior** is action that is consistent with standards of good behavior emanating from the conscience rather than actual evidence. When a person displays good **values,** they are judged as having worthy or desirable qualities. A **belief** is an opinion that is accepted as true or real. **Religions** are organized systems of beliefs and include ceremonies between a group of people and a supreme being. The problem in deciding what is good or evil and right or wrong is who gets to decide. Good or right according to whom?

In the previous chapter, Legal Accountabilities in the Health Care Environment, the fundamental principles of law in the United States were described. Law is important to any discussion about ethics because law often provides the foundation for the argument. Legally defined biological terms are one application that affects health care. The definition of the beginning of life causes concerns when ethical issues such as abortion (*Roe v. Wade,* 1973), stem cell and embryonic research (Cohen, 2005) are raised among the public. Does life begin at conception? Although scientists believe that stem cells from embryos can dramatically affect health care by changing into a variety of cells to replace those damaged in spinal cord injuries or lost during myocardial infarction, is it appropriate to generate embryos for the purpose of conducting research?

Because the law serves as a foundation, there is need for discussion.

Cultural beliefs also have a significant effect on the moral values of individuals and groups. Culture may determine how people view death, and that may also affect end-of-life and organ donation decisions. Some cultures celebrate the life of the deceased in religious services whereas others gather family and friends for social gatherings. The Irish are stereotyped for their boisterous celebratory wakes; other cultures seek different approaches. Some Navajo traditions require limited contact with deceased individuals and their belongings, followed by a purification ceremony for the living to rid the body of spirits from contact with the dead. When a person is no longer able to contribute to the Inuit family or the cultural group, traditional practice is to isolate the person on an ice floe. The decision is often made by the individual and supported in practice by other members of the family or culture. For some members of a culture, this action would be interpreted as suicide, assisted suicide, passive or active euthanasia, or violation of the person's right to choose. Some members of the culture will adapt to new ways, but traditional beliefs have a way of lingering on to affect decisions about right and wrong, good versus bad decisions in health care. It is important to recognize that culture has an impact; however, no culture is homogenous, and glimpses into beliefs do not describe the essence of that culture in totality.

THE DEVELOPING APPLICATION OF ETHICS IN NURSING

Founding nursing leaders have long been interested in providing nurses of good personal virtue to the profession (Robb, 1900). In 1926 the American Nurses Association (ANA) began to show an increased interest in codes useful to solving professional-nursing problems (ANA, 1926). By 1940 nursing leaders wanted to unite professional ethics and personal growth through early discussions about moral virtues and moral responsibilities. The first Code for Nurses (Committee on Ethical Standards, 1940) was presented for this purpose to the ANA House of Delegates. Although there have been numerous revisions and amendments, the title changed to Code of Ethics for Nurses in 2001 and remains so today (ANA, 2001). The eleven statements guide the U.S. nursing profession by providing belief statements about client rights and safety; nursing judgment, responsibility, and accountability; and nursing interaction with other health care providers and the public. The Code of Ethics in nursing represents the rules or standards of conduct of the members of the nursing profession.

In 1980 the ANA published its first edition of Nursing: A Social Policy Statement, which expressed the value of the social contract between society and the profession of nursing (ANA, 2003). Society bestowed trust in the nursing profession and to nurses to govern themselves and at the same time, expected the profession to assure high quality care, always mindful of the public trust (Donabedian, 1976). Self-governance bestows an obligation to act in the public interest. Today this contract between society and nursing continues and is based on the following values and assumptions that provide a foundation for professional nursing:

- The human being and the human experience are valued in their wholeness.

- Health and illness are human experiences that exist on a continuum.

- Nurses and patients have their own values and beliefs that interact with the choices both make as they negotiate the health care to be delivered.

- Decisions made by public policy and the health care system influence the health and well-being of society and professional nursing.

These values and assumptions apply whether the recipient of professional nursing care is an individual, family, group, community, or population.

This social contract and social trust is still widely held and recognized. In popular surveys, nursing remains one of the most trusted groups of professionals, a record we surely want to keep. In 1999 nurses were added to the annual Gallup poll on the honesty and ethical standards of various professions. The most current survey finds nurses at the top of the list, where they have been in all but one year since they were first added to the list (Moore, 2004).

In addition, there are other codes that govern nursing actions, including the International Council of Nurses Code for Nurses, Ethical Concepts Applied to Nursing, and the Patient's Bill of Rights. The Declaration of Geneva and the United Nations Nuremberg Charter require all nurses designing, implementing, and participating in research to use ethical protocols.

SELECTED MORAL THEORIES FOR HEALTH CARE

There is a wide spectrum of moral theories that may be applied to health care ethical dilemmas, and this chapter will review a few of the best known and most frequently used. Many theories have emanated from the writings of philosophers such as Aristotle, Plato, and Socrates. Theories are useful when they provide guidelines that create discrimination and direction in justifying decisions being made. Applied universal theories provide direction and decision making that are more easily used when the nurse is faced with ethical dilemmas.

Moral theories are often divided into the two categories of teleological and deontological theories. Teleological theorists work toward a goal wherein right or wrong action is the result of the goodness of the consequences of an action. Utilitarianism is an example of teleological theory because the moral action is determined by its consequences (Bentham, 1876; Mills, 1961). If the action helps make people happy or gives them pleasure, then it is good. A phrase that is often used with utilitarianism is creating "the greatest good for the greatest number of people." A research study that violates human rights can be justified ethically because the rights of the few do not overbalance the results of the research as a benefit to so many. The consequences of the research study are good because they benefit so many people. Some forms of utilitarianism are based on a particular situation, so that the consequences of a research study are good because they benefit so many people in a particular situation. An example might be human cloning that would potentially benefit a large segment of a population that is affected by specific genetic material.

Deontological theories do not rely on consequences to make a moral choice right or wrong; rather, they focus on a duty or obligation that is owed. Kant (1949) developed the Categorical Imperative, which defines the moral worth of an individual's action as depending entirely on the rule upon which the person acts. Lying is inconsistent with truth telling; cheating is inconsistent with honesty (Beauchamp & Childress, 1994, p. 58). Lying or cheating violates the rules of truth telling and honesty. Furthermore, according to Kant (1949), persons also should not be treated as a means to an end, but rather with the respect and dignity each human being deserves. Each child is born into this world for its own purpose. An infant should not be conceived for the purpose of providing an organ or stem cells to a sibling, because the infant is not a means to an end.

As moral thinking in health care has evolved over time, newer theories are being developed that do not rely on consequences of actions, rules, or obligations. Principled ethics has evolved as one form of moral thought related to biomedical ethics with the four principles of respect for autonomy, nonmaleficence, beneficence, and justice being the most frequent principles named. These serve as guidelines that indicate the rightness or wrongness of actions that fall within the principle (Beauchamp & Childress, 1994, p. 105). The principle of autonomy is one dear to the hearts of Americans. It means rights of privacy, individual rights, self-choice, self-control, freedom to choose, and asserting one's own rights. Respect for autonomy means allowing or enabling the person to have and express these rights. Specifically, it means practicing informed consent so that patients know what procedures will be performed, as well as what side effects

and prognoses may be encountered. It also allows a person the right to participate in or refuse treatment. Conflict can arise when the competence of the individual is in question. If patients are found to be incompetent, they will not be allowed to make their own health care decisions. Under autonomy, nurses need to consider whether the use of electronic medical record keeping devices protect their patients' right to privacy (Implantable Chip, 2005; Miniature Records, 2005; Privacy Issues, 2005). These devices can speed access to medical information and provision of care, but may also be compromised by persons who should not have access to the privileged information.

In 1998 Oregon passed a law allowing physician-assisted suicide, supporting the rights of some citizens to choose their time of death. In recent years the U.S. Attorney General has challenged the law. Oregon's law lets patients with less than six months to live request a lethal dose of drugs after two doctors confirm the diagnosis and determine the person's mental competence. Physicians in Oregon believe the Attorney General is attempting to limit medical practice (Oregon Sues, 2001; Assisted Suicide, 2004). In 2006 the U.S. Supreme Court is expected to review the challenge (Oregon Suicide Law, 2005). This is one example of the conflict between law and the patient's autonomy. Conflicts can also arise between principles. Autonomy often conflicts with principles of justice and beneficence.

Nonmaleficence means to do no harm, a long-held statute in health care. When health care decisions need to be made, it is comforting to the health care provider to make decisions that will not cause harm. However, defining harm is more difficult than at first appearance. Does it cause harm to insert a nasogastric tube or does it cause greater harm not to implement this treatment? Inserting a nasogastric tube is an uncomfortable procedure, which is stressful to the patient, reduces energy reserves, and causes irritation to the nares and dryness to the mucous membranes. It can also decompress the stomach, reducing pain, and remove fluids and other material from the upper gastrointestinal tract so that fluids are less likely to be diverted into the airway passages. The decision for the nurse is which procedure causes less harm, inserting or not inserting the tube.

The third major principle is **beneficence,** which means to act in the interest of others, to defend their rights, help them get better, and protect those persons most vulnerable. Vulnerable populations may include children, mentally or physically impaired individuals, persons of low socioeconomic status, prisoners, and others who are not able to represent themselves. It is understandable then that withholding or withdrawing life-sustaining treatments is often an area of ethics discussion under the principle of beneficence. Just as beginning-of-life situations can cause ethical dilemmas, so can end-of-life decisions. The landmark case of Karen Quinlan helped establish what constituted good treatment when a person was in a persistent vegetative state. The discussions helped establish the ability of health care workers and families to disconnect respiratory ventilators and promoted major discussions in health care communities concerning death with dignity (Angell, 1993). Determining quality of life versus quantity of life was the ethical dilemma—death with dignity versus passive euthanasia or physician-assisted suicide. The case of Nancy Cruzan also set a precedent by allowing the cessation of food and fluids through artificial means and again allowing death with dignity (*Cruzan v. Missouri,* 1990; Crigger, 1990). The results of discussions evolved into the development and acceptance of the Living Will and Advanced Directives, wherein patients state their choices for treatment when and if they become terminally ill. The case of Terri Schiavo also centered on the placement or removal of a feeding tube, but differed due to conflicts of opinion among family members about her wishes (Wolfson, 2005; Dresser, 2005; Cassell, 2005; Schneider, 2005). Her husband believed she had made statements early in their marriage that indicated she did not want to live if it meant existing on artificial feedings. Her parents and brother did not accept the idea that she was in a persistent vegetative state and thus requested full treatment. The lack of clear directives from the patient in this case underscored the importance of establishing Advanced Directives for use by family members who are charged with making decisions about health care.

Following Do Not Resuscitate (DNR), patient choice is another example of beneficence for the nurse. The nurse carries out the patient's choice as an advocate for the patient. However, in beneficence, there is a weighing between risk taking and cost benefit. How much treatment must be provided to an ill family member before the family decides to terminate treatment? Although there is encouragement to act through the goodness of one's heart, in beneficence there is no obligation to act. This is an important distinction. Thus, a family member may choose when to act and is not obligated, for instance, to donate a kidney to another family member.

The fourth major principle is **justice,** which refers to the fair and equitable distribution of goods and opportunities. At first consideration of these principles, most people in the United States would agree with their value and think these are inalienable rights granted by the Constitution and Bill of Rights. Yet, within justice is a belief in the right to a decent minimum level of health care often lacking in the U.S. health care delivery system. Many working people in the United States do not have an equal opportunity to access health care, and thus come in conflict with the principle of justice. With high incomes, some people are able to purchase health care whenever needed from boutique doctors (Zuger, 2005). Because there are limitations in resources, decisions about health care access and treatment have been made based on varying considerations. Who has the greater need? Who will benefit most? Who has the greatest potential for benefit? Who can make the greatest contribution to society? What interventions are worthy of reimbursement? These considerations often bias results by making the choice unequal and not fair to all. People experience harm because they have health care needs that go unmet. Figure 13.1 illustrates the extensive use of resources for a neonate and Figure 13.2 demonstrates how difficult end-of-life decisions are for both the patient and family members.

Scientific advances in transplantation of organs have provided life-saving events for many people. The use of organs has positively affected many people

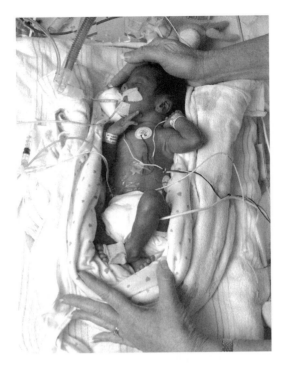

Figure 13.1 **Care for this preterm infant in the neonatal intensive care unit requires extensive resources.**

who would not have had a chance at life. Yet ethics questions persist. If an individual can receive a face transplant (Doctors in France, 2005) or transplanted ears, should there be discussion about transplantation of a head? Should people with financial means be able to purchase organs in other countries? What is the impact on the world's poor when offered more money than they make in a lifetime to sell a kidney? What is the future impact on the donor's health and lifeline? Is this justice?

Principles in ethics often come in conflict with one another, requiring a balance of the attributes of each principle to determine a course of action when trying to resolve an ethical dilemma. Examples of these conflicts include a nurse who acts in what she believes is the patient's best interest, or defending the rights of the patient, and thus produces an action of maternalism/paternalism. Who decides that the nurse

knows what is best for the patient? Paternalism, as a threat to beneficence, conflicts with autonomy because the decision maker overrides the client's right to choose. One example of paternalism is an attempt to protect the patient (beneficence) by keeping health care information from the patient (overprotection). In doing so, the nurse prevents the patient from having information needed to make an informed health care decision. Autonomy often conflicts with beneficence and justice. When the rights of one conflict with the rights of many, then autonomy has the potential for conflict with justice. Utilitarian theory may also conflict with autonomy when the benefits of the "greater good" outweigh the benefit to the single individual. Beneficence conflicts with nonmaleficence when the balance between doing harm and not doing harm is not clear.

RESOLVING ETHICAL DILEMMAS

When does a situation or issue become a dilemma? An ethical dilemma occurs when there seems to be no clear choice between conflicting principles. An ethical dilemma in nursing is often a situation of moral conflict between unsatisfactory alternatives. Ethical dilemmas force a search for values that work.

Ethical dilemmas often elicit the most basic of emotions from broad segments of society. Discussions about ethical issues and situations can and often are emotionally charged events. The fifteen-year legal struggle (1990–2005) in the Florida case of Terri Schiavo represents this well. Family members, the U.S. President, the Governor of Florida, religious organizations, newspapers, and other media organizations were a few of the individuals and groups with concerns about her ethical treatment. As members of society, health care workers also share the concerns of the greater population, while at the same time serving as advocates for the patient. The professional nurse must learn how to dissect these difficult events *and* manage the care of the

CASE STUDY 13.2 | Violence in the Emergency Room (ER)

The patient transported initially by air flight was whisked into Trauma 1 with massive bleeding into the chest cavity. Blood pressure had dropped precipitously in spite of intravenous lines in all extremities. A decision was made by the trauma surgeon to open the chest in an attempt to stabilize the patient prior to transport to the operating room. At just the moment the vessels were clamped and bleeding was controlled, chaos broke out in the rest of the ER. Shots were fired, people were shouting, and one security guard fell injured just outside the Trauma 1 door. The nurse saw him writhing in pain while a pool of blood formed on the floor under him. Decisions needed to be made about transporting the patient to the OR, closing off

Trauma 1 to keep everyone inside safe and secure, and tending to the newly injured persons. The ER nurse has an obligation to provide quality care.

Case Considerations

1. Does the ER nurse have an obligation to place him/herself at risk?
2. Should the nurse try to save the security guard and others who are in danger of being shot?
3. Should the nurse attempt to move the stabilized patient to the OR?
4. Should staff and security be given preferential treatment in the ER?

patient. The task is to identify and resolve moral issues that occur in nursing practice and nursing research. As can be seen in the examples in this chapter, there is no shortage of issues to address.

Ethics decisions in health care can sometimes lead to a "slippery slope." The following example will show how subtle the slope can appear. Genetic engineering has opened a new world in the area of ethics. There is hope that there will be accelerating discoveries in cystic fibrosis, sickle-cell disease, the thalassaemias, fragile-x syndrome, Duchenne muscular dystrophy, hemophilia A, Huntington's disease, neurofibromatosis, and adult polycystic kidney disease, among others. Although it would seem that few would disagree that disabling diseases should be treated genetically, groups so afflicted believe they alone can determine the quality of their lives. Would the world be a better place if there were no persons who are hearing or sight impaired or no one with Down's syndrome? Murray and Livny (1995) project the scenario of the use of currently available genetically engineered human growth

hormone to increase athletic prowess and promote advantages of height in certain cultures. Parents would want to give their child every advantage to earn more income in the United States. These decisions are on a slippery slope because some may seem right and some wrong; but where and who draws the line between such decisions?

Some of the worst ethical decisions about health care are made when humans are objectified, which often takes the guise of making a person less than human. Use of subtle labels such as "those people" or "them" are used to separate groups. The term *eugenics* was first used by the English scientist Francis Galton, who processed mathematical equations of heredity to "improve" human beings (Galton, 1883). Building on Galton's ideas was an American, Charles Davenport, who had a teaching history at Harvard and the University of Chicago, significant financial support from the Carnegie Institution, and who was director of the Biological Laboratory of the Brooklyn Institute of Arts and Sciences in New York. In his influential position, he

WRITING EXERCISE 13.1

Using the case study and the items above, complete a written ethics assignment by adding one additional item:

- State the courses of action with rationale applied correctly from a Utilitarian and a Principled ethics point of view.

espoused that races were very different and ascribed behavior to each. He favored intellectuals in the middle class and the white Protestant majority. After years of northern European emigration into the United States, in the early 1900s the influx changed to include more southern Europeans, who were thought by many to be inferior. Davenport believed that these people would change the American population by making it "darker in pigmentation, smaller in stature, more mercurial . . . more given to crimes of larceny, kidnapping, assault, murder, rape, and sex-immorality" (Galton, 1906; Kevles, 1985, p. 47). By April of 1924 there were new immigration laws established under President Coolidge to restrict numbers of immigrants from eastern and southern European regions. Davenport expanded his ideas to include pronouncements about procreation in families with Huntington's disease and determined that the institutionalized mentally ill and criminals with antisocial behavior should be dealt with by physicians and eugenicists rather than judges (Kevles, 1985). Popularity of these ideas spread. Soon after, there were new marriage laws that prevented interracial marriage and later, sterilization laws to control even further the promulgation of "undesirables" who were called insane, imbeciles, and handicapped persons (Kevles, 1985).

Most people identify eugenics with Nazi Germany just before and during World War II. In the early years, fitter families in Germany were financially rewarded for the birth of babies, whereas those who were designated a menace were sterilized. The German Eugenic Sterilization Law of 1933 went far beyond American laws by being "compulsory to all people, institutionalized or not, who suffered from hereditary disabilities, feeblemindedness, schizophrenia, epilepsy, blindness, severe drug or alcohol addiction, and physical deformities that seriously interfered with locomotion or were grossly offensive" (Kevles, 1985, p. 116). Based on their decisions about people during World War II, Nazi Germany segregated, isolated, and caused genocide to large populations of gypsies, blacks, disabled persons, and Jews in many European countries in order to promote what they considered to be the superior Aryan race. Medical genetic experiments conducted on large numbers of individuals in the name of science were found to lack all scientific rigor and merit (Holocaust Museum, 1997). More recently, genocide has continued under the term *ethnic cleansing* in Uganda, Rwanda, Bosnia Herzegovina, and against the Shiite Muslims in Iraq.

MAKING DECISIONS

Making decisions about ethical dilemmas requires careful critical thinking. It also requires an understanding of the opposing point of view. The following steps will help make the dilemma more manageable:

- Clearly summarize the complete and relevant parts of the case.
- Identify and seek needed missing information.
- Identify moral components.
- State the dilemma correctly.
- Identify a course of action.

APPLICATIONS TO HEALTH CARE IN THE UNITED STATES

Vulnerable populations such as children, the aged, prisoners, and persons with mental or physical disabilities have been categorized as less than the average or not worth saving or salvaging and thus are to be discarded as worthy of experimentation research and health care interventions. When they have not been allowed to speak for themselves or when there is no one to speak for them, they have suffered.

Another group often disadvantaged in moral choices are people of low socioeconomic status. In 1932 the U.S. Public Health Service began a study, known as the Tuskegee study, of the progression of syphilis. The study used a sample of 400 poor black males, who did not receive informed consent and were denied treatment even after penicillin was discovered and known to cure syphilis. The U.S. government supported this study for almost 40 years. Public outrage and the media were responsible for its final demise. The conduct of this study changed the complexion of medical research and experimentation, the exploitation of vulnerable subjects, and emphasized the value of informed consent and the need for the ethical oversight of health care research. President Clinton created the National Bioethics Advisory Commission (NBAC) in July 1996 to provide guidance to federal agencies on the ethical conduct of current and future human biological and behavioral research (Washington FAX, 1996). Today, hospital internal review boards and confidentiality laws further help to protect the

CASE STUDY 13.2

Betty (23 years old) and Edna (25) are sisters who have seen many of the women in their family die at young ages. Their grandmother died at age 47, a maternal aunt died at 41, their mother (45) is currently receiving chemotherapy as treatment for her breast cancer. She does not want her daughters to have to experience the struggles and therapies she has had to endure and thus is encouraging them to get genetic testing. The sisters are trying to decide if they should be genetically tested for the breast cancer marker. In addition to their concern about having the marker, the sisters are concerned about the effect the results of testing will have on their relationship. Genetic testing can threaten even strong family bonds.

Case Considerations

1. What will be the future effect on either sister with the marker?

2. Will she withdraw, feel singled out, angry, or lonely?

3. Will either sister with the marker believe she has a future?

4. Is it ethically more appropriate to be honest or to decrease hope?

5. What will be the effect on either sister who does not have the marker?

6. Will she be relieved of concern and ready to plan her future?

7. If one sister is tested, should the other be cajoled into testing?

8. What ethical principles are used here?

9. How would the Utilitarian theory be applied here?

RESEARCH APPLICATION: ARTICLE 1

Davis, D. S. (2004). Genetic research and communal narratives. *Hastings Center Report.* 34(4), 40–49.

An essay by Davis (2004) focuses on the difficulty of obtaining the appropriate type of informed consent in research wherein large groups of individuals form the sample. In genetic research, it is often advisable to use groups of individuals who are homogenous in order to emphasize genetic patterns and markers. Although it may seem advantageous to seek community-informed consent for these large groups, it is likely the individuals do not speak with one voice. The author warns that community consent doesn't always guard the rights of subjects.

public from overzealous and self-focused researchers (Cloning Guru, 2005).

The completion of the Human Genome Project and ensuing research has and will continue to present new ethical questions. Genetic testing offers the public new information about their health status, which may be welcomed or not welcomed. Consider the following ethical case study:

Utilization of resources is another large area of ethical concern. Whether the discussion is about organ harvest and transplantation, the availability of hospital beds and other equipment, availability of intensive-care beds, or simply primary access to the health care system, the questions remain the same. Who gets treatment and who does not? Sometimes people become discouraged in their attempts to seek health care when appointment times are changed or repeatedly delayed while their symptoms continue and sometimes get worse. In the United States we are far from an equitable distribution of health care and the principle of justice.

Informed consent is based on the principle of autonomy. The patient has the right to choose and make decisions about health care. For these decisions to be made, the patient must receive full disclosure about the advantages and disadvantages of a treatment or procedure, including the most extreme in each category. The person performing the procedure is the one responsible for obtaining the informed consent. Usually this is a physician. Most institutions prefer that employees do not witness an informed consent because it can be viewed as a conflict of interest. When a patient decision is made, it should be followed independent of how it coincides with any health care worker's beliefs.

End-of-life decisions can be made before there is a need with Living Wills, Advanced Directives, and the naming of a Health Care Power of Attorney. Again, the principle of autonomy is being used to allow individuals to state their choices should the need arise. Without this guidance, someone else will make the health care choices for the patient. Some people are afraid to make a Living Will because they believe they will not receive adequate treatment if an accident occurs. It is important to understand that a Living Will states the desires of the patient when and if the person becomes incapacitated, is deemed terminally ill without hope of recovery, or is in a persistent vegetative state. Ethicists are also concerned that some elders make Living Wills to avoid being a burden to the family. Are the persons who are demoralized or depressed able to make their own decisions (Ganzini & Prigerson, 2004)? Although often viewed by many as a necessary procedure for the elderly, a Living Will may be even more important for young adults, who may take more chances in life and are exposed to greater physical challenges. Making a

RESEARCH APPLICATION: ARTICLE 2

Cohen, J. C. (2004). Pushing the borders: The moral dilemma of international Internet pharmacies. *Hasting Center Report, 34*(2), 15–17.

U.S. pharmaceutical firms price medications at market value, producing inadequate availability for many. To many citizens, the use of Internet pharmacies in Canada at lower costs makes good economic as well as moral sense, because people believe U.S. firms are price gouging U.S. citizens. Canadian pharmacies are beginning to rebel against this practice, citing safety concerns, decreasing relationships between patients and health care workers, violations of local and international law, and the creation of a threat to the Canadian drug supply and drug prices for Canadian citizens. The use of these Internet pharmacies has created threats to Canada without solving the problem in the United States.

Living Will can involve an attorney, but is not necessary. Each state has different forms that can be accessed through a variety of organizations such as the U.S. Living Will Registry, Aging with Dignity, and (your state's) Agency for Health Care Administration. Advanced Directives will stipulate in greater detail the procedure that you desire. Perhaps you want to have full treatment in any situation. If this is the case, your Living Will should state that choice. If you do not wish to have artificial tube feedings, be

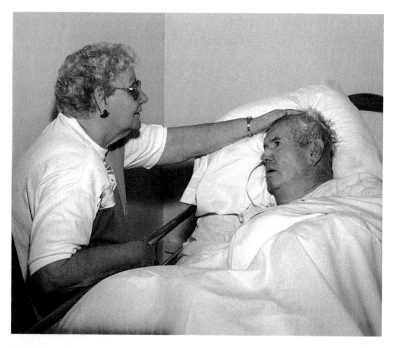

Figure 13.2 End-of-life care is emotionally difficult for both the patient and the significant other.

placed on a ventilator, and so on, the Living Will with Advanced Directives offer this opportunity. A health care surrogate, health care proxy, or health care Power of Attorney will make the choices you have written in your Living Will. If no one is named, the physician will probably make the decisions, but this also changes from state to state. Copies of your forms should be distributed to your physician and family.

CHAPTER SUMMARY

Ethics and moral behavior permeates all of health care and is an increasingly important area of practice. The way people think and react to ethical situations is interdependent with local, state, federal, and international laws as well as cultural beliefs and practices. Knowing some ethical theories and how they apply to the variety of ethical dilemmas that occur will provide a guide in understanding ourselves and other health care professionals. Theories further help us by providing a guide to critical thinking in order to justify and state rationale for moral choices and help in making decisions about the value in a research design, patient decisions about treatment, end-of-life decisions, utilization of resources, and informed consent.

Other sources are available to assist in managing health care ethical dilemmas. Acute-care institutions often have ethics committees composed of a variety of professionals and created for the purpose of reviewing dilemmas and coming to an equitable decision. Internal review boards protect the public by reviewing research designs in order to maintain balanced confidentiality, informed consent, and appropriate treatments. Other sources for seeking answers to questions about ethics include the ANA Center for Ethics and Human Rights, Hastings Center Reports, the National Bioethics Advisory Commission (NBAC), and the Ethical, Legal, Social Issues Committee (ELSI) associated with the Human Genome Project.

The decay of decency in the modern age, the rebellion against law and good faith, the treatment of human beings, as the mere instruments of power and ambition, is without a doubt the consequence of the decay of the belief in man as something more that animated by highly conditioned reflexes and chemical reactions. For, unless man is something more than that, he has no rights that anyone is bound to respect, and there are no limitations upon his conduct which he is bound to obey.
—Walter Lippman (1889–1974)

REFERENCES

Aging With Dignity. Five wishes. www.agingwithdignity. org.

American Nurses Association. (1926, August). A suggested code. *American Journal of Nursing, 26*(7), 599–601.

American Nurses Association. (2001). *Code of ethics.* Washington, DC: Author.

American Nurses Association. (2003). *Nursing's social policy statement* (2nd ed.). Washington, DC: Author.

Angell, M. (1993, Winter). The legacy of Karen Ann Quinlan. *Trends in Health Care, Law & Ethics, 8,* 17–19.

Assisted suicide law challenged. (2004, November 10). The Associated Press.

Beauchamp, T. L., & Childress, J. F. (1994). *Principles of biomedical ethics* (4th ed.). New York: Oxford University Press.

Bentham, J. (1876). *An introduction to the principles of morals and legislation.* Oxford: The Clarendon Press.

Cassell, E. J. (2005). The Schiavo case: A medical perspective. *Hastings Center Report, 35*(3), 22–23.

Cloning guru: Sorry for ethics violation. (2005, November 25). The Associated Press.

Cohen, J. C. (2004). Pushing the borders: The moral dilemma of international Internet pharmacies. *Hastings Center Report, 34*(2), 15–17.

Cohen, J. C. (2005). Stem cell pioneers. *Smithsonian, 36*(9), 78–87.

Committee on Ethical Standards. (1940, September). A tentative code for the nursing profession. *American Journal of Nursing, 40*(9), 977–980.

Crigger, B. (1990, January–February). The court and Nancy Cruzan. *Hastings Center Report, 20,* 38–50.

Cruzan v. Missouri, 497 U.S. 261, 281 (1990).

Davis, D. S. (2004). Genetic research and communal narratives. *Hastings Center Report, 34*(4), 40–49.

Doctors in France do partial face transplant. (2005, December 1). The Associated Press.

Donabedian, A. (1976). Foreword, in M. Phaneuf, *The nursing audit: Self-regulation in nursing practice* (2nd ed.). New York: Appleton-Century-Crofts.

Dresser, R. (2005). Schiavo's legacy: The need for an objective standard. *Hastings Center Report, 35*(3), 20–22.

Galton, F. (1883). *Inquiries into the human faculty.* Macmillan.

Ganzini, L., & Prigerson, H. (2004). The other side of the slippery slope. *Hastings Center Report, 34*(4), 3.

Holocaust Museum (1997). Washington, DC: Author.

Implantable chip speeds care, raises concerns. (2005, November). The Associated Press.

Kant, I. (1949). *Fundamental principles of the metaphysics of morals.* New York: Liberal Arts.

Kevles, D. J. (1985). *In the name of eugenics: Genetics and the uses of human heredity.* New York: Alfred A. Knopf.

Mills, J. S. (1961). *The utilitarians: An introduction to the principles of moral and legislation.* Oxford: The Clarendon Press.

Miniature medical records boosted. (2005, November). The Associated Press.

Moore, D. W. (2004). Nurses top list in honesty and ethics poll. Gallup Organization. Retrieved July 19, 2005, from http://www.gallup.com/poll/content/login.aspx?ci=14236.

Murray, T. H., & Livny, E. (1995). The human genome project: Ethical and social implications. *Bulletin of the Medical Library Association, 83*(1), 14–21.

Oregon sues U.S. government over assisted suicide. (2001, November 8). The Associated Press.

Oregon suicide law goes to top court. (2005, September 29). The Associated Press.

Privacy issues raised over tracking diabetes. (2005, July 26). The Associated Press.

Robb, I. H. (1900). *Nursing ethics.* New York: Teachers College.

Roe et al. v. Wade (1973). District Attorney of Callas County. No. 70–18 Supreme Court of the United States. 410 US.113; 93 S. Ct. 705; 35 L. Ed, 2d 147; 1973 U.S.

Schneider, C. E. (2005). Hard cases and politics of righteousness. *Hastings Center Report, 35*(3), 24–27.

Washington FAX. (1996, July 23). *Life science president names members to the national bioethics advisory commission* [Online]. Available: washfax@methenyl.tiac.net.

Wolfson, J. (2005). Erring on the side of Theresa Schiavo: Reflections of the special guardian ad litem. *Hastings Center Reports, 35*(3), 16–19.

Zuger, A. (2005, October 30). For a retainer, "boutique" doctors lavish care. *The New York Times.*

THREE

Leading
the Profession

CHAPTER 14

Teacher/Learner

Cathleen Schultz

Here is a magical secret we all need to know; People change. No one is stuck who chooses not to be. No one is without infinite potential for a radical turnaround.
—Marianne Williamson

LEARNING OBJECTIVES

At the completion of the chapter, the learner should be able to do the following:

1. Recognize opportunities to effectively teach patients.
2. Discuss the basic elements of each learning theory.
3. Specify teaching strategies for patient learning in clinical situations using more than one learning theory.
4. Choose appropriate teaching strategies for individual and group clinical learning experiences.
5. Design elemental instructional materials for patient and employee education.
6. Select effective instructional methods for use in clinical practice and employee teaching.
7. Relate learner characteristics to designing and implementing teaching opportunities.
8. Design a teaching plan for use in clinical practice.

KEY TERMS

Androgogy	Learner developmental stage	Motivation to learn
Educational process	Learning	Pedagogy
Instructional methods	Learning styles	Teacher
Learner	Learning theories	Teaching strategies

Nurses practice in demanding, complex, and rapidly changing work environments. Daily, they are pressed and challenged by professional, organizational, and patient expectations, many of which are legal in nature. To meet these demands, use of the educational process is an essential part of competent nursing practice.

TEACHING/LEARNING

Although teaching and learning have always been foundational expectations of the nurse's development and care, in recent decades the expectation has been mandated (Gallagher & Rowell, 2003) through professional standards, clinical agency approval, and accrediting processes such as the American Nurses Association Nursing Practice Standards, Joint Commission of Accreditation of Healthcare Organizations (JCHAO), state health departments and offices of long-term care, and national safety initiatives that require documentation of teaching; for example, prevention of patient falls in hospitals, rehabilitation and long-term facilities. Other national initiatives such as Healthy People 2010 (McGinnis, 1993) permeate all aspects of health care as our nation grapples with national health goals to prevent and reduce targeted diseases and promote healthy outcomes.

An additional movement involves outcomes of care. Nurses work with two main categories of outcomes: organizational outcomes (work satisfaction, turnover, average length of patient stay) and patient outcomes (patient satisfaction, rate of reported medication errors and falls) are seriously reviewed in almost all work settings (Mark, Salyer, & Thomas, 2003). By individualizing care, outcomes such as patient satisfaction may increase (Suhonen, Valimaki, & Leino-Kilpi, 2005; Gilleard & Reed, 1998; Dana & Wambach, 2003; Frich, 2003; Ruggeri et al, 2003). Whether directly or indirectly mandated, nurses are expected, through nursing interventions such as the education process, to participate in these initiatives at a quality level.

Reimbursement for care based upon patient outcomes drives the current health care system. Funding for health care treatments, procedures, and custodial care from third-party payers such as insurers and federal and state reimbursement programs depends upon nurses implementing and documenting teaching prior to, during, and following certain procedures such as elective surgeries. At the same time,

nurses are required by agency employment policies and licensing entities to maintain professional competencies. Continuing employment and licensure require acquiring new knowledge and skills that are verified by means such as attaining continuing education units, certifications, and additional degrees.

Teaching skills are as vital to a nurse's practice as the psychomotor skills learned in laboratories and practiced in clinical settings. Like psychomotor skills, teaching skills need to be practiced, evaluated, and refined for clinical application effectiveness with unique individual patients and groups.

Several studies have found a relationship between the nursing workforce and patient outcomes in acute care facilities. Lankshear, Sheldon, and Maynard (2005) reviewed international research published since 1990 that compared patient outcomes with the case mix of staff (Aiken, et al., 1988, 2003; Person et al., 2004). Patient outcomes that have been studied include mortality rate; complication rate (pneumonia, urinary tract infections, nosocomial infections, wound infections); failure-to-rescue; incidence of adverse events (falls, medication errors); length of stay; and patient satisfaction. These large studies strongly suggest that higher staffing numbers and a richer skill mix, especially in registered nurses, are associated with improved patient outcomes. The odds of patient mortality and failure-to-rescue after surgery were decreased in settings with a higher proportion of nurses educated to at least a baccalaureate degree (Aiken et al., 2003). Certainly these trends demonstrate that improving client outcomes through staff education becomes a significant part of a nurse's practice.

The nurse is a continual learner and teacher. Finishing nursing programs at all levels is the first step toward building a nursing career that includes use of foundational teaching and learning information. Although some aspects of learning are highly complicated, particularly from the neurobiophysical sciences (Shultz, 2006), this chapter will address more widely used knowledge that a nurse generally utilizes in multiple clinical settings. Within the profession, beliefs exist that the complex knowledge and skills of teaching and learning belong to clinical nurse specialists and nurse/educators who are prepared at

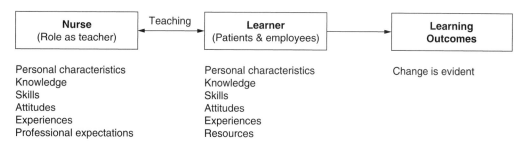

Figure 14.1 Teaching Model for Clinical Practice.

the graduate level. However, regardless of their educational preparation, nurses are challenged to be both learners and teachers in clinical settings. To nursing's credit, nurses attended to patient learning needs in a formal manner decades before most other health disciplines and federal mandates.

TEACHING/LEARNING MODELS

Success in the work environment motivates nurses seeking to grow from a novice to expert as described by Benner (1984). Developing knowledge, skills, and abilities to create and implement expert educational nursing interventions is a continual challenge. Nursing practice is pressed to be conducted within short time periods of actual patient access while using the most cost-effective interventions. Figure 14.1 depicts a model of clinical teaching and learning based upon a synthesis of information from this chapter. As a nurse manages a career, developing teacher skills is critical to promoting and attaining successful patient outcomes.

Benner (1984), based upon the Dreyfus Model, documented five stages as the nurse proceeds on a continuum from beginner (novice) to expert. The continuum is repeated as nurses change units, specialties, and agencies. However, a licensed nurse who has practiced for several years and has been encouraged in the work setting to mature professionally as an expert is well aware of the familiar nursing process, which becomes innate. The nurse can quickly assess complex patient situations and make safe clinical judgments. Inherent in the nursing process is the educational process; the steps are similar (see Table 14.1).

Table 14.1 Comparison of the Nursing Process with the Educational Process

Nursing Process	Steps	Education Process
Determine holistic care needs.	Assessment	Determine learning needs, education level, prior knowledge and experience, readiness to learn, and learning styles.
Develop care plan with mutually developed goals to meet holistic needs; determine expected outcomes.	Planning	Design teaching plan with mutually developed objectives to meet learning needs; determine expected outcomes.
Provide nursing interventions using agency, state and national standards.	Implementation	Teach using teaching strategies and instructional methods and tools specific to the learner.
Review expected holistic outcomes for success. Review nursing process for effectiveness.	Evaluation	Review expected learning outcomes for success (change in knowledge, attitude, or skills). Review educational process for effectiveness.

Table 14.2 **Predominant Learning Theories for Use in Clinical Practice**

Learning Theories
Behavioral Learning Theory
Cognitive Learning Theory
Social Learning Theory
Psychodynamic Learning Theory
Humanistic Learning Theory
Adult Learning Theory

THEORIES

Several theories underpin the educational process. Select theories are summarized along with pertinent references to explore in depth later. For the purpose of relevance to the learner, the theories are explained within the context of nurse/patient relationship learning episodes.

Prior to teaching, the nurse chooses one or more theories that best suit the learning situation; the theories are most helpful in designing instructional materials that facilitate learning. As a complex process, the theories explain how people learn: more specifically, how they obtain, process, and use information to change ways of behaving and thinking (Bastable, 2003). All indicate a need to be sensitive to the learner's uniqueness. Although there is no single best theoretical way to approach teaching and learning, together, the theories provide a wealth of complementary strategies (see Table 14.2).

Behavioral Learning Theory

Developed by behavioral psychologists, behavioral learning theory focuses upon the learner's response to educational stimuli. B. F. Skinner (1974), an early leader in behavior, believed that it could be taught and learned. By breaking down the desired behavior into simple, observable learning tasks, while providing the learner with reinforcement or rewards, the health

behavior can become a permanent habit (Heinich, et al., 1992). Emphasizing only what is directly observable, learning is a product of the stimulus (S), which includes the environment, knowledge, and instructional materials such as educational brochures and the response (R) or result of learning, such as a change in health behaviors.

Behaviorists closely observe learning and responding episodes and then manipulate some aspect of the environment to bring about the targeted health behavior change. Skinner (1974, 1989) mainly developed the Operant Conditioning Model (see Figure 14.2). To modify the patient's health behavior, either alter the environmental stimulus and conditions or change what happens after a response occurs; the latter includes techniques such as reinforcement, which may be positive (reward), negative (escape or avoidance), or punishment; nonreinforcement is the absence of reinforcements. By using the responses, the teacher could increase or decrease the probability of a response or a health behavior occurring.

Caution is encouraged when using punishment as a technique for teaching in that the learner may become highly emotional or may deflect attention away from the behavior due to the perceived threat created by the punishment. Always remember to punish the behavior rather than the person. Skinner (1974) demonstrated that the simplest way to extinguish behavior is to ignore it; this includes both positive and negative learner responses. The goal is to decrease certain unhealthy behaviors and to encourage self-discipline.

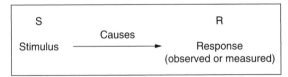

Aim: Manipulate environment, by aligning the stimulus or changing what happens after a response occurs, to bring about an intended change.

Figure 14.2 **Teaching Model Based Upon Behavioral Learning Theory.**

SOURCE: Adapted from Bigge & Shermis (1992) and Skinner (1974).

The use of reinforcement is central to success in using operant conditioning; for example, a learner may not desire all reinforcement. Another issue involves the timing of reinforcement. Initial learning, such as stopping a child from banging his head against a wall, requires a continual schedule to quickly provide extinguishing reinforcement. If the undesired behavior is not presented, then behaviors that approximate or resemble the desired behavior can be reinforced, ultimately shaping the behavior in the direction of desired behavior.

Operant conditioning is a relatively quick and effective way to change health behaviors. Carefully planned educational programs, based upon behavior modification, are effectively used in health care situations such as a smoking-cessation program. An example of operant conditioning for home use is teaching a patient's significant other to ignore any behaviors used by the patient, who remains dependent, complaining, and helpless rather than trying to ambulate or feed himself. In contrast, the significant other can then be taught to reinforce, or pay a lot of positive attention to any patient responses that promote independence, facilitate positive attitudes, and help the patient to return to the highest level of normal functioning.

This learning theory is considered useful when there are complex behaviors to change such as learning to walk again, working with cognitively impaired individuals such as the intellectually delayed; or working with those in early developmental changes of prelanguage, like a six-month-old, or the preskilled language stage of a two-year-old. Skinner's reinforcement theory does not, though, address the internal process of learning; it does, however, aim for the desired optimal behavior. The theory is simple and easy to use, but there is an assumption that the learners are mostly passive, and that manipulation is an acceptable method of working with others. The critical ethical component of this method should be explored prior to initiating the interventions. Also, changed behavior may deteriorate over time, especially when the patient is removed from the therapeutic environment and returned to the same home or work environment in which the undesired behaviors took place.

Cognitive Learning Theory

As contrasted with the behaviorist learning approach, cognitive learning stresses the importance of what occurs inside the learner: the mental processes of learning. The ultimate focus to changing behavior rests with the patient's cognition, described as perceptions, thoughts, memory, processing, and structuring of information. The patient's goals, capabilities, and expectations permeate the motivation, thus creating tension and dissonance, which results in behavioral action. This theory recognizes the myriad characteristics contributing to a patient's individuality; its application also requires a nurse who is skilled at observation and is motivated to determine the patient's uniqueness and assist the patient in acting upon information to change health behaviors. Learner readiness, learning styles, and the ability to assimilate and reorganize information are essential to use the theory.

For the purposes of summarizing this information, three predominant perspectives of cognitive learning theory are presented: first, the gestalt perspective, with three fundamental principles of perception, attention to stimuli, and closure; next, information processing, which involves brain functions during learning; and last is the cognitive-development model, which addresses the learner's maturational changes.

A gestalt view of cognitive learning emphasizes the relevance of perception while learning. One basic gestalt principle holds that patients prefer simplicity, equilibrium, and regularity in their lives. Consider the bewildered look on the faces of patients and their families when they receive detailed medical information; they are unable to relate to these complexities. They desire simple, clear explanations that remove uncertainty and relate to their personal experiences.

An additional gestalt principle is that perception is selective; it acknowledges that a patient cannot attend to all stimuli occurring at the same time. As a result, patients orient themselves to select components of a learning experience while screening out or habituating to other components. For example, patients with severe pain or who are worrying about their minor children while hospitalized have difficulty retaining education materials The nurse who desires to promote retention of information must first address minimizing or relieving the pain or the caretaking situation at home before learners can attend to their present learning needs. Factor into the experience the patient's capacity to choose to attend to or ignore information; this capacity is influenced by numerous elements such as past experiences, present needs, personal attributes, cultural experiences, and the context of the learning situation (Sherif, 1976; Sherif & Sherif, 1969; Sidani & Graden, 1998).

Assessing the learners' processing dynamics strongly influences the nurse's approach to individual or group learning situations. People perceive, interpret, and respond differently to the same learning event; this explains why a teaching approach is effective with one patient and not another.

Another gestalt principle is that patients strive for closure: a psychological desire to complete, end, or conclude a situation that is unfinished. When faced with uncertainty or lack of clarity, patients take action proportionally to the amount of uncertainty or lack of clarity experienced; patient response may be predicted. The more uncertain or unclear, the more patients can be influenced by the suggestions of others, internal needs and motivations, and examination of alternatives rather than what is being taught. Clinical examples of this principle abound. For example, a patient may experience tension and anxiety while waiting for test results. Some patients may create their own explanations and diagnoses. A small number with greater closure needs may pursue expensive quackery methods, deny medical illness or treatment, or pursue suicide. Considering these options, the nurse needs to provide as much structure as possible to patients and families faced with uncertainly in their treatment, recovery, and dying. When a diagnosis is uncertain, tell the patients rather than letting them ponder the test results; those patients with extreme closure needs may require counseling and therapy because further teaching may only escalate their unhealthy responses.

Cognitive- and information-processing views focus on brain functions such as thinking, reasoning, processing, and memory. Reward is unimportant; experience is everything to learners who are encouraged to explore and discover their environment in order to make their own cognitive maps. A common example is that people unfamiliar with a hospital environment are confused and frustrated by the staff's coded language, methods of initiating treatments, and delays in processing procedures. Employees, in contrast, have intricate cognitive maps about hospital environments and view as routine what patients perceive as anxiety producing. This view also recognizes that behavior is not necessarily an indicator that learning has occurred; learning may be demonstrated later rather than immediately following the teaching.

Processing, storing, and retrieving information is useful for patient education (see Figure 14.3). During Stage 1, the patient attends to the situation. If sleepy, distracted, or fatigued, attempt teaching at another time when the patient is more receptive. Delaying a teaching opportunity is a clinical challenge given the time constraints of today's treatment environments.

The second stage involves sensory processing, which is affected by the patient's preferred method of processing information (visual, auditory, or kinesthetic) and the presence of sensory deficits. In the third stage, memory is briefly encoded by transforming the information either into short-term memory, where it is discarded, forgotten, or then stored in long-term memory. The brain organizes the long-term memory by a preferred storage strategy such as imagery, association, rehearsal, or categorizing the information into units.

Long-term memories are lasting. Problems with remembering and retrieving the information may arise, especially with medications or diseases such as the various dementias. The final stage is the action taken by the patient in response to learned information. Should the patient be unable to retrieve or accurately use the information, the nurse should review these stages and coach the patient or family member to reprocess the information into long-term memory. Moments are precious during the learning process because the stages of memory for one fact may take less than a minute to process into memory. Organizing materials and making it meaningful to the patient can accomplish memory enhancement.

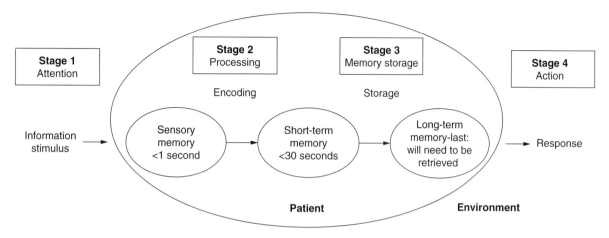

Figure 14.3 Stages of processing information.

SOURCE: Adapted from: Braungart, M. M. & Braungart, R. G. Applying learning theories to healthcare practice. In Bastable, S. (2003). *Nurse as educator: Principles of teaching and learning for nursing practice.* Boston: Jones and Bartlett.

Accurate retrieval of information or skills from memory is essential for accomplishing effective care outcomes that last beyond the teaching event.

Cognitive development is another approach that considers the patient's qualitative cognitive changes in perceiving, thinking, and reasoning as the brain develops and the person matures. Individuals have mental frameworks or schemas that are influenced by their cognitive-development stage. These schemas change drastically throughout a person's lifespan. Readiness to learn is largely dependent upon the learner's stage of cognitive development. These stages were studied and described by two theorists, Jean Piaget (Piaget & Inhelder, 1969) and Jerome Bruner (1966). Both believed that learning occurs as children interact with their environment. Piaget identified two processes of learning as learners: (1) assimilate information to incorporate it into their cognitive schema (e.g., a two-year-old's potty training may be prompted by the ability to watch color changes; place an adhesive blue flower in the bottom of the training potty; as the child urinates, the blue will turn green) and (2) accommodate information by changing the cognitive schema (e.g., a twenty-year-old with a panic response while crossing a bridge in a car due to fear of heights may change that response by consciously going through each step of travel,

then monitoring and altering his response to that step; gradually the response is replaced by an emotional level that tolerates crossing the bridge). Piaget also identified four sequential stages of cognitive development from infancy through adolescence (see Table 14.3).

Of note, researchers have demonstrated that some adults never attain complex, operational cognitive processes (Huyck & Hoyer, 1982). These adults may need highly concrete teaching approaches. Other researchers identified more complex forms of reasoning by adults who learned to work with contradiction, synthesis, and internalization of information (Kramer, 1983; Riegal, 1973). To acquire health education outcomes, the nurse initiates assessment of the patient's cognitive functioning prior to, during, and following the learning experience. Important cognitive-development learning-theory principles are summarized in Table 14.4.

Another aspect is the social cognition or the influence of social factors on cognitive processes. Many explanations are available, but one of considerable interest is attribution theory, which concerns the cause and effect of relationships. Teachers and learners have unique worldviews deeply affected by their cultural values and beliefs. Patient's attributions contribute to their health behaviors. Consider the

Table 14.3 **Cognitive Development Stages***

Sequential Stage	Age	Description
1 Sensorimotor	Infancy	Explores environment and uses motor skills to respond.
2 Preoperational	Early Childhood	Begins to mentally relate to environment, uses symbolization, and egocentrically views the world.
3 Concrete Operations	Elementary School Years	Uses more than one dimension at the same time, incorporates the environment, & understands relationships.
4 Formal Operations	Adolescence	Think abstractly, deals with future, considers alternatives, and reacts to criticism.

*Adapted from Piaget & Inhelder (1949).

patient with a cultural belief that his illness is caused by demon possession, which is removable only by his cultural group's elders or a shaman. These attributions may or may not contribute to healthy beliefs and behaviors. Changing unhealthy attributions takes patience and time.

Social Learning Theory

Incorporating the principles of behaviorist and cognitive theorists, the social learning theory contends that most learning occurs by observation or watching others to see what happens to them. As a social process, others, particularly those considered important to the patient, provide influential role models for thinking, acting, and feeling.

Bandura best illustrates the various aspects of this theory (see Figure 14.4). Role modeling is the central concept along with the principle of vicarious reinforcement. The former supports the use of mentoring new graduate nurses by more experienced nurses during the orientation period. The latter involves watching the behavior of peer nurses to see if they are rewarded or punished for their behavior in work settings. Bandura (1977, 1986) described four discrete stages of internal processes. The first is the attentional phase, with role models most often being those with high group status and recognized

Table 14.4 **Cognitive Development Theory Principles**

Principles of Learning
1. Perception is important to learning.
2. Perception is selective.
3. Each person perceives, interacts, and responds in his or her own way.
4. Information is processed into memory through the senses.
5. Psychological organization of information moves toward simplicity, equilibrium, and regularity.
6. Memory processing and triggering are strengthened by organizing information and making it personally meaningful to the learner.

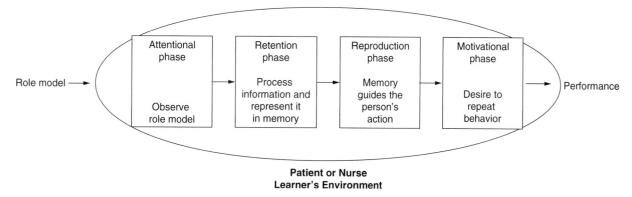

Figure 14.4 **Social Learning Theory Teaching Model.**

competence. Second is the retention phase, involving memory storage and retrieval of the information. Third is the reproduction phase wherein the learner mimics the observed behavior. Techniques such as mental rehearsal and immediate demonstration of the behavior, followed by feedback, greatly strengthen behavioral reproduction. The final phase is motivational, when the learner decides whether or not to perform the behavior. Well-suited to patient education and staff development, particularly in group situations, this learning theory involves attention to the social setting, the expected behavior to be performed, and the learner. Responsibility is required of the educator or leader to be an effective role model and to choose socially healthy learning situations. Also, one-time exposure to a role model does not ensure that learning occurs.

Psychodynamic Theory

Although not usually considered a learning theory, the work, originating with Freud, provides nurses with rich elements that influence learning and changing patients' behaviors. A key principle is that behavior may or may not be conscious, and people operate from a primitive motivation source known as the id (primitive drives), based upon libidinal energy composed of the eros (life source) and thanatos (death wish). The latter explains why patients who are predicted to die from or to survive

a diagnosis do the opposite. The id operates on the pleasure principle: to seek pleasure and avoid pain. An example of this would be a reading presentation of health information without much enthusiasm or emotion by the teacher doing little to inspire a patient to accept or use the information.

The patient's id and superego (internalized values and standards) are mediated by the ego, which operates on the reality principle that a person can choose delayed gratification. Healthy ego development spurs patients to undergo painful procedures and long-term discomfort and pain in order to achieve healthier outcomes. Weak ego strength may affect patients' choices to participate in immediate pleasure fulfillment that delays or stops healing and recovery. Helping patients, especially those with chronic health problems or long-term recoveries, to strengthen ego function promotes needed adjustments to changed body images or lifestyle altered by disease, treatments, and disfigurements. Table 14.5 correlates learner developmental stages and characteristics with sample teaching strategies.

Another important principle is the use of defense mechanisms to protect the self when the ego is threatened. Use short-term, defense mechanisms permits patients to adjust to their reality; however, overuse or retaining them overlong allows patients to avoid reality and may become barriers to learning and adjusting. Most health care environments are stressful, and staff as well as patients may use

Table 14.5 Development Stage Characteristics Matched with Selected Teaching Strategies

Learner	General Characteristics	Teaching Strategies
Infancy/Toddlerhood Approximate age: Birth–3 yrs Cognitive stage: Sensorimotor Psychosocial stage: Trust vs. mistrust (Birth–12 mo) Autonomy vs. shame and doubt (1–3 yrs)	Depends on caregiver Needs security Explores self and environment Displays natural curiosity Has short attention span	Teach the caregiver Use repetition and imitation Stimulate all senses Provide physical safety and emotional security Allow play and manipulation of objects
Preschooler Approximate age: 3–6 yrs Cognitive stage: Preoperational Psychosocial stage: Initiative vs. guilt	Is egocentric Thinking is precausal, concrete, and literal Believes illness self-caused and punitive Has limited sense of time Fears bodily injury Cannot generalize Has animistic thinking (objects possess life or human characteristics) Centration (focus is on one characteristic of an object) Has separation anxiety Is motivated by curiosity Has active imagination, prone to fears Play is his/her work Has short attention span	Use warm, calm approach Build trust Use repetition of information Allow manipulation of objects and equipment Give care with simple explanation Reassure not to blame self Explain procedures simply and briefly Provide safe, secure environment Use positive reinforcement Encourage questions to reveal perceptions/feelings Use simple drawings and stories Use play therapy with dolls and puppets Stimulate senses: Visual, auditory, tactile, motor Use technology
School-Aged Childhood Approximate age: 7–11 yrs Cognitive stage: Concrete operations Psychosocial stage: Industry vs. inferiority	Is more realistic and objective Understands cause and effect Uses deductive/inductive reasoning Wants concrete information Able to compare objects and events Has variable rates of physical growth Reasons syllogistically Understands seriousness and consequences of actions Has subject-centered focus Has immediate orientation Has short attention span	Encourage independence and active participation Be honest, allay fears Use logical explanation Allow time to ask questions Use analogies to make invisible processes real Establish role models Relate care to other children's experience; compare procedures Use subject-centered focus Use play therapy Provide group activities Use drawings, models, dolls, painting, audio- and videotapes, and technology

Table 14.5 (*Continued*)

Learner	General Characteristics	Teaching Strategies
School-Aged Childhood (*Continued*)		Use age-appropriate books, DVDs, and brochures Use games
Adolescence Approximate age: 12–18 yrs Cognitive stage: Formal operations Psychosocial stage: Identity vs. role confusion	Has abstract, hypothetical thinking Can build on past learning Reasons by logic and understands scientific principles Has future orientation Motivated by desire for social acceptance Peer group is important Has intense personal preoccupation, appearance extremely important (imaginary audience) Feels invulnerable, invincible/immune to natural laws (personal fable)	Establish trust, authenticity Know their agenda Address fears/concerns about outcomes of illness Identify control focus Use peers for support and influence Negotiate changes Focus on details Make information meaningful to life Ensure confidentiality and privacy Arrange group sessions Use audiovisuals, role play, contracts, reading materials Provide for experimentation and flexibility Use technology, Web sites, DVDs, and brochures
Young Adulthood Approximate age: 18–40 yrs Cognitive stage: Formal operations Psychosocial stage: Intimacy vs. isolation	Autonomous Self-directed Uses personal experiences to enhance or interfere with learning Intrinsic motivation Able to analyze critically Makes decisions about personal, occupational, and social roles Competency-based learner	Use problem-centered focus Draw on meaningful experiences Focus on immediacy of application Encourage active participation Allow to set own pace, be self-directed Organize material Recognize social role Apply new knowledge through role play and hands-on practice Use technology including Web sites, blogs, DVDs Encourage support groups
Middle-Aged Adulthood Approximate age: 40–65 yrs Cognitive stage: Formal operations Psychosocial stage: Generativity vs. self-absorption and stagnation	Sense of self well developed Concerned with physical changes At peak in career Explores alternative lifestyles Reflects on contributions to family and society Reexamines goals and values	Focus on maintaining independence and reestablishing normal life patterns Assess positive and negative past experiences with learning Assess potential sources of stress due to midlife crisis issues

(*Continues*)

Table 14.5 **Development Stage Characteristics Matched With Selected Teaching Strategies (*Continued*)**

Learner	General Characteristics	Teaching Strategies
Middle-Aged Adulthood (*Continued*)	Questions achievements and successes Has confidence in abilities Desires to modify unsatisfactory aspects of life	Provide information to coincide with life concerns and problems
Older Adulthood Approximate age: 65 yrs+ Cognitive stage: Formal operations Psychosocial stage: Ego integrity vs. despair	<u>Cognitive changes</u> Decreased ability to think abstractly, process information Decreased short-term memory Increased reaction time Increased test anxiety Stimulus persistence (afterimage) Focuses on past-life experiences <u>Sensory/motor deficits</u> Auditory changes Hearing loss, especially high-pitched tones, consonants (S, Z, T, F, & G), and rapid speech Visual changes Farsighted (needs glasses to read) Lenses become opaque (glare problem) Smaller pupil size (decreased visual adaptation to darkness) Decreased peripheral perception	Use concrete examples Build on past life experiences Make information relevant and meaningful Present one concept at a time Allow time for processing/response (slow pace) Use repetition and reinforcement of information Avoid written exams Use verbal exchange and coaching Establish retrieval plan (use one or several clues) Encourage active involvement Keep explanations brief Use analogies to illustrate abstract information Use technology, DVDs Provide support group information Speak slowly, distinctly Use low-pitched tones Face client when speaking Minimize distractions Avoid shouting Use visual aids to supplement verbal instruction Avoid glares, use soft white light Provide sufficient light Use white backgrounds and black print Use large letters and well-spaced print Avoid color coding with blues, greens, purples, and yellows Increase safety precautions/provide safe environment

*Adapted from Bastable, S. (2003).

defense mechanisms. The patient's use of the defense mechanism of denial is frequently the first response to the news of being told that death will occur in a certain time frame; maintaining a state of denial may result in the patient not taking treatment and care. Staff might employ the defense mechanism of intellectualization rather than approach a situation with an accompanying emotional response.

A central component is that psychological development happens in overlapping stages with most of adult behavior built upon childhood experiences. Erikson (1968), a prominent personality-development theorist, delineated eight stages of life, each with a psychosocial crisis to be resolved. The stages are major considerations in achieving effective care and outcomes. For example, when working with adolescents (the psychosocial crisis of identity), they need support in order to adjust to a changed body image or forced social isolation to promote recovery and healing as well as to work through this stage's identity crisis.

Throughout life, personal difficulties and conflicts arise. Problems with learning ensue when patients fail to move through earlier development stages and become fixated or stuck. Before further maturation is possible, the patient must work through the previously unresolved crisis. Fixation with a stage may occur over years. For example, an elderly patient who is 80 years old lost her mother due to cancer when the patient was seven years old. The patient has never resolved her yearning for her mother's love. While in a skilled-care facility and experiencing the loss of her independence, the patient needed inordinate nurturing from family and staff during her rehabilitation. Understanding her fixation in the school-age child stage helps develop necessary strategies to promote learning and independence for this patient.

Past conflicts, particularly during childhood, may interfere with learning. When resistance to teaching or treatment is encountered, it usually indicates unresolved emotional conflicts that must first be addressed. For example, if, when teaching a teen-aged mother about her infant's nutritional needs, she is giggling or disengaged from the learning, then she may have personal feelings needing attention before she can attend to her infant's needs.

Another psychodynamic concept is transfer. Transference is the projection of past feelings, conflicts, and reactions to significant others onto current relationships such as authority figures or caregivers. Therapeutic relationships, such as that between a nurse and patient, may be distorted or altered because of these previous biases. For example, when sick and dependent, the patient might view the nurse as a mother figure and support system. Although a nurse may be flattered by these responses due to unmet personal needs, the relationship becomes unhealthy for both unless the nurse initiates strategies to promote patient recovery and independence. In contrast, patients may remind nurses of someone from their past, creating the process of countertransference. Awareness of these concepts enables nurses to more effectively promote and obtain desired healthy outcomes from learning.

Humanistic Learning Theory

The humanistic perspective is mainly a motivational theory, which views a person's needs, subjective personal feelings, and the desire to grow as reasons for motivation. Major factors in learning are emotions and feelings, spontaneity, creativity, the right to make choices, and the respect of individuality.

Maslow (1954; 1987), an early humanist, developed the well-known hierarchy of needs, which assumes that basic-level needs must be met before an individual can address learning or self-actualizing needs. For example, postoperative patients in pain must have the pain minimized or relieved before they can learn about home care. Although the theory is widely used, research has been unable to consistently support the constructs and principles.

Rogers (1961, 1994) believed that people want unconditional positive self-regard and, in caring situations, it is essential that the nurse respects patients as individuals regardless of their circumstances. A nurse who is prejudiced against drug users will have little, if any, therapeutic effect on

Table 14.6 Relevant Adult Learning Principles

Adults learn best when

1. Learning relates to a felt need or problem.
2. Learning is voluntary, self-initiated, self-controlled, and self-directed.
3. Learning is person centered, problem centered, and pertinent.
4. The teacher's role is as a facilitator.
5. New material draws on past experiences and relates to something the learner knows.
6. The threat to self is minimized during the educational process.
7. The learner participates actively in the learning process and learns in a group.
8. The learning activities change often and are reinforced by application and prompt feedback.

SOURCE: Adapted from Burgireno (1985) and Bastable (2003).

patients seeking recovery. Also, the educator's role is as a facilitator (Buscaglia, 1982; Rogers, 1994). Listening, not talking, is the skill of choice when educators influence learners to make wise choices. Rather than distributing written and audiovisual education materials, an educator who uses humanistic theory would establish and maintain rapport.

Humanistic learning theory has altered education and the role of the educator by attending primarily to the learner's subjective needs and feelings. Critics claim that this approach to learning fosters self-centered learners who are unable to take criticism or compromise.

Adult-Learning Theory

Unless working with infants and children, most patients and all employees are considered adult learners. Adult learning characteristics differ from those of children (Lee & Owens, 2000). Knowles (1990), a prominent adult-learning theorist, developed the theory of androgogy (the study of how adults learn) as contrasted with pedagogy (the study of how children learn). Specific characteristics that enhance learning in adults include their need to be active in the educational process; they participate and learn best when learning directly applies to their personal situations.

Adults bring unique varieties of experiences to learning situations. Their strengths are their goal orientation, self-reliance, and independence, which lead to high levels of motivation. They prefer to self-pace because many have complex life-styles, responsibilities, and commitments. While teaching adult learners, Shultz (2006) found that assessing their levels of anxiety about the learning situation, their work and home obligations, ultimate learning goals, time and resource commitments, learning styles and writing abilities were powerful influences in instructional design and learner success. Relevant adult learning principles are listed in Table 14.6.

THE LEARNER

The learner is the focus of health-related teaching. Although planning requires knowledge and multiple skills, the learner's perception of the teacher also affects the education process. Consider the caregiver's perceptions of nurses in the next Research Focus. From this study, a nurse-developed teaching model was designed (see Figure 14.5).

Research Focus

Source: Cox, J. A., & Oakes Westbrook, L. J. (2005). Home infusion therapy: Essential characteristics of a successful educations process: A grounded theory study. *Journal of Infusion Therapy*, *28*(2), 99–107.

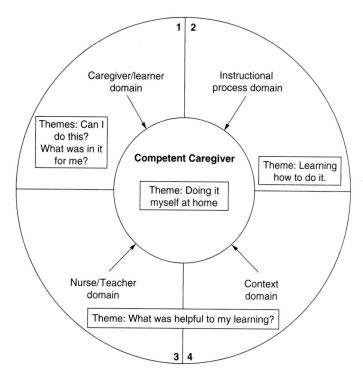

Figure 14.5 **Domains and themes of the teaching-learning process for home IV therapy administration.**
SOURCE: Cox & Westbrook (2005), p. 101. Used with permission.

Purpose

To identify, from the family caregiver's point of view, the characteristics of an education process that results in learners' competence with home infusion therapy (HIT).

Overview

Infusion therapy, a complex care procedure, is presently commonplace in home care due to the Medicare prospective payment reimbursement system. Private insurers also adopted similar reimbursement systems. Home infusion therapy enables hospitals to save money by not going over the reimbursable rate.

Research Design

Using a qualitative research design, the researchers sought to obtain the caregivers' perceptions of the nurses while in an educator role. The sample was adult caregivers who had been independently administering home infusion therapy for family members belonging to a metropolitan HMO. All seven participants had a minimum of a high school education and no previous HIT experiences; they learned the procedure for a spouse or a child. HIT included total parenteral nutrition, hydration, anti-infective, miscellaneous medications, and central catheter care. Data were collected in face-to-face interviews. Qualitative analysis procedures were followed.

Findings

A picture emerged of a successful education process for caregivers administering home infusion therapy. The defining factors were clustered into five themes, which are in the boxes of Figure 14.6. The factors occurred across four domains placed in each quarter of the circle of Figure 14.6. The results supported the importance of using adult learning theory and

Title of Media: _____

Resource Contact Information: _____

Price: _____ Type of Media: _____

Year Produced: _____ Length: _____

Content	YES	NO		Presentation	YES	NO
Accurate?	___	___		Image sharp & clear?	___	___
Relevant?	___	___		Text legible for room?	___	___
Current?	___	___		Audio clear & understandable?	___	___
Organized?	___	___		Distractors present?	___	___
				Appropriate pace?	___	___
				Holds interest?	___	___

Support to use				Additional		
Equipment available?	___	___		Easy to use?	___	___
User's guide?	___	___		Awards?	___	___
Script?	___	___		Recommend?	___	___
Evaluation materials?	___	___				

Reviewer: _____

Figure 14.6 Selecting media for instructional use.
SOURCE: Adapted from Discenza (1993).

the concept of self-efficacy (belief in one's ability to execute a given behavior) in teaching a new skill. Also, the findings emphasize the nurse demonstrating caring from the learner perspective and augment specific practice guidelines and researching findings in the professional literature. In addition, the caregivers gave advice to nurses teaching HIT, which validated the themes and domains. These include

Simplify the training.

Explain all the steps, even the small ones.

Let the learner touch everything at every step.

A return demonstration is imperative.

Understand the anxiety

Do not presume the learner [knows anything].

Understand where we're coming from.

Meet individual learning styles.

Keep it relaxed, low key, not drastic or melodramatic.

Go to an area outside the hospital room.

[Avoid] checkout time.

Update the printed material. A checklist and a single-sheet, large, bold-faced, fill-in-the blank would be helpful.

When teaching, nurses are encouraged to incorporate the needs and concerns voiced by learners as well as the principles and practices advocated by expert clinicians. These will support competence in designing an education process that promotes successful learning outcomes. Figure 14.6 is a nurse-developed education model, which is foundational for future research.

Learner Characteristics

When planning teaching strategies, the nurse as educator carefully considers learner characteristics known to be legally required and to be effective as documented by evidence-based educational research findings (Shultz, 2006). Some agency accrediting groups such as the Joint Commission on Accreditation of Healthcare Organizations (JCAHO) require that patient teaching plans address stage-specific learner competencies. Age alone does not determine the patient's capacity to learn because it is not a reliable indicator of abilities. However, other characteristics such as the patient's developmental stage promote the uniqueness of each person and more than likely ensure individualization of the teaching plan.

Developmental stages have been studied for decades, and useful information exists that affects how, when, and what the nurse will teach. Within each developmental stage are predictable physical, cognitive, and psychosocial elements and tasks to be achieved. Table 14.5 summarizes lists of evidence-based learner characteristics that affect the learning process.

A major element of planning for an educational experience is determining the most appropriate time to teach. When a staff development class or support group is scheduled for a class such as weight loss or for caretaking a person with Alzheimer's, the time element is settled. However, most teaching in clinical settings is conducted one on one, such as when the patient asks a question or a discharge time is known. The best time for teaching is when the patient is ready; this is known as the teaching moment (Havighurst, 1976). Also, a more experienced nurse knows when and how to prompt those teachable moments by peaking the patient's interest or introducing a health topic.

Before making education intervention choices, assessment is a must. Numerous learner characteristics have been studied and researched to demonstrate their effect on the learning process. Following the assessment of present knowledge and skill levels, the nurse matches the teaching plan with the client's developmental level.

As part of the teaching plan, the nurse considers motivational strategies as part of learning theories and the results of evidence-based education research findings. Knowing the unique learner's needs and desires is helpful in matching strategies with the patient's learning situation. Strategies appeal to patients' motives but do not create them; usually these are generated external to the patient through the use of incentives. To improve learner motivation, an application of Maslow's (1943) hierarchy of needs could be useful. Removing or reducing barriers to obtaining changed health behaviors is important in maintaining short- and long-term motivation.

Learning theories are discussed earlier in this chapter. Examples of developmental-level characteristics matched with sample teaching strategies are in Table 14.5. At the risk of promoting an oversimplification of the information by preparing succinct tables of usable information, the nurse aspiring to an expert practice level is referred to resources considered the gold standard for in-depth education information for nursing practice (Bastable, 2003). In addition, recent research findings on the science of nursing education have been synthesized (Shultz, 2006). This publication discusses educational research trends, trends and gaps in research findings, and recommended areas for future research. Although geared toward nurse/educators, many findings parallel nursing-practice educational findings.

Learning Styles

Learning is a complex process, and in health care, results in behavior (such as eating and exercise habits), attitudes (such as valuing care of oneself), or measurable changes (such as blood glucose level). With patients and employees, assessment of the learner's determinants of learning guides the approach to learning and verifies the learning needs. Hoggard (1989) identified three determinants of learning, listed here in order of their assessment priority.

1. Learning needs (what)

2. Readiness to learn (when)

3. Learning style (how)

Assessment of learning needs is essential. If the learner perceives no need for learning (what), the other two determinants are not needed. For example,

Table 14.7 Evidence-Based Learning Style Principles

1. The teacher's preferred teaching style and the learner's preferred teaching style can be identified.
2. Through awareness of their preferred teaching style, teachers can change predominantly teaching in their preferred learning style.
3. Teachers best facilitate teaching when assisting learners to use their own learning style preference.
4. Teaching methods should encourage learners to use their preferred learning style.
5. For increased flexibility in learning situations, learners should be encouraged to diversify their learning styles.
6. Teachers can develop learning activities that reinforce learning styles.

education does not always solve and identify the problem. If an employee has completed an orientation that covers policies and procedures but has a pattern of being late and unorganized, reteaching the policies is not the accurate response. A management technique involving confrontation and documentation of a warning would be an appropriate strategy.

Once learning needs are identified, a prioritizing of the needs assists all who are involved in the education process to attain realistic goals. The Healthcare Education Association (1985) lists three prioritizing categories:

1. Mandatory: Necessary for survival when the learner's life or safety is threatened.
2. Desirable: Not life dependent but does relate to well-being or the ability to provide quality care.
3. Possible: Information that is "nice-to-know," but not essential or required.

Once a knowledge deficit is identified, the next step is timing. Lichtenthal (1990) proposed four types of readiness to learn: Physical, Emotional, Experiential, and Knowledge, or PEEK.

A learning style is the way a person processes information (Guild & Garger, 1998), and each person has a distinct learning style preference. Understanding these styles helps match the learner with the instructional design and teaching approaches. For example, many practicing nurses have had at least one assessment of their learning styles while

completing a nursing program. When hired in different settings, the nurse could share that learning style in order to assist in selecting a mentor.

Learning styles can be identified; no learning style, though, is better than another. The learning style will determine how a learner masters the knowledge and its application. Six prominent principles, identified through research (Friedman & Alley, 1984), are important to using the information in an education process. These are listed in Table 14.7.

The nurse can determine learning styles through observation, interviews, and giving learning-style instruments. Some learners take ample notes, some take none, and some list only major concepts. Learners can be asked when they learn best, with or without noise in the background, and individually or groups.

In using learning-style instruments, some precautions are indicated. None of the instruments measure all learning domains (cognitive, psychomotor, and affective). Using more than instruments contributes to a more holistic view of the learning style. The instruments are not diagnostic; they validate the learner and teacher's perception and, as such, should be used in unison with perceptions. Consider the instrument's validity and reliability before using. Some frequently used learning-style instruments are discussed in Table 14.8.

It is important not to stereotype learners into any of the many categories of learning styles. Use of an instrument to determine learning-style preferences may not be feasible due to costs, time, literacy level, or the context of learning. But by using observation and interviewing, the nurse can

Table 14.8 **Learning-Style Instruments and Their Uses**

Learning Style Instrument	Use
Brain Preference Indicator (BPI)	Determines brain hemispheric dominance bases on brain functioning (Wonder & Donovan, 1984).
Embedded Figures Test (EFT)	Measures how the person's perception of an item is influenced by its context and the person's ability to do something (Bonham, 1988). Best for measuring field in dependence.
Dunn and Dunn Learning Style Inventory	The learner self-reports preferences for functioning, learning, concentrating, and performing educational activities (Dunn and Dunn, 1978; Dunn, 1984).
Myers-Briggs Type Indicator	Not specifically a learning style instrument, but measures differences in personality types that influence how people behave and relate to each other (Myers, 1980).
Kolb's Learning Style Inventory	A self-reporting instrument that identifies learning styles based upon dimensions of perception and processing (Kolb, 1984).
4MAT System	Based upon learning styles and brain functioning, this instrument describes four types of learners within four sequential quadrants of learning (McCarthy, 1981).
Gregorc Style Delineator	A self-analysis depth instrument that measures learning patterns (Gregorc, 1982).

identify basic learning-style information in order to adjust learning environments and experiences that encourage all learners to succeed at learning goals.

Motivation

The concept of motivation also affects learning outcomes (health behaviors). When motivation is set in motion, some internal element moves the patient toward action (Richards, 2003). Readiness is evidence of motivation (Redman, 1993), although behavior can result from influences other than motive, and numerous motives can lead to one behavior. Redman (1993) best summarizes theories of motivation, which address motivation based upon need satisfaction, a stable personality characteristic, and expectancy theory, which includes values and perceived chance of success, relieving the discomfort of cognitive dissonance, and humanistic emphasis on personal choice. The concept is vague and elusive to study but is certainly a determinant of health behaviors. Some well-known motivational factors such as personal attributes, environmental influences, and supports systems, as well as some motivational

axioms or rules that set the stage for motivation (Richards, 2003) are summarized in Table 14.9.

Mishel (1990) views uncertainty as a natural and necessary part of life. Uncertainty motivates people to seek alternatives to life's situations. Premature uncertainty reduction can be counterproductive to learner problem solving.

A comprehensive assessment of learner motivation to change health behaviors may be unlikely in present clinical settings due to the short time patients spend in clinical settings. However, a knowledge of available indicators of motivation is invaluable as the nurse develops and implements the individualized teaching plan. Assessment involves the judgment of the nurse using subjective and objective information. For example, a patient who states, "I really want to lose weight" indicates an energized desire to change behavior.

Although tools for assessing learner motivation have been lacking in the literature, there are some known areas of motivational assessment that could guide design of the educational process. These assessment guidelines are identified in Table 14.10.

Table 14.9 **Motivational Factors and Axioms**

Motivational Factors	Categories
Incentives or obstacles to obtaining results from learning. The teacher role is to minimize blockers and strengthen facilitators to learning.	A. Personal attributes: physical, developmental, and psychosocial. Examples: developmental stage, gender, age, values, beliefs, emotional readiness, cognitive abilities, educational level, health state, severity or chronicity of illness, health care-seeking behaviors, natural curiosity, information process, and memory.
	B. Environmental influences: perception of the environment, noise level, confusion, lack of privacy, accessibility and availability of resources, sensitivity of learning to learner's needs, educator attitudes toward learner, rewards/punishments, and learner comfort.
	C. Relationship systems: support systems such as family/significant others, spiritual relationships and beliefs, cultural identity, work, school and community roles, teacher/learner relationship.

Motivational Axioms	Rules
Premises on which understanding of experiences is based. These rules motivate and promote learning.	A. State of optimum anxiety: Learning occurs best in a state of mild learner anxiety. Techniques to reduce high anxiety include guided imagery, humor, and relaxation techniques.
	B. Learner readiness: Can be externally influenced by reinforcements; rewards; providing encouragement; making learning stimulating, relevant, and accessible; and moderating the environment.
	C. Realistic goal setting: Ones that are reasonable and possible to achieve. To promote, reduce frustration, and be organized.
	D. Learner satisfaction and success: Learners are motivated by success, which feeds self-esteem. Evaluations can be valuable tools in promoting learner success. Self-esteem and success are closely related.
	E. Uncertainty reducing or maintaining dialogue: People have continued internal dialogues (self-talk) that can affect their certainty levels.

Literacy

Determining the employee's or patient's literacy level is not easy because no clear agreement exists about what it means to be literate in the United States. Certainly exploring the person's cultural expectations about reading and writing as well as the educational level is helpful information; however, the latter is an inadequate indication of a person's reading and writing abilities (Adams-Price, 1993; Doak et al., 1996; Matthews et al., 1988). People are most often considered literate if they can read and understand or interpret information at the eighth-grade level or above. Illiteracy is the total inability to read or write; about 5 percent of the U.S. population is illiterate (Doak et al., 1985). Low-literacy or marginally illiterate adults read, write, or comprehend between the fifth- and eighth-grade level of ability; they have difficulty with everyday functioning, such as taking a phone message, reading a newspaper, reading label instructions, or completing an application form. Functional illiteracy involves skills below the fifth-grade level;

Table 14.10 **Selected Assessment Areas of Learner Motivation**

Assessment Area	General Characteristics
Psychomotor Domain	Ability to perform desired behavior
Affective Domain	Emotional state Valuing learning Mild to moderate level of anxiety Attitude Curiosity
Cognitive Domain	Readiness to learn Capacity to learn Thinking and memory abilities Level of certainty/uncertainty
Learner's Environment	Appropriate Social support systems Spiritual support Resources: presence and accessibility Teacher/learner relationship

these people are unable to function. They may read simple instructions such as "take one pill in the morning; take one pill in the evening; take the pill with food," but they will be unable to comprehend the meaning and sequence of instructions in order to enact the directions. These grade levels are approximate, and reading levels are not indicators of intelligence. A person may be illiterate or low literate and still have a normal IQ.

Comprehension and readability affect literacy levels, too. Readability is the ease with which material can be read. Comprehension is the ability to understand the meaning of what is read. These may complicate the ability to transfer information between teacher and learner. For example, the patient or employee may be literate at the eighth-grade level but be unable to read complex instructions or comprehend a teaching session if the teacher uses unfamiliar words. Demonstration may be a very effective instructional method to consider.

The United States has considerable literacy problems, with the mean reading education level at approximately the twelfth grade and the mean literacy level at or below the eighth grade. Most people read 2 to 4 grades below their education level. Also, reading levels, if not practiced, may deteriorate over time, particularly after completing high school (Miller & Brodie, 1994; Mead & Wittbrot, 1988).

Of major concern in health care is that at least one in five Americans don't have literacy levels with which to cope day to day. Driving manuals require a sixth-grade reading level, frozen dinner directions require an eighth-grade reading level, and aspirin bottle instructions require a tenth-grade reading level (Doak et al., 1985). Most people do not readily admit their reading difficulties. Dave Thomas, a prominent businessman and founder of Wendy's International, publicly admitted his illiteracy years after his company was established. He then completed a GED (high school equivalency test) and became an advocate for improving the literacy levels of Americans. He was also a prime example of the "skilled actor" (Fain, 1994b) who covered up his illiteracy.

Illiteracy has been called an "invisible handicap" (Fleener & Scholl, 1992), but most illiterates have had some high school. Many live in metropolitan areas and are unemployed. The groups at risk for low literacy are low-income people, older people, racial minorities, and people who have English as a second language. Most, though, are white, born in America, and English speaking.

Literacy levels can truly make a difference in a person's health status or employment success. Most health information is written. For example, food labels, over-the-counter and prescription medications, environmental or chemical safety warnings, preoperative and discharge instructions, consent forms, party-payer reimbursement forms, and other printed material are important to the success of treatments, prevention, and health promotion. Most printed health care publications are written at above the eighth-grade level, with the average level being between tenth and twelfth grade, well above the reading level of most patients. One could conclude that written patient-education materials are useless unless adjusted to the patient's reading and comprehension levels.

Table 14.11 **Commonly Used Measures of Reading Levels of Written Materials and Patients' Comprehension and Reading Skills**

Type	Purpose	Example	Population
Reading Formula	Tests reading level of written materials	Spache Grade-Level Score	Children in elementary grades from one to three.
		Flesch Formula	Grade levels five to college.
		Fog Index	Fourth grade to college level.
		Fry Readability Graph-Extended	Grade one through college level.
		SMOG Formula	Grade four to college level. Note: Considered more accurate (most valid) of readability.
		Computerized readability software programs	Varies. Take an average of several programs due to readability issues (Maillox et al., 1995).
Standardized Tests	Tests patient comprehension and reading skills	Cloze Procedure (Tests patient's ability to understand what was read.)	Administer to patients who will receive the written information.
		Listening Test (Tests what low-literate patients understand and remember when listening.)	Administer to patients who will receive the written information.
		WRAT (Tests patient's ability to pronounce words and the ability to recognize and pronounce words out of context.)	Scores are converted to an equivalent grade level. Level 1: Children 5 to 12 yrs. Level 2: Testing over age 12 yrs. Scores are normed on age.
		REALM (Tests patient's ability to read medical and health-related information.)	Raw score is converted to a range of reading grade levels.

Nurses who prepare health-related patient education materials (PEM) need to become familiar with evaluating reading materials. Several methods exist that fall into one of two categories: vocabulary difficulty, assessed by mathematical reading formulas; and standardized tests, which measure patient comprehension and reading. The more familiar and simple-to-use tests are listed in Table 14.11. Remember to use a readability formula that is valid for the reader population for whom the PEM is intended. Nurses are encouraged to use these while initially designing health information; the standardized tests can be used individually with patients and better ensure a match between instructional materials and learner.

INSTRUCTIONAL METHODS

Teaching effectively is a learned skill that must be practiced. Dynamic and effective learning experiences are designed, not accidental. The nurse who teaches must be familiar with the educational process,

Table 14.12 Important Educational Terms and Definitions

Education Term	Definition
Learning	A mental, emotional, or behavioral knowledge, skills, or attitudes change due to exposure to experiences.
Learning Theory	A framework with constructs and principles that describe, explain, or predict how people learn.
Teaching	A deliberate intervention involving planning and implementing instructional activities with the goal of producing learning according to a teaching plan. Can be spontaneous and reciprocal.
Instruction	A component of teaching that involves communication of information about a skill in the cognitive, psychomotor, or affective domain.
Learning Needs	These are gaps between a person's actual level of knowledge, attitudes, and skills and the desired level. Between 90% to 95% of learners can master a topic if given sufficient time and appropriate help (Bloom, 1968; Brunner 1966; Skinner, 1954).
Education Process	A sequential plan of action with two major activities: teaching and learning. Examples in nursing are patient information, developing self competencies, teaching staff, and mentoring.
Client Education	A process of assisting people to learn health-related behaviors (knowledge, skills, attitudes, and values) so that they can include them in their daily lives.
Staff Education	A process of influencing employee behaviors (knowledge, skills, attitudes, and values) to maintain and strengthen competencies necessary for providing quality health care and career development.
Nursing Role of Educator	Primarily to promote or facilitate learning in an environment that is most conducive to learning. This includes enhancing a teachable moment rather than waiting for it to occur (Wagner & Ash, 1998). Teaching and learning are participatory processes.
Motivation	A psychological force that moves a person toward action (Haggard, 1989).

including the available instructional methods and ways to use them in various settings with differing learners and clinical settings. Definitions of important terms are in Table 14.12. The expert nurse knows how to choose instructional methods, use them effectively and efficiently, and evaluate their ability to improve the delivery of instruction.

Unfortunately, many clinical agencies promote the use of scripted written informational materials to give all patients with the same diagnoses; some of these are adapted to cultural beliefs, preferences, learner characteristics, or literacy levels. They ensure, on behalf of the agency, that some information has transpired; rarely is the method's effectiveness documented on the patient's record. Technically, the agency met the letter of the law; unfortunately, the patient may or may not apply the information that was exchanged. Generally, there is no plan to evaluate the effectiveness of the prescriptive teaching episode.

Determining which instructional method to use depends upon how active the learner is in the educational process (active or passive) and the amount of control (student centered or teacher centered) that the teacher uses in the learning experience. Other factors to consider include the budget, learning setting, available technology (Suen, 2005), whether the content is student or teacher centered, developmental stage of the learner, audience size, cultural diversity of the learner, the learner's preferred learning style, and various other learner characteristics. Instructional methods are categorized in numerous ways: traditional, nontraditional, and those most familiar

Table 14.13 **Instructional Methods and Teaching Tips**

Instructional Methods
Lecture
Visual Aids
Group Discussions
Role Play
One-on-One Instruction
Learning Contracts
Demonstration/Return Demonstration
Telecommunications
Posters
Printed Materials
Games
Simulation
Audio-Visual Software
Role-Modeling
Internet Resources
Test/Posttest
Computer-Assisted Instruction
Modules
Graphics

Tips
1. Move the learner through the stages of change.
2. Use examples and stories.
3. Risk using uncertainty along with the instructional method.
4. Use appropriate humor.
5. Be enthusiastic and nonhurried.
6. Reinforce, reinforce, reinforce . . . positively.
7. Seek and give feedback.
8. Be organized.
9. Repeat and pace information.
10. Summarize important points.

to learners. Various methods along with related teaching tips are identified in Table 14.13.

Instructional methods in learning situations may be used by themselves or in combination with other methods. When teaching a group of heterogeneous learners, plan to use several instructional methods to reinforce information use by the learners. For example, when providing follow-up teaching to people who participated in a screening clinic for colon cancer, schedule enough volunteers so that patients with positive results have individual discussions with nurse/educators, prepare written materials that summarize what is discussed, and create posters that reinforce important colon cancer prevention and treatment information. The patient then is exposed to three various instructional methods with planned reinforcement. Hammer (2005) reviewed various nursing interventions used in the recovery of patients with congestive heart failure (CHF). Studies were carefully chosen to meet inclusion criteria; many of them used instructional methods to improve patient outcomes. The synthesis of evidence-based research findings is summarized in the Research Focus. The summary reinforces the nurse's role of educator in improving patients' recovery.

Instructional methods can be creatively developed or purchased. Volunteers, patients with similar diagnoses, survivors of illnesses and tragedies, families of those with similar problems, and others can be rich resources for assisting with much needed learning situations, especially when resources such as money and equipment are scarce. Grassroots efforts have changed health practices of individuals, families, and communities.

Evaluation of the effectiveness of instructional methods is an important step of the educational process. Although evaluation can be complex, there are some basic questions that guide the evaluation of the chosen methods. Was the choice appropriate, well received, efficient, cost-effective, and specific to the learner's developmental stage? Is the instructional method available to the learner? For example, developing a Web site or blog to discuss aspects of hypertension prevention and treatment requires determining if the targeted learners have access to computer technology and the ability to use it. Is the method efficient for the number of learners and the time, energy, and resources

RESEARCH APPLICATION ARTICLE

Hammer, J. B. (2005). Posthospitalization nursing interventions in congestive heart failure. *Advances in Nursing Science*, *28*(2), 175–190.

Congestive heart failure (CHF) is a prevalent, costly disorder affecting 5 million people annually in the United States. Hospitalization from CHF rose annually by 1647 percent from 1979 to 2001. CHF management involves coordinated care including individually determined management support and encouragement of any self-care activities. Nursing's role has involved providing emotional support and teaching self-care to patients with CHF.

The purpose of this study is to systematically evaluate the impact of posthospital nursing interventions in the management of CHF. These interventions include a variety of instructional methods.

Numerous studies related to nursing interventions were reviewed and summarized. Twenty-nine studies met inclusion criteria, and these were categorized into models: home-based nursing interventions, multidisciplinary interventions extending to the home with nurses in pivotal roles, heart failure clinics with nursing as a significant component, and telephone- or technology-based nursing interventions.

Various teaching methods were listed among the nursing interventions including enhanced discharge planning, exercise training, assessment and teaching to improve adherence and response, increase caregiver vigilance, printed materials, education linked to support, CHF-related teaching, reinforcement of education, exercise programs, management of meds, group education, video-based self-care group, self-care and medication compliance, and family teaching. Many interventions were reinforced with home visits, telephone calls, return visits, and so on. Although not thoroughly described, education was a strong component of the studied nursing interventions.

As a total group, the results of these studies suggest posthospitalization nursing interventions in CHF have a positive impact on patient outcomes such as functional status, quality of life, and self-care behaviors, and reduce resource utilization concerns such as costs and readmissions. Strengths and weaknesses of the compiled studies were discussed. The models of intervention with primarily positive outcomes were the heart failure clinics with nursing as a significant component and multidisciplinary interventions extending to the home with nurses in major roles. These approaches were encouraged to be incorporated into practice. Among the specific recommendations found to improve outcomes was comprehensive patient and family education.

The study is a wealth of information about nurses' current roles in working with CHF patients. The study also provides research information for nurses seeking to improve specific CHF outcomes through nursing interventions that use education.

available to prepare the method? Does the method help meet the teaching plan that includes the desired objectives? Can the method accommodate the learners' needs and abilities? Is the method cost-effective considering the nurse's time; attaining optimal patient outcomes as cheaply as possible; and the costs of preparation, development, and evaluation?

Table 14.14 **Select Nursing Educational Intervention Studies**

Children with chronic illnesses (Stewart, 2003)
Coronary heart disease (Deaton & Namasivayam, 2004)
Diabetes (Whittemore et al, 2004; Wong et al, 2005)
Evidence-based assessment (Munro, 2004)
Healing and health status outcomes (Cowling, 2005; Kruen & Braden, 2004)
Mechanically ventilated patients (Burns et al, 2003)
Nursing-sensitive quality indicators (Gallagher & Rowell, 2003)
Outpatient neurosurgical procedures (Zanchetta & Bernstein, 2004)
Pain management (Sterman et al, 2003; Kohr & Sawhney, 2005; Tapp & Kropp, 2005)
Preoperative teaching and hysterectomy outcomes (Oetker-Black et al, 2003)
Psychoeducational interventions and surgical patients (Cook & Devine, 1983; Devine & Cook, 1986; Hathaway, 1986).
Quality of life (Suhonem et al, 2005)
Telenursing (Jerant et al, 2003; Moscato et al, 2003)
Women and spouse caregivers of a relative with dementia (Coon, et al, 2003; Dibartolo & Soeken, 2003)

A growing body of teaching interventions has been studied in the practice setting, with diverse topics and instructional methods. Findings clearly demonstrate the positive impact of individual and organizational outcomes. Although these studies have strengths and weaknesses, they support the need for nurses to fully develop the educator role. See Table 14.14.

INSTRUCTIONAL MATERIALS

Instructional materials, the resources used to help communicate teaching information, help the nurse deliver the message more clearly, access more learning styles, and promote retention of the information. When a nurse teaches, the role goes beyond the dispensing of information; it also includes skill in designing and planning for the instruction. The nurse needs to know what instructional materials are available and how to select and use them and, in some cases, create them. Teaching is not printing something from a Web site without evaluating its usefulness, readability, and fit to the patient or employee. With instructional-material resources,

the teaching can be made more enjoyable, interesting, challenging, and effective for various learners.

Whatever instructional method is chosen, the nurse considers the characteristics of the learner, the task to be attained (which learning domain and the complexity of the teaching), and the media (print or nonprint) available for achieving the objectives. The three components of media delivery system (Weston & Cranston, 1986), content, and presentation (Frantz, 1980) must be considered. The delivery system is both the form of the media and the hardware with which to enact it. For example, a lecture may be enhanced by use of overhead transparencies, pictures, or PowerPoint slides; the hardware to use these methods may include a projector, computer, or classroom wiring. When reviewing content, the nurse considers its accuracy, relevance, appropriateness, readability, and currency. Presentation affects the way in which the content is delivered. For example, a simulation model could be used to demonstrate a procedure such as resuscitation; the employee learner could demonstrate the act of resuscitation to ensure accuracy and application of content. Samples of instructional materials are listed in Table 14.15.

When writing and designing instructional methods, there are guidelines that will ensure their use

Table 14.15 **Samples of Types of Instructional Materials**

Written Materials (most common form of instructional method)	Commercially Prepared Materials
Handouts	Brochures
Brochures	Posters
Leaflets	Pamphlets
Pamphlets	Patient texts
Books	Videotapes
Computer information downloaded from Web sites	Slides
	Audiotapes
	Audio and video teleconferencing
	Television
	Telephone
	E-mail contact
	Cable and satellite broadcasting
	Closed-circuit TV
	Computer games
	DVDs
	Compact discs (CDs)
	Web sites with streaming video

and effectiveness. These guidelines include the following: ensure accuracy and currency; organize the materials; keep information succinct; avoid medical jargon; keep readability levels at least two to four grades below the educational level of the target learners; include illustrations between the narrative; always state information in the positive and not the negative; follow a conversational style; use the second person "you" instead of the third person; use adequate spacing with ample "white space" to rest the eye; use a combination of upper- and lowercase letters, which are easier to read; write in the active voice; avoid detailed rationales that might overwhelm the reader; place most urgent and need-to-know first; move from the more concrete to the more abstract; and end with a review that highlights the important points.

The fastest growing form of instructional method is Web-based materials.

Older learners in particular like handouts that are more effective when combined with oral presentations; remember that visual deficits are common, and that short-term memory may be a difficulty for retaining oral-only information. Haggard (1989) stated that using ample white space is the most important element of improving the appearance of written material. This means double-spacing, leaving generous margins, indenting, bulleting short statements, bolding print, and inserting pictorial representations where possible. Redman (1993) believes that pictorial learning is better than verbal learning for recognition and recall. Pictures of animals, however, may be cute for children, but young children tend to interpret concretely; very young children might believe that real animals would be caring for them and could become frightened (Foster, 1987).

Demonstration media include nonprint media such as models, speakers, actual equipment, displays, posters, diagrams, illustrations, charts, bulletin boards, video presentations and clips, whiteboard/chalkboards, photographs, and drawings. Almost any nonprint media is included. Many Internet resources exist, including online library access, which is invaluable to the learner who has the ability to use it. All represent very unique ways of stimulating the visual senses and maybe the senses of touch, smell, and taste. Figure 14.6 provides easy information to assist in selecting media.

PLANNING INSTRUCTIONAL STRATEGIES

As the nurse develops an educational plan, certain teaching events are essential to success before, during, and after the educational situation. Consider how to capture the learner's attention: examples are presenting a problem, appealing to emotion through a story, using humor, asking questions, or sparking curiosity. Consider this as a "learner hook," or a means to draw him into the learning process. Tell the learners where you are going (objectives) with the learning episode, and remind them at the end of the experience so that material is tied together, and retention of material is promoted.

Encourage recall of previous learning as it relates to current teaching. Assist employees or patients to fit the learning to their schemata. For example, if they are unfamiliar with the terms used to manage their newly diagnosed diabetes, or as employees, unfamiliar with a new piece of equipment, identify these terms; perhaps a handout of terms would strengthen recall of the information.

Determine the teaching strategies that best address the learners, the environment, resources, time, and the objectives to be accomplished (psychomotor, cognitive, or affective domains of learning). Learning

Table 14.16 Retention of Learners

Learners retain:
- 10% of what they read.
- 20% of what they hear.
- 30% of what they see.
- 50% of what they see and hear.
- 70% of what they see and discuss.
- 90% of what they discuss and do.

Adapted from Heinich et al. (1992).

guidance takes many forms: direct telling (lecture), posing problem-solving situations, or creating discovery opportunities in experimental learning situations (facilitating). When choosing the learning modality, consider the known retention levels of learners in Table 14.16.

Learners with higher levels of anxiety seem to need more structured teaching strategies such as lecture and identification and recall-type questions. Less anxious learners are more open about more complex experiences, especially those requiring demonstration in front of peers. Discovery learning, however, is more permanent than a pure lecture method (Gagne, Briggs, & Wagner, 1992).

Performance or application of learning is a higher level of learner expectation than taking a test. Requiring application such as a return demonstration by the patient or employee is more of a challenge to the teacher and the learner. Assessing performance is necessary to ensure that the learner has accurately learned the information; this is especially vital when the information is essential to successful healthy daily living. For example, the diabetic patient needs to correctly inject the accurate dose of insulin. What better way to assess his performance than to watch him draw up and administer that dose. Feedback about his performance could be immediate and reinforced with praise and encouragement when completed accurately. The learner should retain the learning and be able to transfer it to his home or the employment setting. To assure that learning becomes more permanent, Bastable (2003) offers the following suggestions: be organized; pace the learning to accommodate the learner's ability to process information; minimize distractions, and make learning pleasant; help learners use information and skills soon after teaching; and promote retention and recall as frequently as possible.

Although creating nursing interventions that are learning situations is complex, with experience the teaching occurs faster, is more cost-effective, and attains more accuracy in learning outcomes. Consider the following case study introduces case study.

CASE SCENARIO 14.1

An 86-year-old woman, widowed for 10 years, was admitted to the hospital from the emergency room. She fell, and although injuries were limited to contusions, she has previously diagnosed early-stage Alzheimer's disease, a trial fibrillation, and osteoporosis. She also has bilateral lens implants. Earlier in the year her frailty and cognitive impairment caused her family to move her in with one of her middle-aged daughters. Other adult children live hundreds of miles away; they can assist financially and periodically with direct care arranged around their work schedules. The patient's strong church support exists in the city of her former home, about two hours from her present location; her daughter has a different religious belief system.

Initial findings show atypical cardiac rhythm patterns, an elevated ProTime of 14 (she takes Coumadin), gait difficulties, and muscle weakness in her lower limbs. Physical therapy (PT) and occupational therapy (OT) were ordered to assess and improve her mobility. She previously walked with no assistive devices. Her daughter at home managed her meals and medications. Born on a farm in 1919, she received a high-school education and one year of business school. She is health conscious and reads prolifically to maintain her quality of life. She reads the newspaper daily. She is 5'2" and weighs 98 pounds. Since moving to her daughter's home, she has gained 10 pounds. She is now concerned about her weight.

The hospital stay exceeded two weeks. Her heart rhythm and ProTime were stabilized. Due to the hospital's fall-risk program, she was confined to bed unless an employee mobilized her; her weakness increased with the bed rest. She was transferred three times during the hospitalization; each move increased confusion, which further impaired her short-term memory. The family decided that she would be discharged to the daughter's home with arrangements for at-home PT and OT visits. The family believed that her confusion would diminish in the familiar home environment. She is scheduled for discharge in three days.

As a nurse case manager, use the following critical-thinking questions, which came from your assessment information, to meet the patient's teaching/learning needs.

What are the patient's and caregiver's learning needs in these areas: mobility, medical diagnoses, medications, nutrition, safety, cognitive, social, and spiritual?

1. What learning theories and principles would best fit this discharge situation? Why?

2. Develop a teaching plan for the patient and her caregiver.

   A. List the prioritized, collaboratively determined, long- and short-term goals and objectives.

   B. Identify content and resources.

   C. Determine your educator role in the needed teaching, and select your methods of presenting and evaluating the information.

   D. Schedule the teaching sessions. What environmental factors and learner characteristics will you consider in implementing the sessions?

   E. What impact could the patient's caregiver's and developmental stages have on the educational process?

Table 14.17 **Teaching Tips to Improve Effectiveness**

1. Prepare, prepare, prepare.
2. Dress as a professional role model; obtain feedback from colleagues.
3. Use facial expressions when teaching information.
4. Don't read unless to emphasize a point.
5. Practice a presentation in front of a mirror.
6. Practice until the main points are memorized.
7. Use the least amount of written notes; write cues in margins (smile, walk, relax).
8. Minimize the physical barriers between the speaker and the audience; ask for a shorter lectern or table rather than using a podium.
9. Decrease information on slides, PowerPoints, handouts; use plenty of white space and check for accuracy, currency, and spelling. If available, get assistance from media departments for preparation.
10. Engage adult learners in the education process.
11. Be aware when "pet phrases" are used repeatedly (you know, like, well, uh); develop alternative phrases or words.
12. When nonwords (ah, um) are used, stop, take a deep breath, and then go on.
13. Make eye contact.
14. Speak to a large audience as if they were one learner.
15. Prepare, prepare, prepare.

Adapted from Woodring (1995).

THE TEACHER

Expert nurses don't just happen. The goal to be an expert nurse is a lifelong pursuit with a passion to be the most effective and best. This chapter presented an overview and survey of materials designed to focus the nurse's attention on developing the skills of a great teacher.

What are the techniques used by effective nurse/educators with patients and colleagues? Some suggestions are offered in Table 14.17. These enhance verbal presentations and generally may be used with a variety of instructional methods.

The role of educating in clinical practice can be one of the most challenging and important interventions

a nurse uses. To do it well, the nurse must be aware of its complexities and remain current in its evidence-based findings. Nevertheless, the learner is the single most important person in the education process. Learning can occur without an educator, but a facilitator who is prepared and knowledgeable while striving to move from novice to expert can enhance learning (Benner, 1984).

Chickering and Gamson (1987) developed seven principles of good teaching practice (see Table 14.18), which may be useful in teaching staff and patients. These principles ensure the most effective teaching and learning results when there is time to use the information. Not all principles apply to the demands of teaching patients on short notice, but they can guide the teacher in making adaptations.

Table 14.18 Good Practice Principles for Teaching

Good teaching practice encourages:

1. Student/teacher contact
2. Cooperation among learners
3. Active learning
4. Prompt feedback
5. Time on task
6. High expectations
7. Respect for diverse talents and ways of knowing

CHAPTER SUMMARY

As the largest health care provider group in developed countries, nurses can be powerful forces to teach the prevention of and rehabilitation from disease and injuries as well as to promote healthy behaviors and lifestyle changes. An astute nurse develops the expertise to effectively use the educational process. Learning theories and instructional methods were summarized as tools to apply in clinical learning situations that address patients, caregivers, and employees.

Learning theories may be better suited to different learners. Each learner is unique. Some learn through acting and responding (behaviorist), perceptions and thoughts (cognitive), and feelings and emotions (humanistic and psychodynamic). Almost all people learn from demonstration and role modeling (social). Learning is more complicated than any theory describes. Each theory, though, highlights information that affects the total educational process.

Although there is no single best theory, instructional design, instructional method, or teaching strategy, the nurse is encouraged to use an eclectic approach to educational opportunities. By avoiding reliance on any one method and by using a combination of teaching methods to accomplish desired objectives, the nurse/educator will more likely meet the information and skill needs of patient learners.

An evidence base of clinical teaching strategies adapted to learners, environments, special populations, and professional, agency, state and national expectations exists. This research demonstrates the effectiveness of well-designed instruction on improving desired patient and organizational outcomes. The research, however, is foundational. Many studies are unity specific, with small samples and findings that are not generalizable. Clearly, clinical teaching and learning is a wide-open field for future nurse researchers.

The clinical environments that employ nurses require employees to be effective and efficient with practice interventions such as teaching. By meeting learner needs, the nurse not only promotes effective patient outcomes but also ensures that the agency meets state and national mandates for teaching and, ultimately, reimbursement for care. Becoming an effective patient teacher is essential to the future of the health of individuals, families, and communities.

> *Call it prayers, call it what you like, but by saying "Help" and acknowledging our distress, we open ourselves to the vast powers of the universe as well as our own wisdom. And if we don't believe there is a power outside of us to listen, one very important person will have heard the call—you.*
>
> —Charlotte Davis Kasl, PhD

REFERENCES

Adams-Price, C. E. (1993). Age, education and literacy skills of adult Mississippians. *The Gerontologist, 33*(6), 741–746.

Aiken, L. H. (1988). Solutions to the nursing shortage bear repeating. *American Nurse, 20*(3), 4.

Aiken, L. H., Clark, S. P., Silber, J. H., Sloan, D. (2003). Hospital nurse staffing and patient mortality.

Bandura, A. (1977). *Social learning theory*. Englewood Cliffs, NJ: Prentice-Hall.

Bandura, A. (1986). *Foundations of thought and action: A social-cognitive theory*. Englewood Cliffs, NJ: Prentice-Hall.

Bastable, S. B. (2003) (Ed.). *Nurse as educator: Principles of teaching and learning for nursing practice*. (2nd ed.). Boston/Sudbury, MA: Jones and Bartlett.

Benner, P. (1984). *From novice to expert*. Menlo Park, CA: Addison-Wesley.

Benner, P. (1994). *Interpretive phenomenology*. Thousand Oaks, CA: Sage Publications.

Benner, P. (2000). The wisdom of our practice. *American Journal of Nursing, 100*(10), 99–105.

Bennett, J. A., Perrin, N. A., Hanson, G., Bennett, D., Gaynor, W., Flaherty-Robb, M., Joseph, C., Butterworth, S., & Potempa, K. (2005). Healthy aging demonstration project: Nurse coaching for behavior change in older adults. *Research in Nursing & Health, 28*, 187–197.

Bigge, M. I., & Shermis, S. S. (1992). *Learning theories for teachers* (5th ed.). New York: HarperCollins.

Bloom, B. (1968). *Learning for mastery*. Instruction and Curriculum. Topical Papers and Reprints No. 1. National Laboratory for Higher Education. Durham, NC.

Bonham, L. A. (1988). Learning style instruments: Let the buyer beware. *Lifelong Learning, 11*(6), 14–17.

Bower, K. A. (2004). Patient care management as a global nursing concern. *Nursing Administration Quarterly, 28*(1), 39–43.

Braungart, M. M., & Braungart, R. G.(1997). Learning theory and nursing practice. In S. Bastable (Ed.), *Nurse as educator: principles of teaching and learning*. Sudbury, MA: Jones and Bartlett.

Bruner, J. S. (1966). *Toward a theory of instruction*. Cambridge, MA: Harvard University Press.

Burgireno, J. (1985). Maximizing learning in the adult with SCI. *Rehabilitation Nursing, 10*(5), 20–21.

Burns, S. M., Earven, S., Fisher, C., Lewis, R., Merrell, P., Schubart, J.R., & Truwit, J.D. (2003). Implementation of an institutional program to improve clinical and financial outcomes of mechanically ventilated patients: One-year outcomes and lessons learned. *Critical Care Medicine, 31*(12), 2752–2763.

Buscaglia, L. (1982). *Living, loving and learning*. New York: Fawcett Columbine.

Chickering, A. W., & Gamson, Z. F. (1987). Principles for good practice in undergraduate education. *The Wingfield Journal, Special Insert*.

Coon, D. W., Thompson, L., Steffen, A., Sorocco, K., & Gallagher-Thompson, D. (2003). Anger and depression management: Psychoeducational skill training interventions for women caregivers of a relative with dementia. *The Gerontologist, 43*(5), 678–689.

Cowling, W. R. (2005). Despairing women and healthy outcomes: A unitary appreciative nursing perspective. *Advances in Nursing Science, 28*(2), 94–106.

Callen, L., Greiner, J., Bombei, C., & Comried, L. (2005). Excellence in evidence-based practice: Organizational and unit exemplars. *Critical Care Nursing Clinics of North America, 17*, 127–142.

Deaton, C., & Namasivayam, S. (2004). Nursing outcomes in coronary heart disease. *The Journal of Cardiovascular Nursing, 19*(5), 308–315.

Devine, E. C., & Cook, T. D. (1983). A meta-analytic analysis of effect of psychoeducational interventions on length of postsurgical hospital stay. *Nursing Research, 32* (September/October), 267–275.

Devine, E. C., & Cook, T. D. (1986). Clinical and cost-saving effects of psychoeducational interventions with surgical patients: A meta-analysis. *Research in Nursing and Health, 9* (June), 89–105.

DiBartolo, M. C., & Soeken, K. L. (2003). Appraisal, coping, hardiness, and self-perceived health in community-dwelling spouse caregivers of persons with dementia. *Research in Nursing & Health, 26*(6), 445–458.

Dickerson, P. S. (2003). Ten tips to help learning. *Journal for Nurses in Staff Development, 19*(5), 244–250.

Doak, C. C., Doak, L. G., & Root, J. H. (1985). *Teaching patients with low literacy skills*. (1st ed.). Phildadelphia: Lippincott.

Doak, C. C., Doak, L. G., & Root, J. H. (1996). *Teaching patients with low literacy skills*. (2nd ed.). Philadelphia: Lippincott.

Dunn, R. (1984). Learning style: State of the science. *Theory into Practice, 23* (1), 10–19.

Dunn, R., & Dunn, K. (1978). *Teaching students through their individual learning styles: A practical approach*. Reston, VA: National Association of Secondary School Principals.

Erikson, E. (1968). *Identity: Youth and crisis*. New York: Norton.

Fain, J. A. (1994a). Assessing nutrition education in clients with weak literacy skills. *Nurse Practitioner Forum, 5*(1), 52–55.

Fain, J. A.(1994b). When your patient can't read. *American Journal of Nursing, 94*(5), 16B, 16D.

Fleener, F. T., & Scholl, J. F. (1992). Academic characteristics of self-identified illiterates. *Perceptual and Motor Skills, 74*(3), 739–744.

Friedman, P., & Alley, R. (1984). Learning/teaching styles: Applying the principles. *Theory into Practice, 23*(1), 77–81.

Fuzard, B. (1995). *Innovative teaching strategies in nursing.* 2nd ed. Gaithersburg, MD: Aspen.

Gagne, R. M., Briggs, L. J., & Wagner, W. W. (1992). *Principles of instructional design* (4th ed.). New York: Holt, Rinehart and Winston.

Gallagher, R. M., & Rowell, P. A. (2003). Claiming the future of nursing through nursing-sensitive quality indicators. *Nursing Administration Quarterly, 27*(4), 273–284.

Gregorc, A. F. (1982). *An adult's guide to style.* Maynard, MA: Gabriel Systems.

Guild, P. B., & Garger, S. (1998). *Marching to different drummers* (2nd ed.). Alexandria, VA: Association for Supervision and Curriculum Development.

Haggard, A. (1989). *Handbook of patient education.* Rockville, MD: Aspen.

Hammer, J. B. (2005). State of the science: Posthospitalization nursing interventions in congestive heart failure. *Advances in Nursing Science, 28*(2), 175–190.

Hathaway, D. (1986). Effect of preoperative instruction on postoperative outcomes: A meta-analysis. *Nursing Research, 35* (September/October), 269–275.

Havighurst, R. (1976). Human characteristics and school learning: Essay review. *The Elementary School Journal, 77*, 101–109.

Healthcare Education Association. (1985). *Managing hospital education.* Laquana Niquel, CA.

Heinich, R., Malenda, M., & Russelll, J. D. (1992). *Instructional media and the new technologies of instruction* (4th ed.). New York: Macmillan.

Huyck, M. H., & Hoyer, W. J. (1982). *Adult development and aging.* Belmont, CA: Wadsworth.

Jerant, A. F., Azari, R., Martinez, C., & Nesbitt, T. S. (2003). A randomized trial of telenursing to reduce hospitalization for heart failure: Patient-centered outcomes and nursing indicators. *Home Health Care Services Quarterly, 22*(1), 1–20.

Kleinpell, R. M. (2004). Randomized trial of an intensive care unit-based on early discharge planning intervention for critically ill elderly patients. *American Journal of Critical-Care Nurses, 13*(4), 335–345.

Knowles, M. (1990). *The adult learner: A neglected species* (4th ed.). Houston, TX: Gulf.

Kohr, R., & Sawhney, M. (2005). Advanced practice nurses' role in the treatment of pain. *The Canadian Nurse, 101*(3), 30–34.

Kolb, D. A. (1984). *Experiential learning: Experience as the source of learning and development.* Englewood Cliffs, NJ: Prentice-Hall.

Kramer, D. A. (1983). Post-formal operations? A need for further conceptualization. *Human Development, 26*, 91–105.

Kreulen, G., & Braden, C. (2004). Model test of the relationship between self-help-promoting nursing interventions and self-care and health status outcomes. *Research in Nursing & Health, 27*, 97–109.

Kubler-Ross, E. (1969). *On death and dying.* New York: Macmillan.

Lankshear, A. J., Sheldon, R. A., & Maynard, A. (2005). Nurse staffing and healthcare outcomes: A systematic review of the international research evidence. *Advances in Nursing Science, 28*(2), 163–174.

Lee, W., & Owens, D. (2000). *Multimedia-based instructional design: Computer-based training, Web-based training, distance broadcast training.* San Francisco, CA: Jossey-Bass.

Lichtenthal, C. (1990). *A Self-study Model on Readiness to Learn.* Unpublished.

Mark, B. A., Salyer, J., & Thomas, T. H. (2003). Professional nursing practice: Impact on organizational and patient outcomes. *Journal of Nursing Administration, 33*(4), 224–234.

Maslow, A. H. (1943). A theory of human motivation. *Psychological Review, 50*(4), 371–396.

Maslow, A. (1954). *Motivation and personality.* New York: Harper & Row.

Matthews, P. J., Thornton, L., & McLean, L. (1988). Reading-level scores of patient education materials and the effect of teaching special vocabulary. *Respiratory Care, 33*(4), 245–249.

McCarthy, B. (1981). *The 4Mat System: Teaching to learning styles with right/left mode techniques.* Barrington, IL: Excel.

McGinnis, J. M. (1993). The role of patient education in achieving national health objectives. *Patient Education and Counseling, 21*, 1–3.

Meade, C. D., & Wittbrot, R. (1988). Computerized readability analysis of written materials. *Computers in Nursing, 6*(1), 30–36.

Melnyk, B. M., Small, L., & Carno, M. A. (2004). The effectiveness of parent-focused interventions in improving coping/mental health outcomes of critically ill children and their parents: An evidence base to guide clinical practice. *Pediatric Nursing, 30*(2), 143–148.

Miller, B., & Bodie, M. (1994). Determination of reading comprehension level for effective patient health-education materials. *Nursing Research, 43*(2), 118–119.

Mishel, M. H. (1990). Reconceptualization of the uncertainty in illness theory. *Image: Journal of Nursing Scholarship, 22*(4), 256–262.

Moscato, S. R., David, M., Valanis, B., Gullion, C. M., Tanner, C., Shapiro, C., Izumi, S., & Mayo, A. (2003). Tool development for measuring caller satisfaction and outcome with telephone advice nursing. *Clinical Nursing Research, 12*(3), 266–281.

Munro, N. (2004). Evidence-based assessment: No more pride or prejudice. *AACN Clinical Issues, 15*(4), 501–505.

Myers, I. B. (1980). *Gifts differing*. Palo Alto, CA: Consulting Psychologists Press.

Oetker-Black, S. L., Jones, S., Estok, P., Ryan, M., Gale, N., & Parker, G. (2003, June). Preoperative teaching and hysterectomy outcomes. *AORN Journal, 77*(6), 1215–1218, 1221–1231.

Piaget, J., & Inhelder, B. (1969). *The psychology of the child* (H. Weaver, Trans.) New York: Random House.

Pontieri-Lewis, V. (2005), Management of gastrointestinal fistulas: A case study. *Medsurg Nursing: Official Journal of the Academy of Medical-Surgical Nurses, 14*(1), 68–72.

Radwin, L. (2000). Oncology patients' perceptions of quality nursing care. *Research in Nursing & Health, 23*, 179–190.

Redman, B. K. (1993). *The process of patient education* (7th ed.). St. Louis: Mosby.

Richards, E. (2003). Motivation, compliance, and health behaviors of the learner. In S. Bastable (Ed.), *Nurse as educator: Principles of teaching and learning for nursing practice*. Boston: Jones and Bartlett.

Riegel, K. F. (1973). Dialectic operations: The final period of cognitive development. *Human Development, 16*, 346–370.

Rogers, C. (1961). *On becoming a person*. Boston: Houghton Mifflin.

Rogers, C. (1994). *Freedom to learn*. New York: Merrill.

Ruzicki, D. A., (1989). Realistically meeting the educational needs of hospitalized acute and short-stay patients. *Nursing Clinics of North America, 24*(3), 583–587.

Sherif, C. W. (1976). *Orientation in social psychology*. New York: Harper & Row.

Sherif, M., & Sherif, C. W. (1969). *Social psychology*. New York: Harper & Row.

Shultz, C. M. (2006; in process). Affective learning. *In publication yet to be named*. New York: National League for Nursing Press.

Sidani, S., & Graden, C. J. (1998). *Evaluating nursing intervention: A theory-driven approach*. Thousand Oaks, CA: Sage.

Skinner, B. F. (1954). The science of learning and the art of teaching. *Harvard Educational Review, 24*, 86–97.

Skinner, B. F. (1974). *About behaviorism*. New York: Vintage Books.

Skinner, B. F. (1989). *Recent issues in the analysis of behavior*. Columbus, OH: Merrill.

Smith, C. E., Koehler, J., Moore, J. M., Blanchard, E., & Ellerbeck, E. (2005). *Testing videotape education for heart failure, 14*(2), 191–205.

Sterman, E., Gauker, S., & Krieger, J. (2003). Continuing education: A comprehensive approach to improving cancer pain management and patient satisfaction. *Oncology Nursing Forum, 30*(5), 857–864.

Stewart, J. L. (2003). Children living with chronic illness: An examination of their stressors, coping responses, and health outcomes. *Annual Review of Nursing Research, 21*, 203–243.

Suhonen, R., Valimaki, M., & Leino-Kilpi, H. (2005). Individualized care, quality of life and satisfaction with nursing care. *Journal of Advanced Nursing, 50*(3), 283–292.

Suen, L. (2005). Educational innovation. Teaching epidemiology using WebCT: Application of the seven principles of good practice. *Journal of Nursing Education, 44*(3), 143–146.

Tapp, J., & Kropp, D. (2005). Evaluating pain management delivered by direct care nurses. *Journal of Nursing Care Quality, 20*(2), 167–173.

Tiedje, L. B. (2004). Teaching is more than telling: Education about prematurity in a prenatal clinic waiting room. *American Journal of Maternal Child Nursing, 29*(6), 373–379.

Trossman, S. (1999). The professional portfolio: Documenting who you are, what you do. *The American Nurse, 31*(2), 1–2.

Wagner, S. P., & Ash, K. L. (1998). Creating the teachable moment. *Journal of Nursing Education, 37*(6), 278–280.

Whittemore, R., Melkus, F. D., Sullivan, A., & Grey, M. (2004). A nurse-coaching intervention for women with type 2 diabetes. *The Diabetes Educator, 30*(5), 795–804.

Wonder, J., & Donovan, M. (1984). *Whole-brain thinking*. New York: Ballantine.

Wong, F. K., Mok, M. P., Chan, T., & Tsang, M. W. (2005). Issues and innovations in nursing practice: Nurse follow-up of patients with diabetes: Randomized controlled trial. *Journal of Advanced Nursing, 50*(4), 391–402.

Woodring, B. (1995). Lecture is not a four-letter word. *Innovative Teaching Strategies in Nursing.* (2nd ed.). Gaithersburg, MD: Aspen.

Zanchetta, C., & Bernstein, M. (2004). The nursing role in patient education regarding outpatient neurosurgical procedures. *Axone, 25*(4), 18–21.

CHAPTER 15

Change Agent

Cesarina Thompson and Linda Wagner

Be the change that you wish to see in the world.
—Gandhi

LEARNING OBJECTIVES

At the completion of the chapter, the learner should be able to do the following:

1. Discuss the role of the nurse as a change agent.
2. Describe traditional and contemporary perspectives on facilitating change.
3. Demonstrate knowledge of leadership competencies required to facilitate change and participate in organizational growth.
4. Determine own level of leader/change agent competencies.
5. Identify effective leadership/change strategies and resources to implement change.
6. Apply change theories and concepts to practice situations.

KEY TERMS

Change	Deep change	Planned change
Change agent	First-order change	Second-order change
Change theory	Leadership	Servant leadership
Chaos Complexity theory	Learning organization	Transformational leadership

INTRODUCTION

As the health care system grows increasingly complex, professionals who possess the skills to adapt with the environment will be needed. An important reason for developing leadership potential is that nurses can then influence change instead of reacting to change planned by others. One of the greatest challenges to preparing nurses is to redefine the caregiver role to include leadership as a key component. Essential skills such as communication, collaboration, team building, problem solving, and vision

(Allen, 1998; Bondas, 2003; Ward, 2002) allow the practicing nurse to participate in the ever-changing health care organization. One of the most important ways to develop nursing leaders is through reinforcement of self-confidence and mentoring (Wieck, Prydun, & Walsh, 2002). Not only do nurses require patient-care skills to care for their families and patients, but they also must begin to internalize leadership qualities and values early on in their careers.

OVERVIEW OF THE RN AS LEADER AND CHANGE AGENT

Contemporary theories of leadership articulate that leadership is about who we are. There is a strong sense of ethical behavior, values, integrity, and relationship building. One way to begin to develop as a leader is to reflect on everyday experiences and establish a foundation for change (Johns, 2004). The process of reflection supports Goleman's (1998) research on emotional intelligence and leadership. His work found that emotional intelligence proved to be twice as important as intellect or cognitive skills when it came to jobs at all levels. The five components identified in emotional intelligence were self-awareness, self-regulation, motivation, empathy, and social skill. The process of reflection assists in developing self-awareness. Characteristics of self-regulation include comfort with ambiguity, change, and integrity. Goleman's (1998) other traits of motivation, empathy, and social skill are all reflective of current leadership literature wherein relationship building, collaboration, and thoughtful consideration are essential.

Transformational leadership refers to a process whereby the leader connects to followers such that the relationship is empowering, motivating, and intellectually stimulating. Burns (1978) defined transformational leadership as being able to clearly communicate a vision, empower the work group to accomplish goals, and provide mentoring to staff. Johns (2004) believes that transformational leaders

should invest in people and collaborative ways of relating, instead of using people as a means to an end, which is more reflective of transactional leadership. It is important not to sacrifice personal integrity.

Similar to transformational leadership is servant leadership, which was first discussed by Robert Greenleaf (1991) in a text titled *The Servant as Leader*. Greenleaf believed that a priority in leadership was to make sure that other people's needs were addressed first (see Figure 15.1). Based on a philosophy of caring behavior and teamwork, the following characteristics are central to the servant leader: listening, empathy, healing, awareness, persuasion, conceptualization, foresight, stewardship, commitment to growth of people, and community building. Spears (2004) summarizes these as listening to what others have to say, expressing empathy, understanding the lessons of the past and how they influence the future, having an awareness of self and the situation, demonstrating the ability to convince and persuade others, balancing the dream with the day-to-day, building community within the workplace, practicing the art of contemplation, and exerting a healing influence upon others.

Years later, Max DePree (1992) elaborated on Greenleaf's work with several texts, one of which was *Leadership Jazz*. In one of his stories, he describes going into a tennis club and picking up the towels left behind. His friend asked him, "Do you pick up towels because you're the president of a company, or are you the president because you pick up the towels?" (DePree, 1992, p. 219). At the core of his philosophy on leadership is the essence of caring, related so eloquently in his prologue. After visiting his granddaughter in the neonatal intensive care unit, where the nurse instructed him that it was important for him to use touch and his voice to connect, he concluded that "at the core of becoming a leader is the need always to connect one's voice and one's touch" (p. 3).

The work of implementing change is often the work of the nurse/leader. Nurse/leaders who practice from the perspective of servant leadership or transformational leadership value the constituents they work with and consider the ramifications that the change will have on employees or patients and

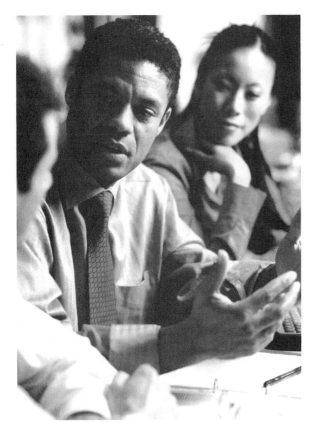

Figure 15.1 Central to the philosophy of servant leadership is caring behavior and teamwork. Photo courtesy of Photodisc.

families. Understanding the context within which people work assists the leader in developing a plan with the least amount of resistance, and one that is the most supported by others.

An example of an area where leadership and an understanding of the change process are important is in the critical-care area. Nurse/managers and staff nurse/leaders must respond to changing economic conditions, high census, and ever-changing technology (Contino, 2004). Contino outlines leadership competencies and highlights the fact that nurses must understand how to anticipate and implement change. It is critical to understand why nurses resist or accept change and to mentor and support them through the change process.

The organization in which one works greatly affects the leader's ability to influence change in a positive manner. A reciprocal relationship is created when the leader is able to create relationships that foster growth, and when the organization supports the leader in doing so (Wagner, 2005). Key components of a synergistic relationship are listening, trust and compassion, caring, and supporting another's growth (Wagner, 2005).

Covey (1991) identifies seven habits of effective leadership that reflect building and sustaining synergistic relationships among members of an organization with the overall goal of enhancing quality. The seven habits are (1) being proactive: be self-aware, have a personal vision, and take necessary actions based on principles that will benefit the organization; (2) beginning with the end in mind: develop a personal and organizational mission that will guide all initiatives and focus more on those activities that will help to achieve the mission; (3) putting first things first: this habit is closely related to the previous one in that it emphasizes the need to focus energy on the bigger picture and on the priorities that are related to the goals and mission of the organization. Covey notes that typically people spend a lot of time prioritizing their day-to-day tasks, rather than focusing on activities related to the long-term objectives; (4) thinking win-win: build relationships that will benefit all stakeholders and foster collaboration; (5) seeking first to understand, then to be understood: try to see the world through others' eyes, mind, and heart by using empathic communication that helps the leader to clearly understand another's ideas; (6) synergizing: a popular idea, reflected in contemporary leadership theories, that the "whole is greater than the sum of its parts." Employees and managers working collaboratively can accomplish much more than by working independently or against each other. Establishing trust and providing appropriate professional development programs enables employees to enhance their capabilities and improve their performance; and (7) sharpening the saw: in order to grow and develop, people must continue to learn and acquire new knowledge and skills in order to continuously improve their performance and ultimately the total quality of the organization.

This last habit is closely related to Senge's (1990) notion of the **learning organization,** "an organization that is continually expanding its capacity to create its future" (p. 14). As the future becomes more complex, change will occur not only in the organizations where we work, but in ourselves as well. Those individuals who are able to reflect on how change affects them personally will make an easier transition in changing times. Another aspect of the learning organization is that we are all connected and part of the larger whole. This concept is the cornerstone, or "fifth discipline," which is systems thinking. The other four key components are personal mastery, mental models, building shared vision, and team learning.

Personal mastery involves a lifelong commitment to learning, being creative, and challenging the status quo. Mental models are "deeply ingrained assumptions, generalizations, or even pictures or images that influence how we understand the world and how we take action (Senge, 1990, p. 8). A shared vision is created when there is a common aspiration that provides energy for learning. Dialogue is essential in team learning and building a shared vision, wherein each supports the other.

A learning organization is created when there is a culture that is open to creating "the opportunities for risk taking and growth, for exploring the total self (mind, body, spirit), and a place to practice and encourage self-care" (Kerfoot & Wantz, 2003). Nurse leaders and change agents will realize that each individual experiences change differently; but with a basic understanding of the change process, open communication, and supportive relationships, growth of both individuals and organizations is possible.

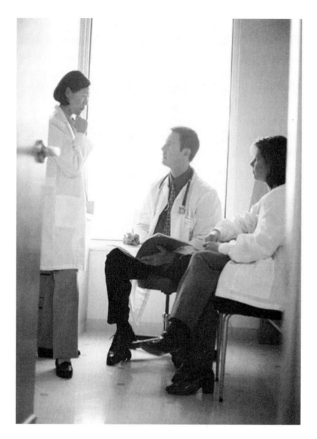

Figure 15.2 In order for change to be successful, all affected parties should be part of the decision-making process.

CHANGE THEORY

Think of a recent change that happened in your life. How did you feel? How open were you to the thought of new opportunities or experiences? Most people do not have positive feelings toward change. We feel more comfortable maintaining the status quo or knowing what our routine is. Change, however, is inevitable and occurs frequently. Technology, biomedical advances, financial constraints, and staff turnover all affect our work environments and patient care. As a staff nurse, adapting an attitude of being open to change and wanting to participate in the process will not only strengthen leadership skills, but the profession of nursing and patient care will be advanced in the process.

There are many definitions and types of **change.** Lippitt, Langseth, and Mossop (1985) commented that "[c]hange lies at the heart of organization development, and it has as its target the elements of growth, effectiveness, and excellence, thus implying that the organization is an open system and capable of improvement on individual, group and organization levels" (p. 28). There is planned change and unplanned change. Change also happens personally, professionally, and organizationally. Learning the skills to recognize, monitor, and facilitate whatever kind of change one encounters in the work area is an important, yet often-complex skill for nurses to learn.

TRADITIONAL CHANGE THEORIES

Lewin's (1951) Force Field Model is often used to illustrate **planned change.** The three stages of unfreezing, movement, and refreezing characterize the process of moving through an anticipated change and what factors should be considered. In the unfreezing stage, participants are motivated to get ready for the change. People often resist change. As one moves through to a new approach, education and support are needed to facilitate the process. A carefully planned process will help create a supportive environment. Providing feedback as well as opportunities to voice concern and encourage the new behavior are positive actions that the **change agent**/leader can make. During the refreezing stage, new behaviors have to be reinforced and assimilated. Evaluating the process and continuing to reinforce the new behavior are important parts of this stage. Essential to the outcome of this process is understanding the dynamics of the group, and what the group member's desires for change are as well as their capacity for resistance to change.

Assessment of the driving and restraining forces of change is ongoing during this process. Driving forces are those behaviors that will facilitate the change, while restraining forces are those behaviors that impede change or make it more difficult. The successful leader or manager will perform a thorough assessment of the environment, culture, and staff

Table 15.1 Comparison of Traditional Change Theories

Lewin (1951) Force Field Model	Lippitt (1958) Phases of Change
1. Unfreezing	1. Diagnose problem
	2. Assess motivation and capacity for change
	3. Assess change agent's motivation
2. Movement	4. Accurate selection of change objectives
	5. Choose an appropriate role for change agent
3. Refreezing	6. Maintain change
	7. Termination of relationship

behaviors and values before beginning to unfreeze the current situation.

Lippitt (1973) expanded on Lewin's model by focusing more on what the change agent must do and described seven stages in the change process. These stages are (1) diagnosis of the problem, (2) assessment of the motivation and capacity for change, (3) assessment of the change agent's motivation and resources, (4) selecting progressive change objectives, (5) choosing the appropriate role for the change agent, (6) maintenance of change, and (7) termination of the relationship.

CONTEMPORARY PERSPECTIVES ON CHANGE

Although the traditional views on leading change as described by Lewin and Lippitt provide what seem to be step-by-step approaches or structures for planning change, the process of actually implementing change is perhaps the more challenging task. Bauman (1998) outlines five requisites for implementing change: (1) cultivate a winning attitude among stakeholders by defining the organization's purpose and mission into something that is of importance to the people involved; (2) use "balanced empowerment" by establishing the overall vision for the organization and outlining the roles of employees, but then having the employees participate in planning and implementing changes; (3) provide continuous learning opportunities for employees to improve processes (e.g., team-building skills); (4) use strategic communication to explain to employees why the change is necessary and how it will benefit them, and (5) incorporate the desired behaviors in performance evaluations or other processes to measure and foster the internalization of the desired behaviors.

Quinn (1996) describes the process of "deep change" that must occur at a personal and an organizational level in order for an organization to be truly transformed. Quinn identifies three paradigms of organizational life: technical, transactional, and transformational. New members in an organization typically see themselves as "individual contributors" who need to achieve "technical" competence for their role to succeed. The focus is more on personal survival than on the overall success of the organization.

As one moves from the role of the individual contributor to that of manager, a new paradigm must be adopted: that of political transaction, to experience success in this new role. Using this paradigm, the manager realizes that one's technical expertise is not enough to bring about change. Rather, the manager must learn to continually negotiate and compromise with others within the organization in order to bring about the desired change.

Although the use of this paradigm requires managers to expand their perspective from an individual to a group level, generally the transactional paradigm promotes a focus on personal role performance that will merit advancement within the organization. When faced with challenges and conflicts, transactional managers typically take the "politically correct" approach by using strategic communication techniques and compromise. As Quinn (1996) explains, this is the type of behavior typically reinforced in organizations.

The most complex of the three paradigms is the transformational. In Quinn's view, the use of the transformational paradigm is what distinguishes a leader from a manager. The transformational leader is more concerned with realizing the vision than with personal survival. As Quinn (1996) notes, "a leader must walk the walk and talk the talk. Every action must be in alignment with the vision" (p. 125). The transformational leader is a visionary and risk taker, who is not necessarily limited by the boundaries of the organization. Transformational leaders are internally driven and guided by morals and values "that are more powerful than the political interests of any particular coalition" (p. 127). The realization of the vision is their most important goal. Obviously, adopting this paradigm is not easy and requires a deep personal change and commitment that will facilitate deep change within an organization.

Quinn (1996) identifies two types of changes: first order and second order. First-order change typically focuses on specific improvements, such as changes in a particular procedure to improve safety. First-order changes might involve only a few people or a small department within an organization. In contrast, second-order change aims to transform processes across departments or across the entire organization. These types of changes require the skills of a transformational leader.

In a more recent publication, Quinn (2004) expounds on strategies for effective change. He identifies three common strategies used by leaders/managers to facilitate change: the telling, forcing, and participating strategies. Although each of these strategies might be effective in certain situations, they are not useful in promoting the type of commitment required for long-lasting, deep change. Using the telling strategies, the leader provides employees with the facts and reasons for implementing the change. This might be an effective strategy when change is desired from a group that is not highly invested in the process. If this strategy is not successful, the forcing strategy might be employed. As the name implies, the leader/manager forces the change by leveraging power or authority. Obviously this is not the most effective strategy to promote long-lasting change and commitment from employees.

The participating strategy reflects a collaborative approach whereby the leader/manager considers feedback and suggestions offered by those who will be affected by the change in order to develop a win-win solution (see Figure 15.2). As Quinn notes (2004), this last strategy has been widely advocated in recent years as a successful leadership strategy. However, even this does not produce lasting effects if it is used as a manipulative technique.

A fourth and more effective change strategy used by transformational leaders is the transcending strategy. Its aim is to transcend self and others and to focus on realizing the vision; not limiting oneself by the current reality, but seeing the emerging possibilities. This is the most difficult strategy to employ because it requires the leader to have a high tolerance for ambiguity and uncertainty and yet still trust that the journey of transformation will be worthwhile.

Even the most gifted leaders, however, should realize that people are, by nature, creatures of habit. Most people do not willingly embrace change. According to Lawrence (1998), an effective leader needs to "create a sense of readiness" for change. This may involve a labor-intensive process to help people recognize the need for change and have them participate in creating the solutions. Similarly, Kotter (1995) states that the first phase of a change process is to establish a "great enough sense of urgency" in order to elicit collaboration. Leaders must provide a compelling argument for the change and outline the threats that can be avoided as well as the opportunities to be gained by implementing the change. Lack of attention to this phase is a primary reason for the failure of transformation efforts (Kotter, 1995).

COMPLEXITY/CHAOS THEORY

Similar in many regards to the nursing process, planned change theories (e.g., Lewin's model) move from one stage to the next and are often linear in nature. They work well for simple planned change; however, they often do not work well in complex, ever-changing organizations. Today's health care organizations are excellent examples of such dynamic and complex institutions. Although traditional leadership and management theories that emphasized planning, organizing, implementing, and evaluating were effective tools for leaders during the Industrial Age, when organizations were hierarchical and linear in nature, they will not be as effective for leaders of complex organizations (Porter-O'Grady & Malloch, 2003).

The developing science of complexity has taught us that everything in our universe is linked in some way. The connections among elements create dynamic patterns that are typically nonlinear and unpredictable in nature (Quinn, 2000; Vicenzi, White, & Begun, 1997). Scientists have identified various types of complex systems, including chaotic, stable, and bounded instability. In a constantly chaotic system, actions are random, and elements behave independently of one another, leading to the eventual failure of the system. Obviously, this is not a desirable state for organizations. In contrast, stable systems are characterized by structure, control, and highly predictable actions. Although this sounds like a more desirable state, it too can eventually lead to system failure as the system becomes stagnant and unresponsive to outside stimuli (Quinn, 2000).

It is human nature to strive for stability in our personal and professional lives. However, the emerging science of **chaos and complexity** suggests that change and creativity cannot occur if we do not experience some form of chaos. A system in the state of bounded instability has structure and boundaries, but also has some instability or chaos. As Quinn (2000) describes, "[a] system based on bounded instability has the capacity to self-organize, and thus to respond to the changing environment and move naturally to higher levels of complexity and integration. Self organizing processes tend to be transformational" (p. 150).

Based on what we have learned from complexity science, leaders cannot rely on the traditional methods of identifying goals and directing all activities toward the achievement of those goals because events are not always predictable. Furthermore, some level of instability is actually desirable within a system or organization in order to foster change and higher levels of functioning. This latter point is similar to Kotter's (1995) idea that a great enough sense of urgency must be created for people to embrace change. A degree of instability, or chaos, may serve as the catalyst for change.

To be effective in complex environments, leaders must not only deal with the present reality, but also live in the "potential reality." As Porter-O'Grady and Malloch (2003) explain, in a chaotic era, leaders cannot rely on traditional methods of leadership by which goals and activities can be easily identified, but must act more as "managers of a journey," in which the goal is not always clear and might change over time. Leaders must be able to "fluidly respond to current demands and changing circumstances, remain open to the messages carried by longer term indicators, and act in accordance with these messages" (p. 4).

MOTIVATION

Whether someone is trying to get staff to change within an organization or to work with patients and families to facilitate change, an understanding of motivation is essential. Changing behaviors or changing values and beliefs involves an assessment of both internal and external factors. An understanding of the cognitive, behavioral, and biological factors of human nature allows both the nurse manager working with staff or the nurse working with patients to utilize strategies to successfully influence change.

Herzberg (2003) conducted studies on what motivated workers in the 1950s. He concluded that "hygiene factors" or external conditions such as salary, benefits, and working conditions lead to job dissatisfaction. Determinants such as achievement, recognition, responsibility and advancement, or "internal" factors motivated workers. This behavioral theory based on need corresponds with Maslow's Hierarchy of Needs, in which basic needs have to be satisfied before higher level needs can be. Creating

an environment in which these needs can be met promotes satisfied and enthusiastic employees.

Breisch (1999) articulates that today's nurse managers must be sensitive to creating a work environment that supports staff through these tumultuous times with an understanding of what motivates or creates dissatisfied workers. Her suggestions are to address staff needs, promote accountability, encourage success, communicate with the group, and ease resistance to change. Hill (2004) expands on Breisch's suggestions by also acknowledging that different generations of employees have different values for what motivates them. For instance, Generation Y (those 22 years old or younger) is motivated by technological advances and expressiveness, whereas the baby boomer population (those 40 to 61 years old) may be motivated by different factors.

Other researchers contend that this view is not as popular today, with other variables such as equity, achievement, and camaraderie becoming more important across generations and types of jobs (Sirota, Mischkind, & Meltzer, 2005). Table 15.2 illustrates the variables that Sirota, Mischkind, and Meltzer found in their research on human motivation in the workplace. Their data were gathered from questionnaire surveys administered from 1994 to 2003 with 2,537,656 respondents.

An understanding of these theories also facilitates a therapeutic intervention plan with patients and families. It is important to assess a client's motivation and readiness to learn, who is available to support them through a change, and if they feel they will be successful. Current research has suggested that individuals can change their behavior if they learn how to set goals and deter self-doubt and anxiety (Franken, 2002).

An alternative theory based on arousal and attention to a specific behavior was first discussed by Easterbrook (1959, as cited in Franken 2002). To facilitate change in individuals, one must create situations in which the individual's state of arousal pertaining to a particular issue is increased. Doing so fosters greater attention to the issue at hand and to behaviors that are congruent with change. When arousal levels become too high, however, a state of

Table 15.2 **Three Factor Theory of Human Motivation in the Workplace**

Equity	Achievement	Camaraderie
Safety	Challenge of the work itself	Relationship between coworkers
Respect	Acquiring new skills	Teamwork within the work unit
Management credibility	Ability to perform	Teamwork across departments
	Perceived importance	
	Recognition for performance	
	Working for a company of which the employee can be proud	

SOURCE: Sirota, Mischkind, and Meltzer (2005).

anxiety is produced and too little attention is placed on change behaviors. Whether or not an individual experiences anxiety has been linked to how they appraise a situation. For example, if a patient is asked to develop an exercise plan to lose weight, an anxious person may not be able to focus on the task, creating a fear of failure and a feeling of being threatened (Franken, 2002). Sensory overload can also lead to high arousal and stress resulting in a shortened attention span. Interventions such as relaxation, eliminating distractions, and setting priorities will all assist in regulating arousal levels so that clients can engage in change and learning.

One additional model on motivating clients to engage in healthy behaviors worth discussing is Prochaska and DiClemente's (1983) Transtheoretical Model of Behavior Change. The six stages of this model have been identified as precontemplation, contemplation, preparation, action, maintenance,

and relapse. In the precontemplation stage, there are no plans for change within the next six months. During contemplation, the individual considers change within three months. In preparation, there is intent to take action within the next 30 days, whereas in action, the change has occurred and there is a risk of relapse. Maintenance indicates that the change has been sustained for at least six months.

Croghan (2005) and Duran (2003) highlight the application of this model with patient care scenarios and interviewing questions. They stress that it is important for nurses to assess motivation and readiness to change.

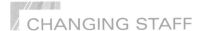

CHANGING STAFF

CASE SCENARIO 15.1

John was hired recently as the new nurse/manager on an adult health unit of a community hospital. He has been a nurse for about

10 years and brings a broad range of adult-health and critical-care experience to his new position. He also recently received his Master's degree in

Nursing with a focus on administration. Most of the nurses on John's unit have been employed there for several years. Although a few of the nurses have a BSN, the majority do not.

At a recent management meeting, nurse/managers and senior administrators engaged in a discussion on evidence-based practice. The consensus among the members of the leadership group was that this model of practice should be the standard throughout the organization in order to improve the quality of care. John and his fellow nurse/managers are given the task of implementing this change in practice on their units.

Case Considerations

1. Identify some of the challenges that John will face in introducing this change to his staff.

2. What strategies can he use to minimize resistance to this change?

3. Select some strategies that he can employ to facilitate this change process.

CHANGING FAMILIES AND INDIVIDUALS

Both planned change theories and the more modern approach to change can be used by nurses to influence change in families and individuals.

Nurses utilize strategies every day to get patients to change diets, stop smoking, exercise more, and lose weight. Evidence-based practice allows nurses to incorporate several theories in order to provide the best care. Knowledge of motivation theory, conflict and negotiation theories, and **change theory** enhance the nurses' ability to provide health education.

RESEARCH APPLICATION ARTICLE

Clark, B., Rapkin, K., Busen, N., & Vasquez, E. (2001). Nurse practitioners and parent education: A partnership for health. *Journal of the American Academy of Nurse Practitioners*. pp. 310–316. Substance-abusing mothers face a host of challenges related to raising their children. Effective parenting requires knowledge of health promotion, growth, and child development. A study by Clark, Rapkin, Busen, and Vasquez (2001) selected substance-abusing mothers currently in recovery to participate in a parenting-education program, entitled Healthy Children, Happy Children, conducted by nurse practitioners. The theoretical framework chosen for this study was Change Theory and Mercer's Theory of Maternal Role Attainment. The education program was the instrument of change as the women experienced an unfreezing of their previous role as an addict, and looked forward to their new role as responsible parent. Thirty-seven mothers participated in the twelve-week curriculum on well-child care and sick-child management. Pre- and posttests revealed that test scores went up after the education sessions, with the average posttest scores exceeding 80 percent. During the "refreezing" process, role modeling continued by the facility and childcare staff, supporting the mothers in adapting to their new role.

CASE SCENARIO 15.2

Margarite is a young Mexican mother with a 3-year-old son and a newborn baby boy. She speaks little English and needs an interpreter for health education and explanation of care. Josue was born four weeks early, with an atrial septal defect and other congenital abnormalities. He was hospitalized for an acute respiratory infection. Margarite is rooming in and breast-feeding Josue. During the course of hospitalization, it was noted that Josue was below the fifth percentile for weight, and the pediatrician and cardiologist wanted to supplement Josue's breast-feeding with formula bottles in order to boost him nutritionally before surgery. Margarite had been reluctant to use the bottle and was often caught by nursing staff breast-feeding when she should be bottle-feeding.

Case Considerations

1. What is the primary issue at hand? Why is this an issue?
2. Select a change theory and work through a plan that will promote weight gain for Josue.
3. Is Margarite being noncompliant?

WRITING EXERCISE 15.1

This chapter has presented various theories and concepts related to leadership and change that are useful in initiating and implementing changes at an individual, group, or system level. The two writing exercises below are designed to help you apply these concepts.

Facilitating change in health behaviors

For this writing exercise (1) identify a client teaching situation in which you were involved (or you observed); (2) select two concepts/theories of leadership/change presented in the chapter; (3) compare and contrast their advantages and disadvantages when applied to this situation; (4) are there other concepts or strategies that would be more effective in this situation? Why or why not?

Facilitating changes in nursing and healthcare practices

For this writing exercise (1) identify an intervention/ procedure/protocol you have observed in the clinical area that you feel should be changed or improved (this could entail a wide variety of procedures/ processes, not strictly nursing interventions, e.g., process for giving/obtaining a shift report, a process for transferring patients from one unit to another, a documentation method, etc.); (2) determine which change/leadership strategies would be most helpful in facilitating this change (e.g., traditional, contemporary, or a combination of both); (3) discuss your rationale for selecting these strategies

CHAPTER SUMMARY

The ability to facilitate change is an important component of the professional nursing role. As health care professionals, nurses might be responsible for initiating, facilitating, or participating in change efforts. The role of nurses as change agents might be limited to individual clients or encompass an entire health care organization. To succeed in this role, nurses must have a working knowledge of and be able to apply theories and concepts of change. They need to develop leadership skills that will engender collaboration from clients and colleagues and motivate individuals to participate in the change effort.

It is important for the nurse to recognize that it is human nature for individuals to strive to maintain the status quo and that generally people do not willingly embrace change. A consequence of this might be that individuals do not fully "buy into the idea" and only make superficial, temporary changes. Transformational leadership skills that transcend self and others and focus on realizing a larger goal are more effective in promoting deep change. Perhaps above all, to be an effective leader/change agent in today's complex and dynamic health care organizations, nurses must be able to tolerate ambiguity, be open to new possibilities, and respond quickly and appropriately to the demands of the environment.

> *Life is intent on finding what works, not what's "right." It is the ability to keep finding solutions that is important; any one solution is temporary. There are no permanently right answers. The capacity to keep changing, to find what works now, is what keeps any organism alive.*
> —Margaret Wheatley and Myron Kellnor Rogers

REFERENCES

Allen, D. (1998). How nurses become leaders: Perceptions and beliefs about leadership development. *Journal of Nursing Administration, 28*(9), 15–20.

Bauman, R. P. (1998). Five requisites for implementing change. In D. C. Hambrick, D. A. Nadler, & M. L. Tushman (Eds.). *Navigating change: How CEOs, top teams, and boards steer transformation.* Boston: Harvard Business School, (pp. 309–317).

Bondas, T. (2003). Caritative leadership: Ministering to the patients. *Nursing Administration Quarterly, 27,* 249–253.

Breisch, L. (1999). Motivate! Create a work environment that brings out each nurse's drive to excel. *Nursing Management,* 27–29.

Burns, J. (1978). *Leadership.* New York: Harper & Row.

Clark, B., Rapkin, K., Busen, N., & Vasquez, E. (2001). Nurse practitioners and parent education: A partnership for health. *Journal of the American Academy of Nurse Practitioners,* 310–316.

Contino, D. (2004). Leadership competencies: Knowledge, skills, and aptitudes nurse need to lead organizations effectively. *Critical Care Nurse, 24*(3), 52–64.

Covey, S. R. (1991). *Principle-centered leadership.* New York: Simon & Schuster.

Croghan, E. (2005). Assessing motivation and readiness to alter lifestyle behavior. *Nursing Standard, 19*(31), 50–52.

DePree, M. (1992). *Leadership jazz.* New York: Dell Publishing.

Duran, L. (2003). Motivating health: Strategies for the nurse practitioner. *Journal of the American Academy of Nurse Practitioners, 15*(5), 200–205.

Franken, R. (2002). *Human Motivation.* Pacific Grove, CA: Brooks/Cole.

Goleman, D. (1998). What makes a leader? *Harvard Business Review,* Nov./Dec. 93–102.

Greenleaf, R. (1991). *The servant as leader.* Indianapolis: The Robert K. Greenleaf Center.

Herzberg, F. (2003). One more time: How do you motivate employees? In *Harvard Business Review on Motivating People.* Boston: Harvard Business School Press, 45–71.

Hill, K. (2004). Defy the decades with multigenerational teams. *Nursing Management,* 33–35.

Johns, C. (2004). Becoming a transformational leader through reflection. *Reflections on Nursing Leadership,* Second Quarter, 24–26.

Kerfoot, K., & Wantz, S. (2003). Compliance leadership: The 17th century model that doesn't work. *Dermatology Nurse, 15*(4), 377–381.

Kotter, J. P. (1995). Leading change: Why transformation efforts fail. *Harvard Business Review,* March-April, 59–67.

Lawrence, D. M. (1998). Leading discontinuous change: Ten lessons from the battlefront. In D. C. Hambrick, D. A. Nadler, & M. L. Tushman (Eds.). *Navigating change: How CEOs, top teams, and boards steer transformation* (pp. 291–308). Boston: Harvard Business School.

Lewin, K. (1951). *Field theory in social science.* New York: Harper & Row.

Lippitt, G. (1973). *A Handbook for visual problem solving.* Bethesda, MD: Development Publications.

Lippitt, G., Langseth, P., & Mossop, J. (1985). *Implementing organizational change.* San Francisco: Jossey-Bass Publishers.

Porter-O'Grady, T., & Malloch, K. (2003). *Quantum leadership: A textbook of new leadership.* Boston: Jones and Bartlett.

Prochaska, J., & DiClemente, C. (1983). Stages and processes of self-change of smoking: Toward an integrative model of change. *Journal of Consulting and Clinical Psychology, 51*(3), 390–395.

Quinn, R. E. (1996). *Deep change: Discovering the leader within.* San Francisco: Jossey-Bass.

Quinn, R. E. (2000). *Change the world: How ordinary people can achieve extraordinary results.* San Francisco: Jossey-Bass.

Quinn, R. E. (2004). *Building the bridge as you walk on it.* San Francisco: Jossey-Bass.

Senge, P. (1990). *The fifth discipline.* New York: Doubleday.

Sirota, D., Mischkind, L., & Meltzer, M. (2005). *The enthusiastic employee: How companies profit by giving workers what they want.* Upper Saddle River, NJ: Pearson Education.

Spears, L. (2004). Servant leadership. *Reflections on Nursing Leadership.* Fourth Quarter, pp. 24–26.

Vicenzi, A. E., White, K. R., & Begun, J. W. (1997). Chaos in nursing: Make it work for you. *American Journal of Nursing, 97*(10), 27–31.

Wagner, L. (2005). Using group process to develop caring leaders. In H. Feldman & M. Greenberg, (Eds.). *Educating nurses for leadership* (pp. 126–135). New York: Springer Publishing.

Ward, K. (2002). A vision for tomorrow: Transformational nursing leaders. *Nursing Outlook, 50*(3), 121–126.

Wieck, K., Prydun, M., & Walsh, T. (2002). What the emerging workforce wants in its leaders. *Journal of Nursing Scholarship,* Third Quarter, 283–288.

CHAPTER 16

Delegator and Decision Maker

Karin A. Polifko

Behind every able man, there are always other able men.
—Chinese Proverb

LEARNING OBJECTIVES

At the completion of the chapter, the learner should be able to do the following:

1. Discuss the notion of delegation as it pertains to the health care setting and the oversight needed by the registered nurse.
2. Compare and contrast the purposes of the State Board of Nursing and the National Council of State Boards of Nursing.
3. Identify at least three key points in delegating.
4. Discuss why the ability to communicate is important to effective delegation.

KEY TERMS

Accountability	Five rights of delegation	Overdelegation
Authority	High-context communication	Underdelegation
Competency	Low-context communication	
Delegation	Nurse Practice Act	

Effective delegation has taken on a new dimension since the surge in the usage of unlicensed assistive personnel (UAP) in health care settings (Feldman & Greenberg, 2005). Long gone are the days when there were only registered nurses on the floors and in the intensive care units. In the last few decades or so, several events have brought the notion of delegation and its inherent issues to the forefront of nursing care. The health care workforce is aging, especially the nursing workforce, with many nurses due to retire within the next decade. The structure of the health care delivery system has changed dramatically from a retrospective to a prospective payment system, altering the reimbursement methodology for hospital and home health agencies alike. Further, the decline in the available numbers of registered nurses—and its rapidly aging population—is a significant worry for health care administrators regardless of the setting. These factors, plus many more, lead to an increase in the UAPs functioning as nurse extenders. It is imperative that the registered nurse not only understands her role and responsibilities, but also that of those whom she supervises, including licensed practical nurses (LPNs) and UAPs.

Patient care delivery is increasingly complex. Tasks such as monitoring a patient's outcomes is now the responsibility of the staff nurse, who needs to learn early on that effective delegation can only help in completing patient care in a timely manner. Today, with the advent of managed care and the need to do more with less expensive personnel, delegation and its ramifications have taken on a whole new perspective and accountability. With a decrease in the number of qualified personnel providing direct patient care, registered nurses are increasingly more liable for the nursing care they assign to LPNs and to UAPs. There are certainly some perceived downsides to delegation; however, there are just as many potential benefits, including the ability to actually get a break while working (a novel thought!), the chance to assist another person to grow professionally and personally, the empowerment of another, and the chance to assist in organizing the care better. And with better organization comes enhanced quality of patient care, and having someone do many of the nonnursing tasks that although important, can lead to frustration, and lower job satisfaction.

DEFINING DELEGATION

Leadership is the art of accomplishing work through the acts of others. Delegation is similar to leadership in that the individual cannot do it, and it takes another individual to achieve the desired end result. Nursing is a complex discipline with multiple tasks that need to be completed within a designated time frame. Given the current state of health care and the

lack of available professional staff, many tasks are reassigned to nurse assistants, with the notion that their work is closely supervised for accuracy, quality, and completeness. The ability to delegate is a learned skill, one that is essential in the daily responsibilities of the professional nurse.

Nursing delegation is the transfer of authority to perform a designated nursing task to someone who has shown competency in a particular area. Specific duties need to be delineated clearly. The National Council of State Boards of Nursing (1990) writes that delegation is "(The) transferring to a competent individual authority to perform a selected nursing task in a selected situation. The nurse retains the accountability for the delegation" (p. 1). Several key words are obvious in both definitions, particularly authority and competency. **Authority** is the official power vested in a position that gives a designated employee the right to perform certain tasks. **Competency** is defined by the National Council of State Boards of Nursing as "the application of knowledge and the interpersonal, decision-making and psychomotor skills expected for the practice role, within the context of public health, safety and welfare" (1997, p. 5).

Part of the challenge surrounding delegation is first defining who can delegate to whom and then what tasks may be delegated as differentiated from the tasks that must be done by a professional registered nurse (RN). All RNs must have a thorough understanding of both their scope of practice and the scope of practice of all personnel with whom they work. Scope of practice is what the person holding a designated license is able to perform legally. For example, an RN is able to legally pronounce a patient expired in a nursing home, whereas this is not within the scope of practice for an LPN. **Accountability** is taking the legal responsibility for an action; RNs are accountable and responsible for their delegation decisions. Responsibility for the profession encompasses concepts such as reliability, dependability, and the obligation to perform professionally and within the designated scope of practice as defined by the individual State Boards of Nursing. The procedure of delegating patient care and duties comes under the assignment-making role of the registered nurse. It is prudent that the RN understands the scope of practice and competencies of those to whom she is delegating patient-care responsibilities. For example, the RN may delegate tasks such as

- Routine vital signs. When there are specific parameters that need to be followed, such as taking a BP after administration of an antihypertensive, the directions such as time and feedback must be clearly given.
- Comfort measures such as bathing, dressing, bed making.
- Transfers, such as ambulation and transportation to procedures.
- Feeding, if appropriate.
- Clearly identified tasks that the UAP has been tested for as competent, such as intake and output measurement, simple dressing changes, simple glucose monitoring.

Examples of tasks that should not be delegated by the RN to the UAP include

- Initial assessment of a newly admitted patient or ongoing assessment.
- Development of a plan of care.
- Evaluation of a task (i.e., how did the patient respond to the two units of blood?).

Figure 16.1 can assist the RN in delegation decisions. This decision-making model provides a decision tree for the RN, LPN, and the UAP in the delegation process, assisting in the determination of whether a task or activity can be safely and legally delegated to another person.

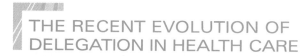

THE RECENT EVOLUTION OF DELEGATION IN HEALTH CARE

As recently as the late 1980s, a popular method of patient-care delivery was the primary-care delivery model. In this model, a registered nurse took care of a small number of patients, performing all aspects of nursing care, including bed baths and treatments as well as more extensive therapies such as ventilator management. On a typical medical/surgical floor, there may have been one nursing assistant who floated among the nurses, assisting them in ambulation of patients or maybe with the passing of food trays. Fast forward to the advent of the prospective payment system, wherein hospitals—and physicians—could no longer charge whatever rate they felt was appropriate based on "usual and customary fees." Instead, the federal government discharged to Medicare providers and facilities a payment that was based upon a predetermined number, which was an average cost per patient day for a particular area of the country. This way of doing business was a radical departure from the previous way that hospitals and physicians were reimbursed, resulting in much angst across numerous acute-care, and later home-care, agencies throughout the United States.

In an effort to minimize expenses, the financial reimbursement system for both hospitals and providers alike became more streamlined regarding the way that care was delivered. Patients are discharged earlier than before; no longer can Grandpa stay in the hospital over the weekend because his family is going out of town and won't be home to take care of him. And rather than rehabilitating in the acute care setting, clients are sent to a rehabilitation setting for "skilled nursing care." Many procedures once done in the hospital sitting are now completed in the outpatient surgical suite: remember the uproar over the proposed "drive-through mastectomies" in the mid-1990s? Diseases are now managed on a timeline, through critical pathways in a case-managed environment. Unfortunately, even though the governmental reimbursement system pays less to health care facilities, the cost of care has not decreased in parallel. With the rapid growth in technology, computerization, buildings and equipment, and salaries for both professionals and nonprofessionals, the cost of health care continues to rise faster than most other industries.

In an effort to assist in cost containment, health care systems began to look at the high labor costs

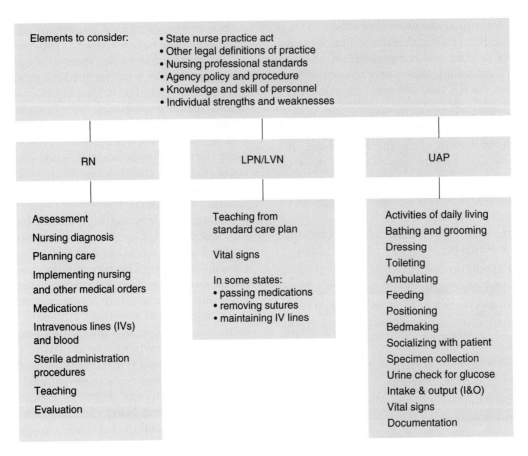

Figure 16.1 Considerations in delegation.

associated with providing quality care. Too many systems decided—wrongly—that because registered nurses are among the highest paid hourly employees, as well as the largest constituent of a hospital's labor budget, administrators would decrease RN positions in order to save money. RNs were also laid off in the early 1990s and replaced by cheaper, less qualified LPNs and UAPs, reverting to a functional model of nursing-care delivery that was popular in the 1950s. Job dissatisfaction grew and thus began the decline of nursing school enrollments, which have only recently begun to turn around. The aging RN population, coupled with the current nursing shortage, has resulted in hospitals, which once turned away RN applicants, not

being able to fill all their vacancies, and therefore using UAPs as substitutes for RNs, thereby stretching those employed RNs even further in their work responsibilities. UAPs hold licenses from the individual State Boards of Nursing: their duties include not only comfort measures such baths and measuring intake and outputs, but can also include sterile-dressing changes, discontinuing IVs, and the pulling of femoral lines post CABG. Although these particular duties used to be done by RNs, many health care agencies have delegated these tasks to the UAPs once they are trained and deemed competent in the designated procedures, which has led to increased vigilance on the part of the registered nurse. Figure 16.1 offers suggested delegation tasks and skills.

DELEGATION: THE FINE POINTS

In order to delegate effectively, the RNs must first know their—as well their subordinates'—job description and scope of practice. The State Board of Nursing is a regulatory body whose primary purpose is to protect the public from unsafe nursing practice by establishing safe nursing care standards. Each Board is responsible for issuing nursing licenses and monitoring individuals in order to ensure that safe nursing care is being provided. If the Board deems unsafe care has been given, it has the authority to take action against that individual in a variety of ways.

The governor of each state appoints membership to the Board, serving for a designated time frame. Each state determines the Board membership, which usually includes registered nurses, licensed practical/vocational nurses, advanced-practice registered nurses, and consumers. There are currently Boards of Nursing in all 50 states, the District of Columbia, as well as the Virgin Islands, Guam, Puerto Rico, American Samoa, and the Northern Mariana Islands. Of these, California, Louisiana, Georgia and West Virginia maintain two Boards of Nursing, one for registered nurses and one for licensed practical/vocational nurses.

One of the common misperceptions that RNs have is that the Board of Nursing regulates their practice; although there are standards of practice that RNs must adhere to, the Board does not look at individual agencies to ensure that the standards are established and maintained. Instead, an organization such as the Joint Commission on Accreditation of Healthcare Organizations (JCAHO), through an extensive self-study process, monitors the nursing care provided to the clients of a particular health care system. When a nurse provides unsafe care, the Board of Nursing is empowered to administer discipline ranging from a written letter of notice to revocation of the nursing license.

The **Nurse Practice Act** of each state delineates the regulations and laws that govern the practice of the registered nurse. This document directs practice, provides the legal groundwork for clinical decision making, and is determined by each state's legislature. It is written broadly rather than with specifics for just this reason: in order for any changes to be made to the Nurse Practice Act, the legislature must first have the recommendation in the form of a bill that is passed by both the House and Senate of the respective state, along with the concurrence by the governor. Many RNs wish that the Act provided clearer parameters for practice, but it is intentionally made general to allow health care institutions their own interpretations and implementations within the limits set forth by the law.

The five rights of delegation

The five rights of delegation are the right task, under the right circumstance, using the right person, with the right direction and communication and the right supervision. A delegation decision-making tree can be found on the Web site of the NCSBN (www.ncsbn.org). Examples of activities under each category for the five rights are in Table 16.1. The primary responsibility for nursing care outcomes, regardless of who actually provided the care, is the registered nurse. The RN should be concerned with the competency of the person to whom she delegates, primarily from a legal perspective. The RN always remains accountable for delegating the task to the UAP. RNs may never delegate nursing tasks that are defined by the individual Nurse Practice Acts, such as diagnosing, assessing, and implementing a strategy of care, establishing and evaluating goals to meet an individual's health needs. Again, it is imperative that an RN fully understands her own Nurse Practice Act with its laws and statutes.

Most states clearly define delegation, putting emphasis on the need to know the delegate's competency in completing the task assigned, and providing subsequent adequate supervision of the delegate. If an RN knowingly assigns a task that the delegate cannot perform due to incompetence or lack of

Table 16.1 **The Five Rights of Delegation**

The Right Task	Is it within the scope of practice?
	Does the hospital include the task in the job description?
	Does the task *not* require assessment or evaluation?
The Right Circumstance	Is the patient complexity appropriate for the delegate?
	Is the patient relatively stable?
	Is the patient in the appropriate setting for this level task?
	Are there resources available in case of difficulty?
	Does there need to be minimal supervision in the completion of the task? And is there a supervisor present?
The Right Person	Is the task within the scope of practice?
	Has the person been trained to complete the task?
	Has the person demonstrated competency?
	Is the task within the job description?
The Right Direction/Communication	Is there a clear explanation of the task?
	Are the expectations clearly explained, along with the timeline needed?
	Are the limits delineated clearly and concisely?
The Right Supervision	Can supervisors give appropriate instructions, outlining their expectations, reporting the mechanisms and parameters of expected patient care?

knowledge, then she not only can be held liable for the resultant actions, but can also be brought up on charges of unprofessional conduct, subject to a hearing by the Board of Nursing. Emphasis is placed on supervision of the individual, with the RN providing guidance and direction. A key component to supervising is the follow-up after a task is completed and its subsequent evaluation. Under delegation law, it does not matter whether an RN is physically present or available by phone: this is known as direct or indirect supervision. Regardless of the place, the RN always needs to be available to the delegate to assist in the planning, assessing, implementation, and evaluation of the care provided. Direct supervision may be in an acute-care setting, where the RN works side by side with the UAP, whereas the RN is available periodically to provide occasional observation and evaluation in the home health setting.

If a UAP performs a task incorrectly, can the RN be held liable? Absolutely, if there are certain parameters that haven't been met, such as assigning a task that the delegate is not competent in, or has not been trained in. Delegates have responsibility for their own actions as well; they knowingly accept an assignment and know whether they have been trained in the assigned task. However, RNs usually have a concern that a delegate can "cause them to lose their license if something happens." The RN must understand the level of competence of delegates; supervise them appropriately by clearly giving directions, outlining expectations and follow-ups; and evaluate the outcome of the task. If there is an untoward effect, the RN must take immediate action to assess the situation and notify the appropriate people of the results. Essentially, if the RN makes a reasonable assignment and continues adequate

CASE SCENARIO 16.1

Due to a shortage of registered nurses, your Vice President of Nursing has decided to place qualified unlicensed assistive personnel (UAPs) lin the high-risk labor and delivery unit (ICU) in which you are the manager. He asks you to develop a job description with appropriate tasks delineated that can be delegated by the registered nurse. This is the first time that UAPs will be utilized in this area.

1. Before beginning, review the potential scope of practice for the UAP.

2. What parameters does your state have for the role of the UAP? For the RN who supervises the UAP?

3. Describe the responsibilities of the RN regarding the delegation of patient-care tasks to an unlicensed person.

4. Identify ten tasks or nursing care functions that you would feel comfortable including in the UAP's job description in the high-risk labor and delivery environment. Why?

5. Identify ten tasks or nursing care functions that you would NOT feel comfortable including in the UAP's job description in the high-risk labor and delivery environment. Why?

6. How does this environment differ from the general medical/surgical floor as far as assigned UAP responsibilities?

supervision and follow-up, then her license is not necessarily in peril, but it is the common misperception by many RNs that regardless of the situation, their licenses are in jeopardy. Patient safety must be the primary concern of the RN, and if she feels that the delegate is not adequately educated in the task, then delegation should not occur.

KEY POINTS TO THE EFFECTIVENESS OF DELEGATION

There are several key points that are important to remember before you delegate anything to anyone.

- Stress results, not details: One does not need the minute-to-minute details of how they completed the task, but you are interested in the results. Setting up a schedule of planned updates when they can give you an overview of what is occurring can be helpful for both the RN and the delegate.

Don't wait until the end of the shift to hear about the intake and outputs or the results of the dressing change, in case there needs to be an intervention by the RN.

- Provide ongoing education for the delegate. If delegates come to you with a question, it is prudent to teach them how to find out the answers to the problem themselves, saving you time in the long run. This can be frustrating in the short term but well worth the effort in the long term.

- Assist delegates with active problem solving as they seek possible solutions. Likewise, if they have questions, ask them for possible answers. For example, if they come to you wanting to know if Mrs. Chou can have a certain item on her diet, teach the UAP where to find the answers to her question.

- Ensure your plan has clear and measurable goals. The more employees have clear and specific objectives the more comfortable they will be acting on their own.

- Develop reporting systems. Again predetermine when and how you would like the delegate to report to you the results of her actions. Feedback is critical, regardless of whether you are on-site or available by telephone. For those who supervise at a distance, set up your reporting mechanisms to ensure timely feedback: this can be monthly, weekly, or whatever way works best for you to get the information that you need.

- Give clear and realistic deadlines. If tasks are left without a completion time, it becomes very difficult to motivate anyone to work on them in a timely fashion.

- Encourage accountability for the results. By not stepping in to assist in the completion of a task, the delegate will have responsibility for his actions.

- Have a delegation log. If you have several employees that you have delegated to, write down who/what/where/when so you can monitor progress and provide feedback as necessary. If you have a number of employees reporting to you, someone's assignment may get lost.

- Understand the talents and personalities of your employees. A clear understanding of delegates' scope of practice as well as their talents and abilities should make assignments an excellent match.

DELEGATION BARRIERS

When first confronted with delegation responsibilities, many new—and experienced alike—RNs offer numerous comments on why they don't want to delegate or increase their level of delegation. Some of the reasons include fear of losing a license; inability to trust the delegate; misunderstanding of the expectations of both the delegator and the delegate; and feeling under/overwhelmed by the entire responsibility, stress, burnout, apathy, anger, confusion and loss of control of the quality they feel only an RN can deliver.

Regardless of the reason behind the emotion, delegation to the unlicensed assistive personnel is a role expectation of the registered nurse in the vast majority of health care agencies, including areas

that were not included earlier, such as the intensive care setting or the emergency department. The ANA Code for Nurses has outlined the parameters of delegation for registered nurses since 1976 (Hansten & Jackson, 2004); and the individual state boards of nursing have their own expectations of delegation by the professional nurse.

There are two opposing categories of delegation that can result in a negative experience for not only the RN and the UAP, but also for the patient. These categories are underdelegation and overdelegation. **Underdelegation** is as common an occurrence in nursing as overdelegation. Underdelegation can happen for a variety of reasons, ranging from the new graduate not feeling that she has the skill level or the experience to make an effective decision in what can or cannot be delegated; or it may occur when an employee does not trust the competencies of those whom they supervise. Or someone may feel that in order to have the task completed—and completed well—they need to do it, rather than giving it to a subordinate. Generally, underdelegation is a negative behavior. By not effectively delegating, the work is only increased, often causing great stress for the RN; and it is ineffective time management.

Overdelegation can likewise occur by the same new RN, who in the spirit of delegation, expects too much from delegates without checking their scope of practice or competency levels. Similarly, experienced RNs can overdelegate; perhaps they have a long working relationship with a UAP that they trust. The RN can then place too much responsibility and accountability on the UAP. This type of behavior can not only overwhelm the inadequately trained person, but it can often place the patient, as well as the RN and UAP, at risk. Again, it is prudent that the person delegating has a good understanding of delegates' abilities, competency in performing a task, and their legal scope of practice.

Other barriers to significant delegation by the registered nurse include

- Uncertainty about what can be delegated and what tasks cannot be delegated. When in doubt, some will avoid the risk, rather than taking the time to investigate.

WRITING EXERCISE 16.1

Jadyn Argoysi, BSN, is a new registered nurse who does not quite know what her limitations and strong points as a leader are yet. Like a typical new graduate, she feels overwhelmed with the myriad tasks, treatments, assessments, and decisions that must be made by the end of the shift. At times, she doesn't really know where to begin, especially when in nursing school she never had more than two patients to provide care for, and now her patient assignment is consistently about 14 patients on the night shift. While feeling incompetent and easily swamped, Jadyn tries to "do it all" without asking for help for fear of appearing a failure to others. Outline what you think is the best way to help Jadyn in her new role, keeping in mind that it is the responsibility of the entire health care team to recognize these behaviors early in a new nurse's career. How would you help her understand how effective delegation can actually improve the efficiency of patient-care delivery, promote positive patient outcomes, and also increase her job satisfaction as well?

- Personal disorganization. Some people are simply better organized than others, and in order to delegate, you first need to have the larger picture in your mind about what needs to be completed, when it needs to be done by, and by what method.

- The perception that only you can complete a task to a certain level of proficiency. Instead of placing your trust in another, you feel that only you can do the job and have it done correctly. This type of thinking will eventually wear everyone down.

- A feeling of loss of control over how a task is begun, carried out, and completed. By delegating, some feel that their role diminishes and they are therefore not providing professional care to their patients. They don't seem to understand that when they delegate certain tasks, they can be freed up to provide more in-depth teaching, assessment, and evaluation of their patients' needs.

- The desire to be recognized as being a "super nurse"—nurses who have a strong need and desire to handle (alone) everything that comes their way. This person may have an ego problem, or just want to be liked. Unfortunately, not many of us can act in isolation, and the results can lead to stress, anger, and, eventually, burnout.

LIABILITY AND DELEGATION

Regardless of the type of licensure held, the licensee is accountable and responsible to the public. Accountability is taking the legal responsibility for an action. The nurse is obligated, by licensure, to provide care that minimally meets the standards of practice as determined by the individual Board of Nursing to regulate that specific practice. Licensed nurses are accountable both for their own practice as well as for the delegation of nursing tasks. Responsibility includes concepts such as reliability, dependability, and obligations to perform professionally.

One frequently hears, "I can lose my license if . . ." Yes, a license can be lost or revoked after the State Board of Nursing has found licensees to be derelict in their duties as a professional nurse, and this can encompass poor delegation skills. However, if the parameters of delegation were correctly met, then the chances of the Board of Nursing—and a jury—finding just cause may become more difficult.

Liability occurs after an untoward event that has caused injury to the patient, and the patient has

CASE SCENARIO 16.2

As the RN team leader on a night shift, you have two UAPs and one LPN working with you to take care of 20 patients. The unit secretary has called in sick. One of the UAPs is a float assistant from the pediatrics floor who admits mostly medical oncology patients. The patients on your floor are all adult general surgery patients. Six of them need preoperative work completed before surgery in the morning.

One patient, Ms. Arez, is four hours post-op after having a total hysterectomy and is apparently having complications with a low blood pressure of 80/68 (her normal is 146/88), and low UOP (only 20 cc's in the last two hours). There is no ICU bed at the moment, so she needs to be taken care of on the floor until one opens up.

Another patient, Mr. Zheng, is also post-op back surgery today, and is beginning to hallucinate, attempting to climb out of bed as well as pull at his IVs and oxygen. His roommate, a 92-year-old man one day post-op for a fractured hip, has dementia and is crying inconsolably for his wife and children to help him "get out of the bathtub." Their room is across from the dirty utility room toward the end of the hallway so as not to wake up all the patients. Additionally, two patients are in need of blood transfusions, and eight need IV push meds. The remaining patients are mostly stable.

Case Considerations

1. What are some critical factors to consider when deciding what tasks to delegate to the team members?

2. What are some of the issues in this scenario that may assist in determining the delegated tasks?

3. Where does one begin in deciding what to delegate and to whom?

4. Identify the tasks that should NOT be delegated and why.

5. Are there any legal ramifications to the delegation decisions?

6. Are there any other options to consider?

---

sustained damages as a result of the injury. Malpractice is often the failure of a professional to act in a reasonable and prudent manner. Negligence is the omission to act in the way that someone in a similar situation would act. In order to prove negligence or malpractice, there are four generally accepted parameters to be met by the plaintiff: (1) a duty or obligation to practice must be established, (2) a breach of duty was found, (3) harm occurred, and (4) harm occurred because of the omission or duty to act.

The most common areas that nursing practice is involved with are failure to monitor, assess, or communicate patient findings and failure to follow the standards of nursing practice. In order to minimize risk from these actions, prudent nurses should adhere to the standards of accepted nursing practice for the state in which they are licensed, for the institution in which they are employed, and for the community in which they practice.

Even if a licensed nurse is found to be liable in a lawsuit involving legal action, it does not mean that the nurse will automatically lose her nursing license. In this case, there are two distinct processes: the determination of malpractice and subsequent damages, and action from the State Board of Nursing on an individual's nursing license. There are actions that the professional nurse can take to reduce risks of liability, perhaps the most important of which is to thoroughly know the scope of practice for RNs and for those whom the RN supervises. Additionally, the RN should know the Board rules regarding delegation. Other actions include the need to apply the appropriate standards of care, maintaining clinical competency, ensuring that those you supervise are competent, and knowing that delegating care is dependent upon the documented skills of licensed and unlicensed personnel alike. Regardless of the situation, judgment by the nurse will always be the key to effective delegation.

IS IT DELEGATION— OR IS IT DUMPING?

Delegation has a fine edge to it: delegate too little, and you can be called controlling, adverse to risk, or simply not wanting anyone else to complete the task at a lower level than you expected. Delegate too much and you place at risk yourself, the delegate, the patient, and the health care setting. How do you find the happy medium that is both comfortable and yet within legal parameters of all scopes of practice? When does delegation become dumping: a situation wherein the nurse simply does not want to do a task and assigns to another without regard for the other's workload or obligations?

One of the first steps that any RN should take in the delegation process is to ensure that delegates understand not only their scope of practice, but also the job descriptions from the institution, which are generally more specific regarding role expectations. Part of the responsibility of the RN is to assist the UAP or LPN in understanding role and job expectations, and to clear up any misperceptions before there are issues. For instance, when the UAP receives her assignment and notices that all 24 patients are assigned to her for bedbaths, ambulation, and vital signs, she may immediately feel like her assignment is too heavy. Is it? Or is this an appropriate assignment given the other members of the health care team and their assignments? Without an explanation, the UAP may feel exploited and dumped on, when in fact, her skills in multitasking and ability to care for the clients on a personal level are very much valued and appreciated by the RN and other team members as contributing greatly to overall patient-care delivery (Cohen, 2004). Curtis and Nicholl (2004) call the delegation of unpleasant tasks "dustbin dumping," and caution against pretending that everything assigned will be desirable; there are always going to be those jobs that are interesting and those that are totally unappealing, but regardless, all need to be done.

It is important to keep in mind that not only is one person delegating to the UAP, but perhaps numerous others throughout the shift. How many times has someone answered a light in a patient's room only to find the patient's perhaps in a compromising condition needing immediate attention, or is stopped by family members who want specific things done "right now"? Sometimes it is helpful to stop for a moment and look at the assignment— and the expectations—through the eyes of the delegate to really get a sense of the responsibility and workload asked of the delegate. Being careful to ensure that the assignments are equally distributed is also a helpful technique: it may be better to assign patients by acuity rather than by rooms. Don't doubt someone's ability to do the task, and to do it well. Asking, rather than always directing, is another helpful technique to aid the UAP in feeling more a part of the team, as well as saying "please." And finally, acknowledging a job well done and saying "thank you" go a long way in promoting job satisfaction and bolstering someone's self-esteem. Admit it: the role of an UAP is often invisible and unappreciated by most, including the RN.

THE IMPORTANCE OF COMMUNICATION, FEEDBACK, AND THE DELEGATION PROCESS

Communication is an essential and necessary skill for the RN. Given a vague message, no two people will interpret it in the same way, leaving plenty of room for mistakes, misunderstanding, and confusion. Oftentimes, you hear and communicate based

RESEARCH APPLICATION ARTICLE

Harrison, S., Dowswell, G. & Wright, J. (2002). Practice nurses and clinical guidelines in a changing primary care context: an empirical study. *Journal of Advanced Nursing, 39*(3), 299–307.

A study took place in England, with its authors, Harrison, Dowswell, and Wright (2002), interested in the manner in which nurses (called Practice Nurses) in the English National Health Service primary-care workforce are delegated work by the General Practitioners. Clinical guidelines are the linkage between the government-driven policy concerns and the movement toward evidence-based practice, with its noticeable outcome measures. The study's purpose is threefold: (1) to seek out the attitudes of the nurses as they worked with the clinical practice guidelines, (2) to examine the relationship between the nurses and the physicians, and (3) to illustrate the challenges of delivering primary care.

Twenty-nine nurses were interviewed three times during a sixteen-month period to ascertain the above information. The authors found that the nurses were generally receptive to the delegation by the physicians, and were more supportive when they were able to somewhat influence the physician's clinical practice in order to adhere to prescribed desired outcomes. Although this research article looked at the interaction between nurses and physicians, with delegation by the MDs, the authors discovered that when the nurses believed they were offering information that contributed determining outcomes of patient-care delivery, they felt better about their role and their subordinate professional status.

on the framework of your world: someone with limited experiences outside of their small community may not have a clear understanding of the directive "offer the client culturally competent care" if their only exposure to someone of a background different from theirs was through television. The critical factor in communication is to be able to truly listen to what others are saying, without filtering the information offered.

Culture, age, religion, race, and gender have great influence on listening and sending communications. We all have bias and communicate it either knowingly or perhaps subconsciously. Some cultures are considered low context, such as peoples from the United States, Canada, and some parts of Europe. In **low-context communication,** words and phrases may be taken literally and directly, with people expressing exactly what they feel without trying to please the other party. Sensitivity to another's feelings may not be kept in the forefront of verbalization to someone from these countries.

On the contrary, **high-context communication** weaves a variety of situations and scenarios together to frame the conversation. The communication is indirect, keeping in mind not only the verbalization, but the nonverbal messages as well. A goal of this type of communication is sensitivity to the other party, not wanting them to misinterpret your intentions, and always speaking in a tactful manner. In Asia, where gender is a strong consideration in the correct verbal and nonverbal styles, people are high-context communicators. Accordingly, issues of space, touch, eye contact, and speaking volume are more carefully considered in high-context countries as compared with low-context countries that value brevity, clarity, and persuasive speech as the hallmarks of a good communicator.

There are two distinct styles that can quickly eliminate the possibility of listening: passive and aggressive speech. In passive speech, the underlying emotions can be guilt, helplessness, fear, anxiety, stress, feelings of inadequacy, and hurt. This person may feel that it is easier to ignore, placate, or diminish the actual issue rather than addressing it straight on. We have all worked with passive personalities who actually get indirect benefits from acting the martyr ("I can take on 30 patients by myself tonight if you feel too tired") or being withdrawn, those who painfully do their work with joy or excitement. The RN must sense this type of delegate and carefully work through this negative communication style by asking appropriate questions and seeking feedback.

On the polar end of the scale are those who are deemed aggressive in their communication methods. Aggressive communicators are full of blame: it is your fault that the patient fell out of bed! The words are riddled with hostility, anger, and criticism. Listening is minimal—if at all—because, after all, the situation is really the other person's fault. The problem with this type of communication is that there is little praise and feedback, except to what is wrong. A person on the receiving end of this type of berating very quickly becomes defensive, hurt, and perhaps vengeful and livid with the accusations by the aggressor. When delegating, it is crucial to keep in mind these two particularly negative communication styles as those that you don't want to inflict on others.

Another consideration to effective communication is that of offering evaluation through effective feedback. As part of the role of delegator, the RN needs to ensure that the task is done to completion, and satisfactorily so. Before you walk away from the delegate, ensure that

- The information was heard in the manner in which it was intended.

- The desired outcome was discussed.

- The method of evaluation was discussed.

- The time needed for reporting back to the RN was discussed.

- The parameters were discussed regarding situations that needed immediate attention by the RN and that can wait until the end of shift until report.

There are several ways to see that you have been successful with your directives, with the easiest one being observation. Verifying with your own eyes the direct outcome of a task completed will allow you

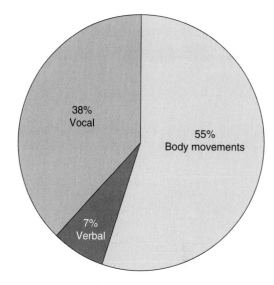

Figure 16.2 How we interpret a message.

to offer feedback that is not secondhand. Nonverbal behavior is also a way to give feedback; and it is not always done in a positive manner. McKay, Davis, and Fanning (1995, p. 53) found that a message's impact is 7 percent verbal (words); 38 percent vocal (volume, pitch, rhythm); and 55 percent body movements, mostly facial expressions (see figure 16.2).

Many find that nonverbal expressions actually reflect the person's real feelings more accurately. Have you ever seen someone who is emphatically stating that he is in agreement with the discussion at hand, yet his hands are clenched, his jaw tight, and speaking in a hurried manner? A key of successful communication is the congruence between what is spoken and what is seen by others. When giving feedback, it is imperative that what you are saying is in synch with your nonverbal expressions. Do you look people directly in the eyes, or do you avoid their glance as they question your statements? Are you speaking calmly, in a fairly even tone, or does your voice rise and get louder while you speak in crisp, incomplete sentences? Are you gesturing wildly, or are you relaxed? Are you touching the person, or are you out of their personal space?

CASE SCENARIO 16.3

Justin is a new nurse on your unit who has difficulty working with his team members. Although he is technically competent and makes good decisions, he insists upon doing everything himself. Those tasks that he does delegate, which are usually vital signs, emptying trash, handing out trays, and performing intakes and outputs, are always double-checked, giving a perception to others that he doesn't trust them, even though most of the staff has been on the unit for over five years. When approached by his manager about his nondelegating style, he simply says, "If you want it done right, you need to do it yourself." You and the others are getting increasingly frustrated with him and decide to speak with him tonight.

Case Considerations

1. What are some of the issues that bring you and the staff to speak to Justin? Why bother?

2. Why do you think that he insists upon doing most tasks himself?

3. Discuss how the staff could approach him.

4. What should one not say to him and why?

5. How can he be helped in understanding how effective delegation can benefit both him and the patients?

6. Outline some suggestions for improving Justin's delegation skills while assisting him in understanding his new role as a registered nurse.

7. Does gender play into this scenario at all? Why or why not?

CHAPTER SUMMARY

Delegation, regardless of one's experience, can be challenging and place registered nurses in uncomfortable situations if they are not well prepared. In order to effectively delegate to others, whether the delegate holds a license, a certificate, or is a nursing assistant, several key factors must be reviewed and established, including

- the scope of practice for the registered nurse and the people to whom she will delegate.

- the job descriptions of all involved.

- the competency of the delegates.

- the ability to carry out the task correctly and thoroughly.

- the consideration of the five rights of delegation: the right task, under the right circumstance,

using the right person, with the right direction and communication, and the right supervision.

Further, the registered nurse should ensure that the directions are clearly communicated, with explicit parameters for reporting back the results. Constant and consistent feedback is desirable and allows both the registered nurse and the person being delegated the opportunity for professional and personal growth, as well as an opportunity to provide optimal patient care while experiencing satisfaction with responsibility and accountability.

REFERENCES

Cohen, S. (2004). Delegating vs. dumping: Teach the difference. *Nursing Management, 35*(10), 14, 18.

Curtis, E., & Nicholl, H. (2004). Delegation: A key function of nursing. *Nursing Management, 11*(4), 26–31.

Feldman, H. R., & Greenberg, M. J. (2005). *Educating nurses for leadership*. New York: Springer Publishing Company.

Hansten, R. I., & Jackson, M. (2004). *Clinical delegation skills* (3rd ed.). Boston: Jones and Bartlett Publishers.

Harrison, S., Dowswell, G., & Wright, J. (2002). Practice nurses and clinical guidelines in a changing primary care context: An empirical study. *Journal of Advanced Nursing, 39*(3), 299–307.

McKay, M., Davis, M., & Fanning, P. (1995). *How to communicate*. New York: MJF Books.

National Council of State Boards of Nursing (1990). *Concept paper on delegation*. Chicago: NCSBN.

National Council of State Boards of Nursing (1997). *Assuring competency: A regulatory responsibility*. Chicago: NCSBN.

CHAPTER 17

Collaborator and Negotiator

Karin A. Polifko

A gem cannot be polished without friction, nor a man perfected without trials.
—Chinese Proverb

LEARNING OBJECTIVES

At the completion of the chapter, the learner should be able to do the following:

1. Define the various types and sources of conflict.
2. Discuss the application of the six sources of power.
3. Give examples of the five stages of conflict staging.
4. Identify and discuss at least five coping strategies to conflict resolution.
5. Verbalize the differences between soft, hard, and principled negotiation.
6. Distinguish between interest bargaining and positional bargaining.
7. Discuss how attitude can affect the negotiation and collaboration processes.

KEY TERMS

Accommodation	Expert power	Legitimate power
Avoidance	Forcing	Negotiation
Coercive power	Information power	Positional bargaining
Collaboration	Interest bargaining	Principled negotiation
Competing	Intergroup conflict	Referent power
Compromise	Interpersonal conflict	Reward power
Conflict	Intragroup conflict	Role conflict
Confronting	Intrapersonal conflict	Withdrawing

Regardless of the setting, the topic, and the people involved, eventually there will be some essence of a conflict. Conflict is inevitable as it is part of the fabric of communication. Yet while this topic has spawned numerous books, articles, and even more research, most people would probably state that they are most uncomfortable in dealing with others with whom they are in conflict, often not knowing what to say or how to converse when they are in this situation. Conflict makes most of us ill at ease, and many of us (actively) try to avoid being placed in a position where conflict exists. Yet to deal effectively with conflict is one of the greatest tools that one can learn as both an employee and leader in nursing, especially with the multiple roles and expectations that characterize the health care setting.

DEFINING CONFLICT

Most would agree that conflict is a given in most situations that involve two or more people. Basically, **conflict** is an expression of differences (Bar-Siman-Tov, 2004). Conflict centers on a difference in values, viewpoints, goals, attitudes, or beliefs between individuals, groups, or organizations. The conflict may be actual or perceived, but regardless of the authenticity, it is treated as real and present and can result in angst and disagreement. Conflict may result from the competition for attention, for scarce resources, or simple incompatibility. Regardless of the source and whether it is real or imaginary, conflict can have positive or negative effects on the people involved.

FUNCTIONAL AND DYSFUNCTIONAL CONFLICT

Until the 1960s the very thought of conflict was to be avoided. Early management theorists and writers believed that conflict in any fashion was to be avoided for its negative—and destructive—impact, regardless of the situation and circumstances involved. During this period, organizations shared these perceptions about conflict:

1. Conflict was always perceived as a negative influence indicating that something was wrong. Because of this, the goal was to eliminate (or avoid in the first place) all conflict situations. Conflict is bad.

2. If conflict exists within an organization, there must be something wrong with the organization.

3. Those who are causing the conflict are somehow inherently emotionally ill.

4. The job of the manager is to eliminate all conflict, even if it means discharging the employee. The situation surrounding the dismissal was usually not discussed publicly, but other employees were encouraged to keep up the facade that everything was fine while abiding by the rules without question.

5. Conflict results in less productivity for the organization.

Since then, organizations and their managers have made a 180-degree turnaround on the nature of conflict within the organization, resulting in the following thoughts:

1. Conflict is inevitable.

2. Conflict can be as productive for an organization as it is destructive and inhibiting; it all depends on how the conflict situation is managed.

3. Most conflict can be successfully managed in order to maximize the potential and minimize the expected losses.

4. Conflict can actually lead to a higher level of performance and other positive outcomes if addressed appropriately.

5. Some say that in the absence of conflict, ambivalence could potentially result, leading to

lack of motivation, lowered productivity, and apathy. A positive side effect of conflict could be heightened creativity in order to solve problems.

So who is to say what is functional conflict and what is dysfunctional? Depending on the situation and the people involved, it could be either scenario, with very different outcomes. Essentially, if the conflict restricts the organization from achieving its desired goals, then it could be classified as dysfunctional. On the other hand, if the conflict assists the organization in moving forward with more creative problem solving and reaching a higher level of excellence, then constructive or functional conflict exists. Constructive conflict can also result in increased unity and the "team" pulling together toward a common goal, oftentimes with surprising leadership within the ranks. Conversely, dysfunctional or destructive conflict may result in the organization pulling apart, with obvious—or even subliminal— arguing along with a decrease in quality and performance level. Whether something is identified as functional or dysfunctional is dependent upon the setting, the players involved, the desired goals, and the methods used to employ the conflict resolution.

FINDING CONFLICT—OR HAVING IT FIND YOU

The potential for conflict is never too far away. Whenever there is more than one person, there is an opportunity for a disagreement based on past experiences, values, beliefs, and attitudes. Cultural differences are real aspects to consider when communicating, and it is in these differences that the potential for the divergence of ideas and conclusions runs the highest. Take the simple notion of time, for example. There are cultures, like the American culture, that expect promptness and preparedness at the mutually agreed-upon time, and if expected to be more than a few minutes late, a phone call is made. Conversely, other cultures, such as the Filipino culture, are more relaxed about promptness, and accepting late arrivals without

repercussions. Without an understanding of cultural differences, there is potential for misunderstanding and miscommunication. There are numerous examples of cultural misunderstandings; therefore, in order to value another's culture, the first step is to understand and appreciate the differences, while hopefully decreasing the prospect of a disagreement.

Conflict can also occur when snap judgments are made, or a decision is made without all the facts, or the facts are distorted. A problem may have several components, and those who are trusted with solving the problem may not have agreement on which section is the more critical one, based on individual values, personal agendas, or outside influences. Ethical perspectives also may cloud decisions that need to be made, with divergence in the route that is necessary to take while making the decision.

Regardless of the background, there are numerous sources that may lead to a conflict situation, especially in a complex health care organization. The potential for conflict increases as the complexity of the organization increases, both in scope of practice and the sheer number of employees at various levels of education and experience. In addition, people with diverse backgrounds have just as varied behavioral expectations, many of which are not always clearly defined or expressed, leading to a potential for misunderstanding. The potential for a misunderstanding due to a different—not better, not worse—set of values is huge, especially in light of today's multicultural society. Health care systems mimic the larger society, with positions ranging from hourly, nonbenefited jobs, to salaried executives, to privileged providers. Unfortunately, it is difficult to state which value set is the correct one: ideally, values are not viewed as right or wrong, but simply different. Each party views themselves as having the right value set, with the other party wrong. This type of thinking is dangerous because it can lead to egocentric thinking, remarks, and behaviors.

One of the first areas encountered that may have a value difference is between an employee and the organization's value sets. There are religious health care systems that do not perform certain procedures, and there are health care systems that actively seek private-pay patients almost to the exclusion of those without insurance. If an employee's belief set is in opposition to the larger organization, then there is potential for conflict as everyday work is performed. If the purpose of the organization and the purpose in being part of the organization are not in concert, again, there is a more than a passing chance of conflict developing.

The change process (actual or merely perceived) has great potential for causing conflict among people—managers and subordinates alike. Although there are some who relish the idea of something new and different and see change as exciting, there are just as many who view change as damaging, harmful, and maybe even hurtful. Although the various change theories have already been discussed in the text, there are several steps to effecting a successful change process:

1. Do your homework on the issues and the actual need for change.

2. Gather as much information as possible about potential alternatives for the change.

3. Involve those who will be affected by the change early in the process because they will be more likely to embrace and rally behind it than if they were just told about it at the last minute.

4. Acknowledge that change can be scary for many people, and that one goal of the process is to decrease the potential for conflict situations.

5. Ensure that all the affected stakeholders are kept in the communication loop during the change process.

6. Clearly define preferred outcomes.

7. Be able to evaluate the new outcomes.

8. Acknowledge the new change and be ready to tweak the results if they are not producing the outcomes that are desired.

Change can be a catalyst to conflict, regardless of the setting, the rationale for initiating, and the possible outcomes (both desired and actual). Even the most flexible person can become a little frazzled when encountering change. Although some people appear to thrive on the new, believing that the same thing over and over again is boring, the vast majority of people like to have routine in their lives. When that routine is disrupted, life changes, and conflict may result.

Regardless of the planning process of change, there is always potential that a facet of the project will be reorganized, revamped, or reengineered, not once, but several times during the process. These changes can lead to misunderstandings, misunderstandings to miscommunications, and miscommunications to mistrust and conflict. Even though much emphasis is placed on the minute details of the proposed changes, less time is spent contemplating the effects on the staff and employees. These particular effects are much harder to predict, control, and redirect than the non-people-oriented results. It takes careful and strategic planning by all those affected to consider the potential side effects of the change process, with one of the goals to address concerns before they become a conflict.

The fight for limited and often scarce resources is found increasingly in health care settings. Regardless of the resource desired, competition generally increases as the resource becomes more restricted. The competition for limited resources is ripe for conflict situations, because everybody generally wants more and better than their coworker, neighbor, or friend. In a work situation, one of the first issues is that of personnel resources: who has more, who is better educated, and who has the highest educational levels? With the current nursing shortage, competition for newly hired RNs can be intense, with some specialty areas more popular than others.

Rare is the hospital today that doesn't eagerly recruit qualified and competent registered nurses, and many times, actively and obviously recruit from neighboring facilities. Fortunately, RNs have become a desirable commodity once again, given that the profession of nursing has had its swings in employment. If there is a potential that a local hospital is wooing a group of RNs, the home institution often goes into high gear in retention strategies. Other personnel are also in short supply, such as nursing faculty and geriatric nurses, as well as unlicensed assistive personnel (UAPs).

Like personnel, space is limited and often cannot be expanded easily. Space—or the lack thereof—can be a subliminal conflict source. The corner office has always given the impression of power, as do windows, size, and location. It is certainly preferable to be located near the unit manager rather than in a small, cramped area in the basement!

Competition for equipment and other paraphernalia also increases the potential for conflicts. Have you ever known anyone who "hid" the IVACs in the clean utility room so that there were enough for the patients? Also, most people need the newest tool, the flashiest model, and the one piece of equipment that will certainly lead to increased patient revenues. Remember how every hospital had to have its own MRI and CAT scanner when they were first developed, rather than sharing cooperatively with the area facilities? Computers and the need for updated software can also make life much easier, especially because many hospitals have gone to paperless systems. Technology is great when it works; and when it doesn't, it can increase tenfold the time needed to perform a simple function.

Jealousies and conflicts can arise when one area is treated as what is perceived as special: perhaps Unit A receives new cardiac monitors over Unit B, even though Unit B's monitors are older. Unit A attracts the highly profitable invasive cardiology patients, whereas Unit B houses the hemodialysis patients, many of whom are on Medicaid. While the purchasing of the new equipment makes logical sense from one perspective, how can one rationalize this purchase to the hemodialysis staff who have been waiting for their new monitors for several years?

The previous scenario leads to another point of conflict: a clash of personal values. With the majority of our values determined by the age of seven, we are a product of our environment: social and family structure as well as genetics. A clash in values is incredibly common in the workplace, both individually and collectively. Many of us work where we do and in a particular line of work because we believe in at least the core values and belief sets. Couple the numerous possibilities for values along with ethical

and moral parameters, and there is a huge potential for conflict scenarios at every turn. Many nurses enter the health care field with the notion of service and wanting to help others. These values at times may be in direct conflict with the organization's business values, which may involve the patient not always being the primary focus in decision making, leading many nurses to experience conflict within themselves as well. In addition, with a complex organization, there are increasing opportunities to have value clashes with others who believe they are right regardless of the situation, perhaps because they have been placed in dominant roles within the organization. Our own values cannot be projected onto another, nor can we expect others to understand our values that differ from theirs. Given the increasing cultural and racial diversity in the United States, there is a rising probability that conflict situations will also intensify, primarily based on misunderstandings, differing values, and inadequate communication skills.

POWER: THE ROOT OF ALL EVIL?

The quest for power, success, and recognition can place one at odds with others who are trying to achieve the same accomplishments. Regardless of the scenario, there will always be people who want what you have, despite how the outcome was achieved, or the purpose behind the outcome. Everyone is watching everyone, just to make sure that one person doesn't get more than the other, who similarly believes he is just as deserving. One only has to observe toddlers who haven't quite learned to share to see this picture unfold, as they jockey for the biggest slice of cake or a parent's attention.

Power is simply processing the ability to get people to do what you want them to do or having a controlling influence over someone else. Power can be used in both positive and negative manner, and either through influence or coercion. Hershey, Blanchard, and Johnson (1996) believe that power is an influence that a leader can use to obtain either commitment or compliance from others. Unfortunately, power is something that can be easily abused, and it takes extra care to ensure that the effective leader and manager learn how to use it carefully and for beneficial purposes. Oftentimes, people believe that desiring power is a bad thing; however, it is critical to note that the desire for power can mean different things to different people. For example, power, if used to influence rather than control, can be the impetus for change. Regardless of the reason, power can be exerted only by someone *on* someone else: power cannot be established in isolation.

There are two basic types of power: personal power and expert power. Individuals have personal power when they feel sure of themselves—hence the overused term *empowered*—knowing exactly what they want and how to achieve their goals through their own abilities. Leaders with charismatic power have no trouble finding followers: people willingly join their causes. Similarly, those who use expert power are using their professional knowledge to achieve a power base that acknowledges who they are and what they contribute to the workplace.

French and Raven (1959) assert that there are five primary sources of power, plus another that is common in the literature (see Table 17.1). The first two, reward and coercive, are polar opposites.

1. **Reward power** is given in return for a behavior. For example, the nurse/manager can grant a three-day weekend in exchange for working overtime when short staffed.

2. **Coercive power** is associated with threats if a behavior or results are not accomplished. Using the above example, if the staff nurse does not agree to work overtime when the manager asks, then the opportunity for a three-day weekend disappears. Coercive power can also be viewed as punishment and pressure to force a person to perform under the threat of negative consequences.

3. **Legitimate power** is the most common power that is linked directly to a person's position (it is also called positional power by some). A Vice President of Patient Care Services has certain powers due to the authority vested in this role and like other types of power, can

be used for both positive and negative consequences.

4. **Expert power** is obtained due to someone's expert knowledge, skill, and competence in a certain role. Perhaps there is one nurse on the unit to whom everyone goes when there is a difficult IV stick to perform, or another nurse who understands wound care better than the rest of the staff. These nurses are recognized for their depth of knowledge and ability to share with others.

5. **Referent power** is somewhat linked to expert power, but has more of the nuances involved with leadership and charisma. A staff member may be recognized for her ability to get others to rally around an idea because of her informal leadership abilities, as well as her ability to inspire, motivate, and influence others. This type of power is more difficult to measure, but will involve others who readily follow another.

6. **Information power** is not one of French and Raven's original types; however it is well known in the literature that information power is indeed critical. It is possessing knowledge about a certain topic that is of value to others. Information is power; just think of the staff members who know exactly how many patients are going to be discharged on the evening shift. When the supervisor calls to ascertain staffing patterns for this shift, he needs to know accurate numbers in order to staff accordingly. The staff has the correct information: if are a lot of patients to be discharged, it may lower their staffing numbers, and they may not be staffed as well as they would like.

TYPES OF CONFLICT

Intrapersonal conflict occurs when there is an internal conflict between a given circumstance and a person's morals, values, or belief sets. Although someone may understand the scientific rationale for

Table 17.1 Types of Power

Reward:	Given as an incentive
Coercive:	Associated with threats, used as power over someone
Legitimate:	Linked by position
Expert:	Held due to knowledge
Referent:	In addition to knowledge, also has an element of charisma
Information:	Holding certain facts that others do not know

withdrawing life support, and may have assisted in the discussion surrounding the withdrawal, this enormous decision takes on a whole different light when it is someone related. A person may have conflicting viewpoints between what is scientific and what is personal.

Interpersonal conflict becomes an issue when there is a concern between two or more people.

For example, a newly hired person may have all the academic and work-related qualifications necessary for a designated position, but unless there is a fit between the person and those that he or she are expected to work with, the relationship may be doomed. Personality conflicts are quite common in the workplace, and unfortunately, they cannot always be predicted—or fixed. Sometimes it is just easier to acknowledge the differences and to see if mutual agreement can be achieved.

When a group's perspective or activities are altered due to external challenges, **intragroup conflict** is at risk of occurring. This can happen, for example, when there are two opposing viewpoints to an issue, such as a best practice technique that is introduced after a new research has been presented: half of the staff wants the original method because it "worked," and the other half wants to institute the new methodology because of the research findings. **Intergroup conflict** is quite common in health care because many groups compete for limited resources. For example, there may be overt competition for new

WRITING EXERCISE 17.1

Think about the types of power that some of your colleagues exhibit. For each type or source of power, identify someone who easily uses this power. Is the power used in a positive or negative manner?

Why does power often lead to conflict? Remembering that power needs to involve at least two people, there are always going to be circumstances that lead to discussion, disagreement, and predictable conflict of interests. Power is dependent on a relationship, with not all relationships being equal in nature; many have a dominant/subordinate association. When ascertaining the potential for relationship conflict, it is often helpful to carefully and critically assess the relationship at hand, reviewing several key factors:

1. Who is the most powerful? Why?

2. How is the power exhibited? Is it power through coercion, exploitation, manipulation, or competition?

3. Oftentimes the person with the most interest in maintaining the relationship has the most to lose in a conflict situation and will tend to accommodate more than the more powerful person.

4. People who tend to maintain the status quo—as compared with those who challenge the system—are generally more protected in their power base, weakening those who are attempting to challenge an organization's more established ways.

cardiac monitors. The diagnostic cardiology floor just received all new cardiac monitors, even though the ones replaced are only 3 years old, because of the increasing revenues brought in by the patients, the majority of whom have private insurance. In contrast, the dialysis unit, which has 14-year-old cardiac monitors, again was denied monitor replacements due to the decrease in revenues, as the vast majority of these patients are Medicaid patients whose reimbursement just decreased. It is human nature to have envious feelings that can result in obvious intergroup conflict.

A role as explained by Roy (Roy & Andrews, 1999) is composed of a set of expectations that others in society have toward one another. A role set consists of those multiple roles that someone holds simultaneously, such as mother, wife, social activist, or career professional. **Role conflict** occurs when there is tension that results from multiple role expectations and may further cause internal symptoms, such as headaches or stomachaches, or external symptoms, such as anger or withdrawal. Role conflict may also be initiated by incongruence between internal and external role expectations—the feeling that one is not meeting the role expectations of others. Working parents, particularly mothers, may feel conflicted between wanting and needing to be at work, and wanting to spend more time with their children. Table 17.2 illustrates several types of conflicts.

Table 17.2 **Types of Conflict**

Interpersonal:	Occurs when there is an inner turmoil
Intrpersonal:	Issue between two or more people
Intragroup:	Occurs when members of one group have issues
Intergroup:	Concern between certain groups of people
Role:	Tension within a person due to various expectations

CONFLICT STAGING

Conflict, as a process, manifests in fairly predictable stages. Pondy (1967) and Filley (1975) delineate five distinct stages: (1) the antecedent or latent stage, (2) the perceived conflict stage, (3) the felt conflict stage, (4) the manifest conflict stage, and (5) the conflict resolution or aftermath stage.

There are certain preexisting or initiating conditions that begin the conflict process, such as a power struggle, scarce resources, or intergroup issues. If the problem does not dissipate at this initial point, the process moves on to the perceived phase, wherein the issues are thought about, then to the felt stage, which then becomes emotional. At this point, it may be hard to keep focused, because there may be anger or feelings of defeat. With the scenario now both cognitively and affectively addressed, the conflict moves into the action, or behavioral, phase, wherein one party may verbalize negativity or react in a way that indicates to others that there is a conflict situation at hand. Conflict is then either eliminated by resolution, or it can be suppressed—both of which identify the conflict aftermath stage. When someone expresses himself loudly and negatively, it can disperse the tension and sometimes the conflict, at least temporarily. It is the suppressed aftermath that is more insidious and dangerous, for the actual conflict is never really addressed, but by avoidance and neglect, the person affected hopes that the situation will resolve by itself. The negative feelings may not be resolved, further contributing to the conflict and perhaps even extending it.

WHO WINS THIS ROUND?

Not every conflict situation ends positively, with everyone happy with the results. Filley (1975) identifies three end categories of conflict: win/win, win/lose, and lose/lose. The first one, win/win, is the ultimate goal when there is a conflict scenario; the objective here is to ensure that both parties are satisfied, not only with the outcome, but with the process of achieving the outcome. Generally, both parties are invested in achieving the best possible outcome, so creativity, innovation, and improvement are all at the forefront in decision-making and problem-solving activities. The focus is on goal achievement, with a consensus taken on how to accomplish the mutually set goal. Both parties have their needs met, and no one has to compromise, leading to greater satisfaction about the results.

In a win/lose situation, there is an emphasis on one party winning over the other, who unfortunately has to lose in order for the conflict to resolve. This approach is probably the most commonly seen; most people in organizations are highly competitive and want to win, sometimes regardless of the manner in which the challenge is conducted. A win/lose situation is often seen between supervisor and subordinate, wherein the supervisor is the usual winner because the staff person may be too afraid to challenge the boss. The focus tends to be on the opposing person rather than on solving the problem.

The most difficult situation to be in is lose/lose: nobody gets what they want, no one is happy, and there are probably bitter, resentful feelings that are simmering below the surface of most communications. Compromise is a lose/lose scenario because both parties have to give up what they really want. Both the win/lose and lose/lose arrangement have commonalities, but possibly one of the most important is the lack of a mutual problem-solving atmosphere; instead, both sides are in opposition, attempting to get the better of one another. Goals, values, or belief sets may be in conflict, but regardless of the setting, the attempts made at solving the conflict are minimal. Viewpoints are from only one perspective rather than trying to see things from both side. Also critical to the lose/lose and win/lose situations is the personalization of the conflict; again without the focus being on mutual problem solving but on power or domination, the goals for solving the conflict are not jointly determined.

COPING STRATEGIES

There are several and various strategies in which one can engage in order to cope with conflict situations (see Table 17.3). Not all of the following strategies work in all situations, and some people may be better skilled at applying one or more of the strategies than others. Any number of these strategies may be used at various times in an attempt to diminish conflict, but it is important to carefully choose the method to match the particular conflict; not every situation is actually worth losing sleep over!

Sometimes a conflict is so trivial that it takes more energy to address it than to ignore it. **Avoidance** is used when the potential gain is small, the conflict is temporary, the issue is unimportant, or the goal is to minimize any attention to the issue. Avoidance is lose/lose mainly because it simple does not address the concern, is unassertive, and sometimes uncooperative. I can't see the conflict, therefore the conflict does not exist.

Withdrawing is a form of avoidance that takes one party out of the conflict loop. It may not be a positive thing to remove oneself from conflict, but sometimes it is the best thing to do in order to avoid an argument.

Accommodation is often used in situations wherein there is a power difference, or one person is self-sacrificing to the extent of "the result is not as important to me as it is to you, so I will give up my stance so you can get what you want." Sometimes this is a necessary strategy, such as when the other person is more powerful and therefore likely to win, or when harmony needs to be maintained at all costs. Accommodation is the collection of social credits when there will be favors to accrue in the future for a more meaningful win.

There may be a time when the supervisor directs that an issue be addressed so that one side wins and the other loses. In **forcing**, power is used in a dominating fashion. Taking a vote so there is clear delineation of sides—and a winner—is a method used in forcing.

Table 17.3 **Coping Strategies**

Avoidance	Evading the issue on purpose	Win/lose
Withdrawing	Takes one party out of the conflict loop	Win/lose
Accommodation	Yielding to another	Win/lose
Forcing	Power is used to dominate	Win/lose
Compromise	Neither side gets what it really wants	Lose/lose
Competing	Ensuring that goal is met, regardless	Win/lose
Confront	"I" statements are used to clarify	Win/win
Collaboration	Assertive and cooperative	Win/win

Compromise is a lose/lose situation wherein neither side gets what it really wants. However, when used as a mediation method, it can bring two sides together who are markedly apart, to at least see and appreciate the other's viewpoints. Assertiveness and cooperation are used in this methodology, but there is still some resentment due to the incompleteness of the conflict resolution. In order for this method to be effective, both parties should be fairly equal in power and with achievable, mutual goals.

In a competitive environment, one will always win at the other's expense; there is no middle ground here. **Competing** occurs when there is a clear desire to ensure that the goal will be met, regardless of what is encountered along the way. This is a win/lose situation, and one that should be used sparingly.

Confronting is another method used in conflict resolution and mediation, and when done correctly, can be a win/win scenario. "I" statements are made rather than "you" statements. For example, one would say, "I feel that at the staff meeting, you indicated that I was not able to effectively manage my overtime budget, and I would like to know if there are ways that this can be addressed," rather than "You told me I couldn't manage my overtime budget at the staff meeting." In confronting, the person making the statements is careful to take the responsibility by decreasing defensiveness, allowing the other person to hear the message instead of simply reacting to it.

Collaboration is both assertive and cooperative in a win/win way. Both sides work together to achieve mutually set goals, without personalizing the process. It is clearly the most desirable win/win scenario among all the strategies, but sometimes it is one of the most difficult to attain, because it requires both sides to want to work together for mutual problem solving. Creativity and innovation are encouraged, yet a side effect of collaboration is that it takes a fair amount of time, in that all alternatives are studied for their potential effectiveness. Collaboration will be discussed in more depth later in the chapter.

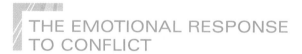

THE EMOTIONAL RESPONSE TO CONFLICT

Ask people if they enjoy a conflict, and the vast majority will emphatically state, "absolutely not"! Although it may be easy to logically analyze the conflict situation, what caused it and how to solve it, the first response will more than likely be an emotional one: either a fight response or a flight response. In a fight response, anger and resentment are exhibited, perhaps punctuated with caustic words. The flight response brings on silence, avoidance, and an ignoring of the problem in the hopes that it might go away. In both situations, the conflict is passed over or pushed down, but never effectively addressed, solved, and dispersed.

CASE SCENARIO 17.1

Gerri is the charge nurse on the 7 a.m. to 3 p.m. shift of a busy medical/surgical unit. Predictably, there is a phone call from the Emergency Department (ED) at 2 p.m. with four patients who need to be transferred before the end of the 7 to 3 shift due to the ED being swamped. Likewise, the medical/surgical unit is trying to discharge six patients to receive four post-op patients, who are due within the hour. Both the ED and medical/surgical nursing are frustrated and angry with the situation, and no one wants to budge.

1. Identify the conflict.

2. Who is involved with the conflict? Who are the leaders to help with the resolution?

3. What stage is the conflict in? What can predictably occur in the next stage?

4. Using at least four conflict strategies, give a way that the conflict scenario can be addressed.

The key to handling a conflict with emotional control is to first understand what personal bias a person holds, then to realize that self-control is needed regardless of the emotional triggers. It is essential to first understand personal bias, values, and belief sets and how they may differ from those of another person or group. Though it may not be easy to always understand another's viewpoint, it is crucial to control emotions and to recognize bias when there is conflict.

With increased self-understanding, one may be better able to have more emotional control and oral restraint in an uncomfortable encounter. The old adage, "Take a deep breath and count to ten" before saying anything goes a long way toward stopping a verbal barrage of insults and hurt to another person, especially those comments that are immediately regretted. Conflict, like power, does not exist in isolation; there is always another side to the situation. Both sides should take responsibility for the cause and effect of the conflict situation. Likewise, both parties are accountable to each other for the resolution of the issue at hand while seeking a common intention. People cannot elicit change in another's behavior, but they can change their own.

In a conflict, we immediately feel there is a need to have the other person hear our side of the story first in an attempt to defend our position. Pettry (2003) believes that we "Listen with the intent to reply, not to understand" (p. 21), rather than practicing active listening wherein we want to hear—and actually do hear—the other person's perspective on the situation first. She continues to assert that another key factor to controlling emotionalism is to identify mutual needs, interests, and goals. Listening can be an effective technique in controlling a rising conflict. Again, one of the key factors in a truly collaborative process is to understand what the common objectives are between parties and to jointly work together in achieving the optimal results.

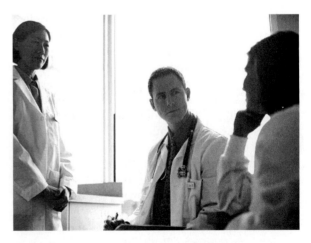

Figure 17.1 **Effective negotiation requires carefully listening to others' concerns.** Photo Courtesy of Photodisc.

RESEARCH APPLICATION ARTICLE

Van Ess Coeling, H. & Cukr, P. L. (2000). Communication styles that promote perceptions of collaboration, quality and nurse satisfaction. *Journal of Nursing Care Quality, 14*(2), 63–74.

All of us know that collaboration between physicians and nurses is the key to successful conflict management, but this technique is not always successfully applied in the workplace due to a variety of reasons, including the lack of reasonable skills. In a study by Van Ess Coeling and Cukr (2000), specific skills are identified that are necessary contributors to effective, a high quality of care, and nursing satisfaction. Additionally, the authors discuss three specific behaviors that increase the perception of nurses with collaboration, quality, and satisfaction in a health care setting. Norton's Communicator Styles was the primary instrument used, along with author-developed tools.

The logic in the findings lies in the validation by the authors that when there is an attentive versus dominant or contentious communication style usage by physicians, nurses perceive an increased level of collaboration, care quality, and satisfaction with the communication episode. Likewise, it was found that when nurses use the attentive communicator style as compared with the dominant or contentious style, there is a similar perception by their peers. The higher level of significance was found at the physician level as compared with the nurse level, further suggesting that nurses may be more sensitive to the MD's communication style than their own. The authors suggest that in order to enhance collaborative work relationships, particular attention to the communication style is essential between physicians and nurses.

TECHNIQUES THAT ADDRESS CONFLICT

Because of human nature, there are bound to be disagreements, misunderstandings, miscommunications, and the inability to always completely understand another's perspective consistently and accurately. Conflict is inevitable in many situations, but it does not necessarily have to result negatively. One of the more useful strategies to learn, regardless of role, is that of successful negotiation and collaboration. Nurses consistently negotiate on behalf of their clients and their families, whether it is with an insurance company (longer hospital stay), a physician (better pain control), or enhanced services (home health services). Due to the multi- and interdisciplinary nature of health care, negotiation and collaborative skills are crucial to successful relationships and achievement of work goals.

Negotiation

Negotiation is the gentle art of having the opposing party not only understand your position, but also to be able to come to a compromise in some fashion about theirs. However, it is in being able to see that the problem is the issue, not necessarily the person, that will make a negotiation successful. Birmingham and Anctil (2002) define negotiation as the "means to finding ways to achieve a particular goal within the circumstances that exist at any given time" (p. 74). Debate and negotiation are processes that start out similarly, but have diverse processes. In debate, there are two dichotomous viewpoints, with the goal of having one side prevail over another. Although there are two sides to consider in negotiation, the primary goal is not for one side to unequivocally win, but for both sides to reach a compromise that will help both sides achieve their goals. Negotiation is a skill that can be learned, but just as there are many sides to one issue, there are also many techniques one can use in successful negotiation.

Positional bargaining is similar to debate: both sides present their positions (identified demands) and gauge success on how many of their *stated* positions are met. The measure of success is how many of the positions are achieved, with the goal of winning the majority of personal positions. This is sometimes known as hard negotiation, wherein

1. There are two clear adversarial sides.
2. The goal is for one side to win.
3. The negotiation process will yield one result, so the need is to look at only one solution.
4. Compromise is not the objective.
5. Neither side trusts the other to be honest and up front.

Instead of attempting to win as many positions as possible and therefore beating the opponent, **interest bargaining** takes a different tack. In this type of bargaining, both parties look to the *actual* needs of their opponents, with the idea of understanding their desires, what will please them ultimately, and mutually satisfying both sides. In an example, a manager with a positional bargaining perspective will bargain down a request by an employee for a long weekend for a family wedding because (1) the unit is not as well-staffed on the weekends, (2) the staff member just had a long weekend off a month before to get married herself, and (3) others had expressed interest in the weekend as well, but had not formally asked. The employee, on the other hand, would most probably either call out, have a loud discussion about the situation to all and anyone who would listen, or perhaps even look for a transfer to another unit. Clearly, the manager has his position and will not move on it, thereby winning. In contrast, if there is interest bargaining, both sides come to a compromise, with as many mutual goals as possible achieved. The nurse may get the long weekend off,

but she will be the one to find staff coverage rather than the manager so that the unit is not left short-staffed; and because the nurse was the one to do the asking, the other staff nurses are more likely to go along with her request being met by the manager. The manager sought to find out why the employee wanted off and worked collaboratively with her toward meeting that goal.

Another type of negotiation technique is soft negotiation. In this type of negotiation, there is a camaraderie that occurs in solving the problem jointly. In addition,

1. There is assumed trust between the two sides.
2. The goal is to have a solution to which both sides readily agree. Whether or not it is the best goal or the one with the highest level of promise is not really as important as it is to get early agreement.
3. There is mutual accommodation—and frequently—so as to keep the other side happy.

The Negotiation Process

Nierenberg (1975) identified three components that must be met before true negotiation can occur:

1. The issue must be one that can be negotiated. Some things are not negotiable, such as how much sick time is earned.
2. Both sides must be interested in achieving their goals by being able to give up something that they deem important; beating the opponent is not the ultimate goal in negotiation.
3. There must be trust by both sides present, and there must be faith in the negotiation process itself; otherwise, the situation turns into arbitration, wherein one side forces the other into a decision.

The negotiation process is just that: a process. The goal is to produce an agreement between two parties who do not immediately see eye to eye or who may have divergent, yet equal, requests. In order to initiate and continue the negotiation process, there must be a relationship; so a primary goal in this process is to maintain a workable and trusting relationship. There can't be a sense of one side already being the winner or one side that is inferior to the other. With the objective to provide creative and viable solutions that are mutually agreeable, there often is a fair amount of work that is done by both parties to reach this accomplishment jointly.

With the goal of negotiating a positive end position, there are several fundamental points to keep in mind during the process:

- Come to the negotiation table prepared. Have a clear picture of what you are willing to negotiate: what you are and are not willing to lose.

- Understand the issue thoroughly before beginning the negotiation process. Having all your facts straight will allow you to be in the best position. Be able to offer facts about the issue if challenged.

- Spell out in clear language the issue, the problem, and the desired result. Being clear in the beginning as to expectations will save time in the end. Clarify the actual problem rather than assuming; and restate using the other party's perspective and words. Use reflective communication: "What I hear you saying is . . ."

- Understand who it is that you are negotiating with. What power do they bring to the table? Are you actually able to bargain, or is it just an exercise? What values does the other party have, what are their goals in this process? Is the person your boss, your subordinate, your peer? The ability to make a decision will change based upon your relationship to the other person.

- Look for solutions to the issue that can be win/win for both sides, rather than one side winning at the expense of the other.

Attitude can make a huge difference in the negotiation process. Some attitude perspectives to consider are

1. Be positive. Believe that there can be a solution to the issue at hand, and that there will be mutual acceptance of the solution. If one goes into the negotiation process with negative, this-will-never-work-out thoughts, there is a high likelihood that the other party will not be motivated to work together collaboratively to mutually solve the problem.

2. Show flexibility in the solutions discussed. Make sure that even if the ideas that are being presented seem a little crazy, at least there is active listening occurring. You never know; there may be a solution hiding in the silliest option, it just might need refining.

3. Be patient. Even the easiest negotiation may take time until both sides can comfortably agree on the solution. Also, choose carefully the battles to fight; not everything needs to be addressed, and it is better to stick to the issue at hand.

4. Be true to your word. If a solution is agreed upon, don't go back on it. Restate the commitment so that both parties understand without questioning the solution, and get it in writing if possible.

5. Show mutual respect. It doesn't help the situation if you come into the negotiation process wanting to "put one over" on the other side, or belittle them behind their backs. There needs to be genuine respect for the other party's opinions and their suggestions at solving the issue. The goal for respectful negotiation is to have sensitivity for the person and to value each other's differences. Active listening—wherein both sides hear, without emotion, the other's viewpoint—is a skill that takes some work. Remember, it is the "I" language, rather than the "you" language that can quickly turn a negative situation into a positive one. People want to be heard, not placated.

Principled Negotiation

Principled negotiation is a term that was coined by Fisher, Ury, and Patton (1991) in their book, *Getting to Yes: Negotiating Without Giving In.* With negotiation being a back-and-forth process in which both sides may have to accommodate, principled negotiation results in a "wise agreement . . . which meets the legitimate interests of each side to the extent possible, resolves conflicting interests fairly, is durable, and takes community interests into account" (Fisher et al., 1991, p. 4). Unlike hard and soft negotiation, principled negotiation has four primary principles as outlined by Fisher and colleagues (1991):

1. In solving the issue at hand, only objective data should be utilized.

2. Focus should be on the mutual interests as opposed to the positions of each side.

3. The person(s) needs to be separated from the issue or problem; keep personalities away from the equation.

4. Look at those alternatives that have mutually acceptable solutions.

5. Both sides, with compromise, assume trust as a real alternative.

Lens (2004) goes on to say that principled negotiators continue to advocate for their clients, seeking to maintain positive relationships for both parties.

One of the strengths of utilizing the principled negotiation technique is the focus on mutual problem solving, with the goal of ending with a solution that is creative, agreeable, and makes both sides feel as if they are winners. Needs are considered, communication channels are effective, and change is facilitated without relationships being harmed. Principled negotiation can be used in almost any situation wherein there is ongoing rapport, with those involved wanting to work together as partners rather than as adversaries, and both sides mutually agreeing to a fair conclusion.

Collaboration

Collaboration is another technique that has been reviewed extensively in the literature as a method to achieving conflict resolution. Collaboration has components that are quite similar to principled negotiation, and yet it has additional pieces that set it apart. Negotiation is sometimes perceived as a win/lose scenario, whereby one party succeeds at the expense of the other. On the other hand, collaboration is thought of as a more equalizing process, wherein problems are brought into the open. The goal is to

CASE SCENARIO 17.2

You are the undergraduate student representative on the Academic Affairs Committee of the College of Nursing. One of the agenda items is particularly contentious: that of raising the grading scale for passing to an 82; the old pass was a 75. The faculty's rationale is that the pass rates for the NCLEX examination are approximately 83, and that they want students to graduate and be prepared to successfully pass the exam. Students feel that the number is too high and would place undo hardship on them; after all, the University's passing grade is 65.

1. What is the identified conflict?

2. Who are the stakeholders involved, and what is their perspective?

3. Using hard, soft, and principled negotiation techniques, outline potential outcome scenarios for all three. Which one has the greatest possibility for a positive result that is mutually agreed upon?

4. What are some of the basic rules to use when negotiating?

5. How does attitude affect the outcome of the negotiation process?

6. What is the desired end result of this scenario?

bring the issues that cause the problem to the conversation, and to focus on identifying the underlying causes in an effort to find a solution that is mutually acceptable. Collaboration is an intricate process, with knowledge exchange that is intentional and focused on the problem at hand, with both sides taking responsibility for the achievement of the goal (Lindeke & Sieckert, 2005). The collaborative process has the potential for the highest success in an organization where there are two parties of somewhat equal power, a mutual need to achieve a satisfactory outcome, an expectation of interdisciplinary work, and a high probability of outcomes that are beneficial to both the organization and to both parties.

Thomas, Sexton, and Helmreich (2003) state that collaboration and teamwork are often used synonymously within context, which gives an interesting twist to conflict resolution. Although negotiation ensures that there is a problem that needs to be solved, there are various methods and processes to achieving resolution, including hard, soft, or principled negotiation. In collaboration, the process of conflict resolution is important, but it is in partnership with others that the goal is achieved. Teamwork is emphasized, with various stakeholders being involved in the process during the problem-identification phase, the decision phase, and the resolution phase. Gardner (2005) views collaboration as both a process and an outcome, but the need to work with others effectively is tantamount to successful achievement of collaboration. The collaborators' opinions and viewpoints are considered as well as all perspectives.

Kramer and Schmalenberg (2003) believe that effective professional collaboration involves mutual trust and respect, not simply one person directing another; instead it consists of an open communication wherein information is exchanged and understood. This point is especially significant; the health care field is so intricate that with so many levels of personnel at the professional, staff, and administrative levels, even basic communication can be easily misinterpreted. Successful collaboration involves simple common sense, yet the dynamics for achieving mutually desired objectives without having I-win-you-lose results are challenging.

Where there is successful collaboration, there is another situation that does not achieve mutually satisfying goals. What can cause a well-intentioned collaboration to become ineffective?

1. Hidden agendas. In collaboration, honesty should reign, with the goal of delving into the problems at hand in order to solve them. If there are hidden agendas, honesty cannot prevail, communication will be stifled, and there may be lack of trust and respect.

2. Lack of homework. For a collaborative experience to be successful, there should be preparation into the causative factors that generated the problem at hand. One can't solve a problem without an understanding of the events leading to the situation. Information is power, and when one side has all the information, the power base is obviously shifted.

3. Poor communication skills. Not everyone can say negative statements in a respectful, kind manner, and this particular skill takes practice. In collaboration, communication skills are emphasized, with the goal of effective messages that are received as they were sent. Open-ended rather than yes or no questions should be utilized in seeking responses. Likewise, both parties need to practice active listening, reflecting upon the communication sent.

4. Time issues. Collaboration is not a quick process of decision making; instead it is a back-and-forth exchange of ideas and acceptance. Having too little time to fully understand the issues and solve the problems will only result in frustration and poor outcomes. True collaboration can be intensely time-consuming, requiring much patience, because both sides may struggle to reach the same conclusion, but at different times. Similarly, not everyone has the same concept of time. At the very beginning of the collaborative relationship, expectations for time and responses need to be developed and mutually agreed upon. It can be extremely frustrating to have the necessary information

Table 17.4 Elements of Collaboration

Effective Collaboration Elements	Ineffective Collaboration Elements
Equal power status	Unequal power status
Trust and respect	Mistrust and hidden agendas
Enough time to work	Limited time to devote to the process
Research done about issues	Lack of information about issues
Shared responsibility	Refusal to take responsibility
Positive, can-do attitude	Negativity about process and goals
Cooperation	Antagonism
Good communication skills	Limited communication skills
Want to problem solve	Want to win the fight
Goal is to reach mutually acceptable end	Goal is to win at any cost
Many alternatives to problem exist	Only one right way to solve problem
Willing to compromise	Refusal to compromise any aspect
Plays well in the sandbox with others	Takes toys and goes home

needed for a mutual decision while the other party has not completed its fact-finding.

5. Power is used against the other side. Collaboration should be an equating of power bases, not an abuse of them. Dominance is not an aim in this type of relationship; it precludes shared goals. Conflict resolution is often thought of as a win/lose situation, wherein the individuals with the least power acquiesce to those in authority over them.

Collaboration involves many different elements, as shown in Table 17.4 with their opposites.

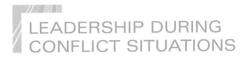

LEADERSHIP DURING CONFLICT SITUATIONS

One of the key responsibilities of the leader during a conflict situation is to quickly acknowledge the conflict and begin working immediately on resolution strategies. The goal in any organization should be to minimize the conflict; however, it is important to note that conflict is inevitable in any organization, yet there are leadership steps to take that can minimize any negative side effects.

A leader should model a positive negotiation strategy by having both parties attempt to work out a mutually satisfying agreement. The leader should get both sides to identify the problem; discuss possible alternatives; explore the issues, including the sensitive ones; and encourage each side to see the other's viewpoints. They should be positive that a mutually beneficial solution can be worked out, to the betterment of both parties and the organization. Honest and open communication should be stressed, along with equal respect, patience, and flexibility. By the same token, the leader should be able to facilitate successful conflict resolution in an environment that is conciliating, not antagonistic and negative. It is simply not acceptable for a leader to avoid all conflict, because conflict does not go away.

CHAPTER SUMMARY

The leader's viewpoint on the successful management of conflict has changed dramatically since the topic was first written about in management literature. The current thoughts are that conflict is inevitable, and that while uncomfortable for many sides, it can be a productive growth opportunity for an organization— or it can be destructive and divisive. The end result depends heavily on the manner in which the leader manages the conflict. The possibility for conflict increases in direct proportion to the complexity of the organization, with a tremendous potential for misunderstandings due to varying personalities. Differing expectations, multiple levels of power, and the constant change of the health care environment itself can all lead head-on into conflict.

Although an organization will have conflict situations, there are methods to employ that can result in a win/win situation for both sides, rather than a win/lose or lose/lose scenario. Several coping strategies are useful techniques to apply, including accommodation, compromise, and collaboration. Collaboration, as a nonmanipulative technique, is the only true assertive and positive stance to take in conflict resolution. Negotiation and collaboration are acquired skills, but even though they are commonly used, they may take a concentrated effort to refine. Negotiation has some fairly simple rules: both sides need to be honest, respectful, and want to achieve a mutually beneficial outcome; but it can be a difficult process to maneuver during a crisis or confrontational circumstances.

REFERENCES

Bar-Siman-Tov, Y. (2004). *From conflict resolution to reconciliation*. New York: Oxford University Press.

Birmingham, J., & Anctil, B. (2002). Managing the dynamics of collaboration. *Case Manager*, May/June, 73–77.

Filley, A. (1975). *Interpersonal conflict resolution*. New York: The Free Press.

Fisher, R., Ury, W., & Patton, B. (1991) *Getting to yes: Negotiating without giving in*. New York: Penguin Books.

French, J., & Raven, B. (1959). The bases of social power. In D. Cartwright (Ed.), *Studies in social power* (pp. 150–167). Ann Arbor: University of Michigan, Institution for Social Research.

Gardner, D. B. (2005). Ten lessons in collaboration. Retrieved June 28, 2005, from http://www.medscape.com/viewarticle/499266.

Hershey, P., Blanchard, K. H., & Johnson, D. E. (1996). *Management of organizational behavior: Utilizing human resources* (7th ed.). Upper Saddle River, NJ: Prentice-Hall.

Kramer, M., & Schmalenberg, C. (2003). Securing "good" nurse/physician relationships. *Nursing Management*, *34*(7), 439–440.

Lens, V. (2004). Principled negotiation: A new tool for case advocacy. *Social Work*, *49*(3), 506–513.

Lindeke, L. L., & Sieckert, A. M. (2005). Nurse-physician workplace collaboration. *Online Journal of Issues in Nursing*, *10*(1), 92–103.

Nierenberg, G. (1975). *Fundamentals of negotiating*. New York: Hawthorne.

Pettry, L. (2003). Who let the dogs out? Managing conflict with courage and skill. *Critical Care Nurse*, February.

Pondy, L. (1967). Organizational conflict: Concepts and models. *Administrative Science Quarterly*, *12*, 296–320.

Roy, C., & Andrews, H. A. (1999). *The Roy adaptation model* (2nd ed.). Stamford, CT: Appleton & Lange.

Thomas, E., Sexton, J., & Helmreich, R. (2003). Conflict and conflict management. In M. D. Dunnette (Ed.), *Handbook of Industrial and organizational psychology*. Chicago: Rand McNally College Publishing Company.

Van Ess Coeling, H., & Cukr, P. L. (2000). Communication styles that promote perceptions of collaboration, quality and nurse satisfaction. *Journal of Nursing Care Quality*, *14*(2), 63–74.

CHAPTER 18

Evaluator

Amy Barlow Britt

The purpose of evaluation is to improve, not to prove.
—Daniel L. Stufflebeam

LEARNING OBJECTIVES

At the completion of the chapter, the learner should be able to do the following:

1. Describe the types of evaluations nurses are expected to perform.
2. Discuss the importance of evidence-based practice in nursing.
3. Compare formative and summative program evaluation.
4. Compare formal and informal processes of self-evaluation.
5. Compare and contrast evaluation of peers and subordinates.
6. Describe how different standards of evaluation are applied in nursing.
7. Discuss the factors contributing to the need to measure nursing-specific outcomes.

KEY TERMS

Evaluation	Formative evaluation	Self-awareness
Evidence-based practice	Nursing-sensitive outcomes	Summative evaluation

Evaluation is a fundamental part of nursing and means to examine and judge, or to appraise. In relation to nursing and health care, evaluation is defined as the rating or assessment of the accuracy of a diagnosis, the effectiveness of a plan of care, or the quality of care; or a clinical judgment (Taber's Cyclopedic Medical Dictionary, 2005). Accordingly, nurses tend to think of evaluation in terms of patient care or clinical research. However, it is a process that occurs within many different contexts and situations. Thus, evaluator is one of the most important roles of nurses, who must have strong evaluation skills that can be applied in any setting.

Many nurses confuse evaluation with research. The two are closely related because evaluation is an essential component of research; however, they are not one and the same. There are some key differences between evaluation and research (Fain, 2005; Isaac & Michael, 1995). The purpose of evaluation is to determine whether goals have been achieved or needs met. The purpose of research is to gain new knowledge and provide results that can be generalized to other populations, conditions, or times. The outcome of evaluation is a decision based upon a judgment regarding how effective an intervention is. The outcome of research is a generalizable conclusion. Therefore, research has the additional burden of examining the context within which the intervention is provided.

The act of evaluating involves making a judgment regarding what is effective, appropriate, or adequate (Isaac & Michael, 1995). Dowding and Thompson (2003) assert that the actual process of evaluation in nursing is not well understood. They discuss ways of measuring the quality of judgment and decision-making processes of nurses. They define a judgment as using different clinical data about a person to arrive at an evaluation of his current health status. A decision is described as making a choice between alternatives based upon the evaluation.

There is an increased need to understand decision making in nursing (Cader, Campbell, & Watson, 2005). The Cognitive Continuum Theory has been applied to the decision-making process of many professionals in the fields of engineering, social policy-making, medicine, and nursing (Cader et al., 2005). Traditionally the decision-making process has been viewed as a dichotomy; that is, it involves either of two types of thought processes—analytical or intuitive. An analytical way of thinking is a slow, deliberate, and consistent review of facts and information. An intuitive style involves rapid data processing that occurs almost unconsciously. The Cognitive Continuum Theory places thought processes on a continuum from analytical to intuitive. The premise is that professionals utilize both types of thinking—how much of each depends upon the situation.

Under the Cognitive Continuum Theory, tasks are also viewed on a continuum from well structured to ill structured. An example of a well structured task is the review of a patient's medication orders by a nurse, who compares them to the medications the patient brought from home. An example of an ill-structured task is assisting a patient in transferring from a wheelchair to a bed, when the patient falls. The nurse has to assess, diagnose, and intervene very quickly in this dynamic situation. The Cognitive Continuum Theory links different types of situations and tasks to different types of thought processes. The researchers believe this theory is especially appropriate in nursing, because clinical situations are complex, and as a result nurses use different types of decision-making processes. Cader et al. (2005) assert that nurses who incorporate this theory into their practice will be able to increase the accuracy of their evaluations by utilizing the most appropriate type of thought process for the situation. The theory can also help nurses explain their evaluations to others, thus enhancing their credibility as professionals.

The types of evaluations that nurses perform can be classified in one of three ways: evaluation of patient care (the term *patient* refers to either an individual or group), evaluation of the process by which the care is provided (through evidence-based practice or health care programs, policies, and protocols), or evaluation of the personnel providing care (the nurse, peers, or subordinates), see Table 18.1.

EVALUATION OF PATIENT CARE

A key function of nursing is gathering information about patients, evaluating it, and making decisions about the plan of care (Bakalis & Watson, 2005). Nurses are constantly evaluating patients, because this is the final phase of the nursing process, wherein the nurse determines how the client has

Table 18.1 Types of Evaluation in Nursing

Focus	Subjects
Patient Care	Individual or Group of Patients
Patient Care Processes	Evidence-Based Practice
	Health Care Programs
	Policies
	Protocols
Personnel Providing Care	Nurse
	Peers
	Subordinates

progressed toward previously identified goals and outcomes. Evaluation also involves reassessing nursing interventions. During evaluation, the nurse will either decide to terminate the plan of care when outcomes are achieved, modify the plan of care as needed, or continue it if more time is needed to achieve the outcomes (Taylor, Lillis, & LeMone, 2005).

Effective evaluation requires that the preceding steps in the nursing process have been completed accurately. Patient goals must be appropriate and realistic; outcomes must be measurable. Without clearly defined goals and outcomes, it is difficult for the nurse to measure what has been achieved. An effective evaluation forces the nurse to address all pertinent questions (Kapborg & Fischbein, 2002). In this phase nurses must (1) identify criteria and standards; (2) collect data relative to these standards; (3) interpret the findings; (4) document their judgment; and (5) terminate, continue, or modify the care plan (Taylor et al., 2005). Nurses need to recognize that the decisions they make have a significant impact on the outcomes and experiences of patients (Dowding & Thompson, 2003).

There are two common misconceptions about evaluation and the nursing process. First, evaluation is not something the nurse unilaterally does to a patient; it is a collaborative process. The nurse and client are the primary participants in the evaluation, but other people such as the client's family and other health care personnel may be involved as well. Second, evaluation is frequently thought of as an endpoint. Evaluation

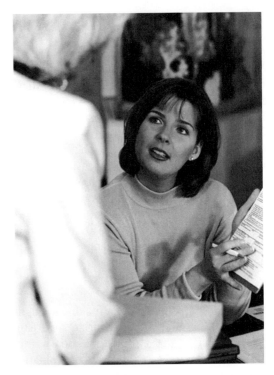

Figure 18.1 The evaluation of patient outcomes is a key nursing responsibility. Photo courtesy of Photodisc.

provides not only valuable information relative to the status of previously identified criteria but also serves as a starting point for further care. The results of this evaluation then either serve as a termination point for the identified unmet need or provide more assessment data to continue the process. Evaluation is not an end in itself (Kapborg & Fischbein, 2002).

EVALUATION OF PATIENT-CARE PROCESSES

When evaluating patient care processes, the nurse examines the structure and manner in which the care is provided. If the process is flawed, then the patient cannot receive appropriate care.

Evidence-Based Practice

Evidence-based practice is becoming the standard for providing professional care to patients (Thurston & King, 2004). The rise of evidence-based practice is a response to greater public expectations regarding health care quality and the drive to close the gap between research and practice (Newhouse, Dearholt, Poe, Pugh, & White, 2005). Quality of care can be described as providing the appropriate interventions to the client in a technically competent manner (Boylan, 2001). Other factors that play a key role in quality care include clear communication; an understanding of the patient's desires; and sensitivity to culture, age, and religious beliefs (Boylan, 2001). Nurses have to adapt to the increased emphasis on evidence-based decision making in their practice (Dowding & Thompson, 2003).

Nurses should strive to provide care based upon the most current clinical research. This may involve questioning the status quo. Why are certain interventions performed? This can be a challenging question to answer. There are interventions provided today with little scientific evidence to support their value. Evidence-based practice requires the nurse to keep up to date with current research findings. This can be accomplished through reading current journals and texts, participating in continuing education activities, and using the Internet to access online resources. Although this represents what should happen, it does not necessarily reflect reality. In a recent study, Pravikoff, Tanner, and Pierce (2005) found that a majority of the nurses surveyed had not even heard of evidence-based practice. Many nurses did not know how to access information from research articles and computer databases. One possible reason for this is the age of the nursing workforce. A majority of the respondents in the study were over the age of 40, which mirrors the current overall demographics of nursing. Information technology has changed significantly since most of these nurses graduated from school.

EVALUATION OF PROGRAMS, POLICIES, AND PROTOCOLS

From a broader perspective, nurses are involved with evaluating programs, policies, and protocols. How is care delivered to multiple patients? Is it quality care? The way care is delivered to patients is constantly changing, due to rising health care costs, nursing shortages, and the emphasis on improving quality outcomes for patients (Smith et al., 2005). Nurses are responsible and accountable for evaluating specific as well as overall outcomes of care provided (Cohen & Cesta, 2001).

There are two types of evaluation that can be used when examining a health program, policy, or protocol: while it is being utilized (**formative evaluation**), or after it is complete (**summative evaluation**). Formative evaluation, also known as quality assurance, provides evidence-based rationale for program changes during the implementation phase (Glick & Thompson, 1999). Summative program evaluation provides information for decision making regarding program changes that are introduced after implementation has concluded (Glick & Thompson, 1999). Methods used for both formative and summative evaluations include chart reviews, surveys, and other tools.

Not only can programs, policies, and protocols be evaluated from different points in time but also from different perspectives. They can be evaluated from a scientific perspective in terms of whether or not they meet the standard of care (evidence-based practice) or in terms of whether or not outcomes are being met. Patient care processes should be examined from the patients' perspective. For example, patient satisfaction is an outcome that is frequently measured. Smith and colleagues (2005) examine patient satisfaction scores and other outcome measures after a change in how discharge instructions are given on a hospital unit. Finally, the nurse's perspective should be considered. Interventions with favorable nurse opinions are utilized more frequently, resulting in better compliance.

RESEARCH APPLICATION ARTICLE

Smith, C. E., Rebeck, S., Schaag, H., Kleinbeck, S., Moore, J. M., & Bleich, M. R. (2005). A model for evaluating systemic change: Measuring outcomes of hospital discharge education redesign. *JONA, 35,* 67–73.

In their study, Smith, Rebeck, Schaag, Kleinbeck, Moore, and Bleich (2005) present a model for evaluating patient-satisfaction outcomes following a change in how discharge instructions were given to patients. In their organization, the responsibility for providing routine discharge instructions to patients shifted from the clinical nurse specialists to the allied health personnel under the supervision of the staff nurses. The authors took a formative approach to this and used a precase/postcase design to compare patient-satisfaction scores, knowledge of instructions, and readmission rates for the patients. They found a decrease in patient satisfaction and a lower retention rate for the instructions. The data regarding readmission rates were inconclusive. This article describes a complex research study conducted to evaluate the effects of a redesign in health care delivery on patient care. This study illustrates the importance of evaluating new patient-care processes. It appears to provide some evidence that supports nursing's unique contribution to health care.

EVALUATION OF PERSONNEL PROVIDING CARE

Evaluating health care providers can be difficult. Nurses are taught how to evaluate patients in terms of their response to nursing interventions and progress toward goals and outcomes. However, nurses are not routinely taught how to evaluate personnel, even though this is an expected component of job performance.

Self-Evaluation

Nurses are accountable for the quality of their practice and their role as a member of the health care team (Cohen & Cesta, 2001). Ellis & Hartley (2001) concluded that (1) nurses have an ethical responsibility to evaluate themselves, (2) a careful self-evaluation is a key step toward protecting patients from substandard care, (3) self-evaluation can be difficult and unpleasant at times, and (4) it is an important process that is carried out by individuals who know themselves better than anyone. Nurses can be the best source of information about their performance (Tomey, 2000).

Self-evaluation occurs both formally and informally. The formal process is usually done as part of the performance-appraisal process. Performance appraisals are typically done annually as part of orientation to the organization. The unit director or manager asks the nurse to complete a self-evaluation on a series of performance standards. The nurse may also be asked to identify strengths and weaknesses, and to set professional goals for the coming year.

Informally, reflection on one's practice provides the basis of learning from experience and promotes professional development (Meretoja, Leino-Kilpi, & Kaira, 2003). Developing **self-awareness** is an important part of nursing practice. Knowledge of oneself is essential to a helping relationship. People's behavior is largely determined by their values and beliefs; thus, nurses need to be aware of these values and beliefs so they can behave in a therapeutic way. Self-awareness involves being cognizant of one's self-concept, understanding one's own feelings and how they are handled, knowing one's limitations and strengths, and realizing there are choices in the way one interacts with the environment and with others. It is not just self-awareness of a nurse's values and beliefs, but also whether or not a nurse is meeting the standards of care. Novice nurses tend to focus more on the latter than the former. These two forms of evaluation occur routinely, often without formal recognition that they are happening.

There are several strategies a nurse can use to increase self-awareness. Introspection involves observing one's behavior in various situations and identifying its themes and patterns. It can be accomplished through anecdotal notes, journals, or diaries. Reflecting and writing about one's experience is a good way to analyze behavior. Nurses can also write their own philosophy of practice and identify values that are important to them; they can identify strengths and weaknesses as well as set appropriate goals. In order for these strategies to succeed, nurses must be open and willing to explore their behaviors. They must have a nonjudgmental attitude and try not to be defensive.

Evaluation of Peers

As members of the health care team, nurses have both individual and joint accountability (Cohen & Cesta, 2001). Therefore, they must not only evaluate

themselves but other nurses as well. As with self-evaluation, peer evaluation occurs regularly in nursing, both formally and informally. Many organizations incorporate a peer-review component as part of the nurse's performance-appraisal process. During this process, nurses are expected to evaluate their colleagues on the basis of selected job-performance measures. Peer review is an objective process by which groups of practicing RNs evaluate the quality of another RNs professional performance (Tomey, 2000). Peer review can be intimidating. Friendships may influence results, and peers may not feel comfortable sharing suggestions for improvement (Tomey, 2000).

In one form of peer evaluation, nurses may serve as preceptors for new staff. Preceptors have tremendous responsibility. They are typically experienced staff members who have strong clinical skills and who facilitate learning through various means, including role modeling. They need to be prepared to evaluate and manage a variety of nurses, from the learner who has an unsafe practice, to the learner who does not seem to care, and other challenging situations (Speers, Strzyzewski, & Ziolkowski, 2004). Evaluating clinical performance has serious consequences with regard to protecting patients from unsafe practice (Mahara & Jones, 2005). When evaluating a peer, the preceptor should determine whether or not the nurse is meeting the specified

WRITING EXERCISE 18.1

Describe a situation with a patient that was difficult for you, then answer the following questions:

1. How did you feel after the situation?

2. What specific beliefs or behaviors did the patient display that bothered you?

3. How are these beliefs or behaviors different from yours?

4. What is the benefit to the patient for having these beliefs or behaviors?

5. How did you respond to the patient in this situation?

6. How would you handle this experience differently in the future?

7. What did you learn about yourself from this experience?

CASE SCENARIO 18.1

You are a nurse working on a medical unit, and notice that a colleague, Maria, always seems to be in the nurses' station. You observe after the completion of shift report that she makes rounds on her patients taking only a minute or so in each room. Then she sits down and documents assessment findings and vital signs. Even though you did not observe what went on in each patient's room, you are suspicious because Maria did not spend enough time in each room to obtain the vital signs and physical assessment data she is now documenting.

Case Considerations

1. What are the issues in this case?
2. How would you describe Maria's behaviors?
3. What professional standards are not being met?
4. How would you handle this case?

outcomes. Comments should objectively describe professional behaviors. As part of the orientation, the nurse should have specific performance criteria identified. The preceptor should be able to evaluate how well the new staff person is meeting the criteria.

Informally, nurses are constantly evaluating whether or not their colleagues' practice is meeting the standards of care. If deficiencies are noted, the nurse needs to identify the reasons why. Does the nurse have deficient knowledge of a particular area? Is the nurse working on a unit that she is not typically assigned to, with unfamiliar unit-specific policies and procedures? Is the nurse impaired in some way? Even though informal peer review is constant, most nurses struggle with the follow-up portion. It can be difficult to pull a colleague aside and give honest and constructive feedback regarding performance. Even though this is an informal process, the key is to provide objective feedback. Nurses should limit their critique to what professional outcomes are not being met.

Evaluation of Delegated Care

In addition to peer review, the nurse can be asked to evaluate other members of the health care team to whom elements of patient care have been delegated. These providers can include unlicensed assistive personnel, licensed practical nurses, nursing assistants, and emergency medical technicians. When nurses delegate tasks, they are still responsible for them. They must evaluate each situation to determine the appropriate means of delegation. Nurses should evaluate each person who has been assigned a task in order to make sure the task is within his or her scope of practice and that individuals are proficient in performing the task. Finally, the nurse is still responsible for evaluating the patient's response to the intervention.

STANDARDS OF EVALUATION

Standards, or criteria, are the yardsticks for evaluation (Swansburg, 2002). They represent the levels of performance accepted and expected by other nurses and health care providers (Taylor et al., 2005). Who sets the standards? That is a key issue related to evaluation. Outside stakeholders frequently set the standards for evaluation in nursing.

Just as there are multiple contexts for evaluation to occur in nursing, there are multiple entities setting the standards for evaluation. The standards set for evaluation within the context of the nursing process are the goals and outcomes that are mutually set by the patient and nurse. For example, the nurse working with a patient who is recovering from hip-replacement surgery may collaboratively set the goal of being able to ambulate 50 feet to the nurses' station by the end of the week.

CASE SCENARIO 18.2

You are a nurse working in the emergency department. You have asked an LPN, who has received training in IVs, to start one on a patient who needs intravenous fluids and medication. You prepare the medication that has been ordered, and when you go to give it to the patient you notice there is swelling around the IV site. You immediately stop the fluids and assess the site. You determine the IV has infiltrated and will have to be restarted. You leave and find the LPN to tell her this, but she disagrees with you and even goes back and argues the point with you in front of the patient.

Case Considerations

1. What are the issues in this situation?
2. Was this an appropriate task to delegate? Why or why not?
3. What options does the RN have in this situation?

The fundamental reason for evaluating self, subordinates, and peers is to determine whether or not standards of care and patient outcomes are being met. Nurses need to remember this when giving feedback to others. The feedback should be professional and objective, highlighting the specific standards that are not being met.

Health care organizations and professionals with appropriate expertise identify the standards for evaluation of programs, policies, and protocols. For example, the American Heart Association establishes standards for the emergency care of patients with myocardial infarctions. Nursing organizations such as the American Nurses Association, Emergency Nurses Association, and other specialty organizations set standards for nursing care. Other entities such as the Institute of Medicine (IOM) have identified priority areas of health care that should be targeted in order to improve the quality of health care (IOM, 2003). Accrediting bodies for health care organizations also set standards. The Joint Commission on Accreditation for Healthcare Organizations' (JCAHO) mission is to improve the safety and quality of patient care through performance improvement (JCAHO, 2005). JCAHO evaluates quality of care through its accreditation process for health care organizations such as hospitals.

The government sets standards both as a payor and a regulator of health care through government agencies whose work is to maintain the health of the country. Payors, to the dismay of many health care professionals, play a pivotal role in establishing health care standards. There has been a push to incorporate economic methods into the evaluation of health care delivery (Tahan, 2001). Cost-Effectiveness Analysis (CEA) is one method used to evaluate health outcomes and resource costs of patient care (Tahan, 2001). This method is used by several federal agencies including the Centers for Disease Control and Prevention; however, it has not been readily incorporated into nursing research (Tahan, 2001). This is problematic insofar as these agencies are using this method to make important policy decisions. Nursing needs to be able to describe its contribution to health care delivery in these terms in order to have a greater role in health care policy and decision making.

NURSING-SENSITIVE PATIENT OUTCOMES

Increasing demand for professional and financial accountability as well as increasing concerns about the effects of nursing shortages on patient care have served as the impetus for examining the contribution of nursing to clinical outcomes (Sidani, Doran, & Mitchell, 2004). Nurses are becoming increasingly aware of the need to highlight their important contribution to health care delivery and to have nursing contribute to the standard for evaluation. Members of the profession are concerned with evaluating **nursing-sensitive outcomes.** These are outcomes that are influenced primarily by nursing interventions. By highlighting these, the profession of nursing can demonstrate its value in health care delivery. A notable accomplishment in this area of research is the creation of a language that labels nursing outcomes. Nurse researchers at the University of Iowa have developed a standardized language to describe outcomes of nursing interventions. This language, the Nursing Outcomes Classification (NOC), is officially recognized by the American Nurses Association as meeting its standards for information systems (University of Iowa, 2005). Additionally, it is included in the National Library of Medicine's Metathesaurus for a Unified Medical Language and the Systemized Nomenclature of Medicine, which are standardized languages used for health care delivery, research, and reimbursement (University of Iowa, 2005). The creation of the NOC, as well as other standardized languages in nursing, will help the profession describe and demonstrate its unique and valuable role in health care delivery.

It is important to note that other health care entities are studying nursing-sensitive outcomes. Recognizing that nurses are the primary providers of patient care, the National Quality Forum (NQF) has developed 15 voluntary consensus standards for nursing sensitive care (NQF, 2004). The NQF is a private, nonprofit organization that is working to improve the quality of health care through the development of standards and methods to measure quality care. The standards are divided into three areas: patient-centered outcomes, nursing-centered intervention measures, and system-centered measures. Patient-centered outcomes include eight measures, among which are pressure ulcer prevalence, falls, and use of restraints. Nursing-centered intervention measures include three related to smoking-cessation counseling. System-centered measures include four that address skill mix, nursing care hours per patient day, and turnover.

CHAPTER SUMMARY

Evaluation is a fundamental part of nursing. The types of evaluations nurses can be expected to perform can be classified into three different types: evaluation of patients, evaluation of patient-care processes, and evaluation of personnel who provide care. Various stakeholders set the standards for evaluation in health care delivery. A challenge for nursing is to have a greater voice in the process, thus the importance of studying nursing-sensitive outcomes.

Good judgment comes from experience. Experience comes from bad judgment.
—Jim Horning

REFERENCES

Bakallis, N. A., & Watson, R. (2005). Nurses' decision-making in clinical practice. *Nursing Standard, 19,* 33–39.

Boylan, M. M. O. Quality and outcomes: An overview. In E. L. Cohen, & T. G. Cesta (Eds.). (2001). *Nursing case management: From essentials to advanced practice applications* (3rd ed.) (pp. 525–530). St. Louis: Mosby, Inc.

Cader, R., Campbell, S., & Watons, D. (2005). Cognitive Continuum Theory in nursing decision-making. *Journal of Advanced Nursing, 49,* 397–405.

Cohen, E. L. & Cesta, T. G. (Eds.). (2001). *Nursing case management: From essentials to advanced practice applications* (3rd ed.). St. Louis: Mosby.

Dowding, D., & Thompson, C. (2003). Measuring the quality of judgement and decision-making in nursing. *Journal of Advanced Nursing, 44,* 49–57.

Ellis, C. R., & Hartley, C. L. (2001). *Nursing in today's world: Challenges, issues, and trends* (7th ed.). Philadelphia: Lippincott, Williams & Wilkins.

Fain, J. R. (2005). Is there a difference between evaluation and research? *The Diabetes Educator, 31,* 150, 155.

Glick, D. F., & Thompson, K. M. Program and project management. In J. Lancaster (Ed.). (1999). *Nursing issues in leading and managing change* (pp. 483–504). St. Louis: Mosby.

Institute of Medicine Committee on Identifying Priority Areas for Quality Improvement (2003). *Priority areas for national action: Transforming health care quality.* Retrieved June 29, 2005, from http://www.nap.edu/openbook/0309085438/html/R1.html.

Isaac, S., & Michael, W. B. (1995). *Handbook in research and evaluation* (3rd ed.). San Diego: EdITS.

Joint Commission on Accreditation of Healthcare Organizations (2005). Reference materials. Retrieved June 27, 2005, from http://www.jcaho.org/pms/reference+materials/.

Kapborg, I., & Fischbein, S. (2002). Using a model to evaluate nursing education and professional practice. *Nursing and Health Sciences, 4,* 25–31.

Mahara, M. S., & Jones, J. A. (2005). Participatory inquiry with a colleague: An innovative faculty development process. *Journal of Nursing Education, 44,* 124–130.

Meretoja, R., Leino-Kilpi, H., & Kaira, A.M. (2004). *Journal of Nursing Management, 12,* 329–336.

National Quality Forum (2004). *National voluntary consensus standards for nursing-sensitive care: An initial performance measure set.* Retrieved May 31, 2005, from www.qualityforum.org.

Newhouse, R., Dearholt, S., Poe, S., Pugh, L. C., & White, K. M. (2005). Evidence-based practice: A practical approach to implementation. *JONA, 35,* 35–40.

Pravikoff, D. S., Tanner, A. B., & Pierce, S. T. (2005). Readiness of US nurses for evidence-based practice. *AJN, 105,* 40–51.

Sidani, S., Doran, D. M., & Mitchell, P. H. (2004). A theory-driven approach to evaluating quality of nursing care. *Journal of Nursing Scholarship, 36,* 60–66.

Smith, C. E., Rebeck, S., Schaag, H., Kleinbeck, S., Moore, J. M., & Bleich, M. R. (2005). A model for evaluating systemic change: Measuring outcomes of hospital discharge education redesign. *JONA, 35,* 67–73.

Speers, A. T., Strzyzewski, N., & Ziolkowski, L. D. (2004). Preceptor preparation: An investment in the future. *Journal for Nurses in Staff Development, 20,* 127–133.

Swansburg, R. C. Controlling or evaluating. In R. C. Swansburg & R. J. Swansburg (Eds.). (2002). *Introduction to management and leadership for nurse managers* (3rd ed., pp. 518–532).

Taber's cyclopedic medical dictionary (20th ed.). (2005). Philadelphia: F. A. Davis.

Tahan, H. A. (2001). Case management evaluation: The use of the Cost-Effective Analysis method. In E. L. Cohen & T. G Cesta (Eds.). (2001). *Nursing case management: From essentials to advanced practice applications* (3rd ed.) (pp. 503–524). St. Louis: Mosby, Inc.

Taylor, C., Lillis, C., & LeMone, P. (2005). *Fundamentals of nursing: The art and science of nursing care* (5th ed.). Philadelphia: Lippincott Williams & Wilkins.

Thurston, N. E., & King, K. M. (2004). Implementing evidence-based practice: Walking the talk. *Applied Nursing Research, 17,* 239–247.

Tomey, A. M. (2000). *Guide to nursing management and leadership* (6th ed.). St. Louis: Mosby.

CHAPTER 19

Manager of Information Systems

Nancy N. Menzel

*It is a very sad thing that nowadays there
is so little useless information.*
—Oscar Wilde

LEARNING OBJECTIVES

At the completion of the chapter, the learner should be able to do the following:

1. Identify information management trends.
2. Define informatics.
3. Describe the transformation from data to knowledge.
4. Discuss computer applications in health care.
5. Describe the nurse's role in informatics.

KEY TERMS

Bits
Bytes
Client
Clinical information systems
Computer-based patient
  record
Customers
Data
Data capture
Data integrity
Database

Electronic health record
Electronic medical record
Hardware
Healthcare information
  systems
Information
Information technology
Internet
Intranet
Minicomputers
Nursing classification systems

Nursing informatics
Nursing information systems
Operating system
Server
Software
Standardized nursing
  languages
Telehealth
Telemedicine

INTRODUCTION TO INFORMATICS

Health care depends on information, and nurses are at the command center of the information matrix. Here are just some of the questions others are likely to ask the nurse in a typical hospital setting: "Has Ms. B. had her x-ray?" "Does Mr. N. have an allergy to penicillin?" "Is Ms. Q.'s blood pressure stable?" Whether you observe a modern nurse standing in the center of an intensive care unit interpreting a cascade of visual, auditory, tactile, and olfactory cues or visualize Florence Nightingale doing the same in a Crimean hospital, the common denominator is the processing of **data** and **information** about patients and their environment. Because nurses in hospitals have an around-the-clock presence and physicians usually only an intermittent one, it is nurses who collect and transform data first into information and then into knowledge as the primary function of their job. Nightingale had few tools other than paper and a quill pen with which to augment her cognitive skills and to assist her in organizing data. In today's health care environment, nurses have the tool of **information technology,** which is "the management and processing of information, generally with the assistance of computers" (Hebda, Mascara, & Czar, 2005, p. 5).

Informatics is the process of using cognitive skills and computers to manage information. Many prefixes have been applied to informatics: health care, medical, and nursing, with health care informatics becoming accepted as a term more inclusive of all disciplines. Health care informatics encompasses "the retrieval, storage, presentation, sharing, and use of biomedical information, data, and knowledge for providing care, solving problems, and making decisions" (Shortliffe & Perrault, 2001). The American Nurses Association (ANA) (2001, p. 17) has defined **nursing informatics** as follows:

Nursing informatics is a specialty that integrates nursing science, computer science, and information science to manage and communicate data, information, and knowledge in nursing practice. Nursing informatics facilitates the integration of data, information, and knowledge to support patients, nurses, and other providers in their decision-making in all roles and settings. This support is accomplished through the use of information structures, information processes, and information technology.

The purpose of informatics is to create and acquire knowledge in order to assist patients. As in General System Theory, where "'systems' of various orders [are] not understandable by investigation of their respective parts in isolation" (von Bertalanffy, 1968, p. 37), the output of informatics is greater than and different from the sum of the subsystems. The focus is on the interaction rather than the individual parts.

SIGNIFICANT TRENDS IN INFORMATION MANAGEMENT

The military, the government, and businesses long ago recognized that managing information was crucial to their missions. The first computers used in the United States were introduced in the military in the early 1940s and then in the U.S. Census Bureau. In the 1950s International Business Machines (IBM) began selling computers for businesses. However, health care organizations and providers have been very slow to adopt this new technology for managing health care information.

This lag began to close when Medicare legislation was passed in 1965, and the government began to require documentation of services before it would pay hospitals and physicians, creating a huge paperwork burden for providers. Looking for solutions, institutions and individual practitioners, such as doctors' offices, increasingly turned to computers to help manage financial information. Federal and private insurers and private accrediting bodies (e.g., Joint Commission on Accreditation of Healthcare Organizations) next called for using computerized medical records as tools for improving patient care quality; for example, retrospective chart audits against quality indicators. Most recently, the Centers for Medicare and Medicaid Services (CMS) has linked payment to performance, based on data on quality measures relating to treatment standards for three medical conditions common among Medicare recipients. Hospitals must transmit the data electronically. An emerging trend is the use of **information technology** (IT) to improve patient safety, such as use of bar coding for medication dispensing. With powerful forces mandating the use of information management systems, the nurse of the future will make increasing use of existing technology and devise new ways to use it to support practice.

THE NURSE AS INFORMATION MANAGER

According to Thede (2003, p. 261), "data are elements that have not been interpreted." Consider the number 100; by itself, it is meaningless. Now combine this number with another: 180/100. The nurse then recognizes these numbers (data) as a blood pressure reading, which the nurse collects. The nurse arrays a collection of these data to look for patterns to produce information. The nurse interprets the data in Table 19.1 to mean that the patient's blood pressure is approximately the same in both arms over a 15-minute period. To convert information into knowledge upon which to base action, the nurse must have additional information, that is, the normal range for blood pressure readings. Using the information that normal blood pressures are below 120/80, the nurse can now convert information into knowledge that this patient is exhibiting signs of hypertension and that intervention is needed. The nurse may create new knowledge by observing that other patients in similar

Table 19.1

Date	Time	Blood Pressure	Arm
7/9/06	8:00 a.m.	180/100	L
7/9/06	8:02 a.m.	178/98	R
7/9/06	8:15 a.m.	182/102	L

situations exhibit a similar pattern (e.g., after administration of a particular drug intravenously).

Nurses are inundated with data and information about their patients every day (see Figure 19.1). Key roles for nurses are ensuring that the data are collected on time and recorded accurately, followed by transmission of information as needed to the people who need it, such as immediately notifying a physician that a patient's blood pressure is dangerously high. Thus, these are the main information management roles for nurses: (1) collect clinical data, (2) record data, (3) interpret data to produce information, (4) use information to produce knowledge, and (5) share knowledge and information with those who need it.

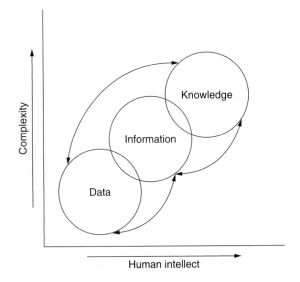

Figure 19.1 **Transformation of data to knowledge.**

SOURCE: From Scope and Standards of Nursing Informatics Practice, published by nursesbooks.org. Reprinted with permission.

To facilitate data capture, many systems for **standardized nursing languages** have been developed; they are called **nursing classifications systems.** The American Nurses Association (ANA, 2005) established in 1995 the Nursing Information & Data Set Evaluation Center (NIDSEC) for the following purpose:

[T]o review, evaluate against defined criteria, and recognize information systems from developers and manufacturers that support documentation of nursing care within automated **Nursing Information Systems** (NIS) or within **computer-based Patient Record** systems (CPR).

As of mid-2005 NIDSEC standards listed 13 terminologies that ANA recognizes as supporting nursing practice:

- North American Nursing Diagnosis Association, Inc. (NANDA)
- Nursing Interventions Classification System (NIC)
- Nursing Outcomes Classification System (NOC)
- Nursing Management Minimum Data Set (NMMDS)
- Clinical Care Classification (CCC)
- Omaha System
- Patient Care Data Set (PCDS)
- PeriOperative Nursing Dataset (PNDS)
- SNOMED CT®
- Nursing Minimum Data Set (NMDS)
- International Classification for Nursing (ICNP®)
- ABC Codes
- Logical Observation Identifier Names & Codes (LOINC®)

The goal of standardized nursing classifications/nursing classification systems is to standardize terminology for clinical problems and nursing responses to permit assessments of quality of care, describe nursing interventions and outcomes, enable research, promote education, predict trends, facilitate comparisons of nursing care across populations, and provide nursing care information for health policy and administrative decisions. Although most of the recognized nursing classifications are hospital based, the Omaha System (see Figures 19.2 and 19.3) is designed for use in community, case management, educational, and long-term-care settings. It includes an assessment component (Problem Classification Scheme), an intervention component (Intervention Scheme), and an outcomes component (Problem Rating Scale for Outcomes) (Martin, 2005).

Data integrity "refers to the ability to collect, store, and retrieve correct, complete, and current data so it will be available to authorized users when needed" (Hebda et al., 2005, p. 65). Although data integrity is a phrase associated with electronic data, it also applies to data stored on paper. The acronym GIGO (garbage in, garbage out) addresses data integrity; if nonsensical material is entered into a computer, the computer will produce nonsense. Another definition of the acronym is Garbage In, Gospel Out, referring to the misplaced belief that if a computer says it's so, it must be. Sophisticated computer systems have built-in safeguards to prevent certain types of errors, such as prohibiting entering text into numerical fields, limiting a field's length (e.g., can enter 10 but not 1000), and offering drop down boxes to restrict entries to valid choices.

Data capture, or the process of encoding real-world health data into digital format, is available through a variety of electronic devices. For example, there are now digital pens, containing a tiny camera, which transmit information to electronic patient records from special paper forms. In addition, many biometric monitoring devices (e.g., blood pressure, intracranial pressure, fetal heart monitors) are equipped to transmit their data directly to the electronic patient record, eliminating the intermediate step of reading the monitor and keying in the results.

A current challenge in nursing is incorporating the rapid proliferation of new knowledge into the evidence base for practice. Fortunately, there are many tools to assist nurses in accomplishing this ongoing activity. Information management tools such as treatment protocols, clinical guidelines, drug databases, and clinical pathways made their first appearances as print documents; however, many have been converted

PROBLEM CLASSIFICATION SCHEME

Environmental Domain

Income

Sanitation

Residence

Neighborhood/workplace safety

Psychosocial Domain

Communication with community resources

Social contact

Role change

Interpersonal relationship

Spirituality

Grief

Mental health

Sexuality

Caretaking/parenting

Neglect

Abuse

Growth and development

Physiological Domain

Hearing

Vision

Speech and language

Oral health

Physiological Domain (continued)

Cognition

Pain

Consciousness

Skin

Neuro-musculo-skeletal function

Respiration

Circulation

Digestion-hydration

Bowel function

Urinary function

Reproductive function

Pregnancy

Postpartum

Communicable/infectious condition

Health-related Behaviors Domain

Nutrition

Sleep and rest patterns

Physical activity

Personal care

Substance use

Family planning

Health care supervision

Medication regimen

PROBLEM RATING SCALE FOR OUTCOMES

Rating	Knowledge	Behavior	Status
1	No knowledge	Not appropriate behavior	Extreme signs/symptoms
2	Minimal knowledge	Rarely appropriate behavior	Severe signs/symptoms
3	Basic knowledge	Inconsistently appropriate behavior	Moderate signs/symptoms
4	Adequate knowledge	Usually appropriate behavior	Minimal signs/symptoms
5	Superior knowledge	Consistently appropriate behavior	No signs/symptoms

(Continues)

Figure 19.2 **Overview of the Omaha System.**

SOURCE: Reprinted with permission from Martin, K. S., *The Omaha System, 2nd ed.* © 2005 by Elsevier, Inc.

INTERVENTION SCHEME
Categories
Teaching, Guidance, and Counseling
Treatments and Procedures
Case Management
Surveillance

Targets
anatomy/physiology
anger management
behavior modification
bladder care
bonding/attachment
bowel care
cardiac care
caretaking/parenting skills
cast care
communication
community outreach worker services
continuity of care
coping skills
day care/respite
dietary management
discipline
dressing change/wound care
durable medical equipment
education
employment
end-of-life care
environment
exercises
family planning care
feeding procedures
finances
gait training
genetics
growth/development care
home
homemaking/housekeeping
infection precautions
interaction
interpreter/translator services

Targets—continued
laboratory findings
legal system
medical/dental care
medication action/side effects
medication administration
medication coordination/ordering
medication prescription
medication set-up
mobility/transfers
nursing care
nutritionist care
occupational therapy care
ostomy care
other community resources
paraprofessional/aide care
personal hygiene
physical therapy care
positioning
recreational therapy care
relaxation/breathing techniques
respiratory care
respiratory therapy care
rest/sleep
safety
screening procedures
sickness/injury care
signs/symptoms-mental/emotional
signs/symptoms-physical
skin care
social work/counseling care
specimen collection
speech and language pathology care
spiritual care
stimulation/nurturance
stress management
substance use cessation
supplies
support group
support system
transportation
wellness
other

Problem
Classification Scheme
Level 1
Domains (4)
• Environmental (includes Income)

    Level 2
    Problems (42)
    • Income

        Level 3
        Modifiers (2 sets)
        ⎡ Individual (who owns the problem)
        ⎢ Family
        ⎣ Community

        ⎡ Health Promotion (most+)
        ⎢ Potential
        ⎣ Actual

        Level 4
        Signs/symptoms
        (low/no income)
        (uninsured)
        ⋮
        (each problem has a cluster of
        s/s that are unique to that
        problem and 1 "other")
    • Sanitation
    • Residence
    ⋮

• Psychosocial (includes Spirituality)
• Physiological (includes Circulation)
• Health-related Behaviors
  (includes Substance use)

Intervention
Scheme

Level 1
Categories (4)
• Teaching, Guidance, and Counseling
  (i.e., range)

    Level 2
    Targets (75 actions and 1 "other")
    • Anatomy/physiology
    • Anger management
    • Behavior modification
    • Bladder care
    ⋮

    Level 3
    Client-specific information
    (not included in the Scheme itself)

• Treatments and Procedures
  (i.e., direct care, technical)
• Case Management (i.e., referral, coordination)
• Surveillance
  (i.e., monitor care over time, compare change)

Problem Rating Scale
for Outcomes

When
• Admission
• Interim
• Discharge

What

	low				high	
• Knowledge	1	2	3	4	5	(what the client knows)
• Behavior	1	2	3	4	5	(what the client does)
• Status	1	2	3	4	5	(how the client is)

Figure 19.3 **Understanding the Omaha System.**
SOURCE: Reprinted with permission from Martin, K. S., *The Omaha System, 2nd ed.* © 2005 by Elsevier, Inc.

to electronic format, and the most up-to-date versions are widely available through computers and other hardware, such as hand-held personal digital assistants (PDAs).

HARDWARE

To access and manage electronic information, the nurse uses various types of **hardware,** the physical equipment of a computer system. An **operating system** (OS) is **software** that provides programmed instructions to the computer to control various resources, such as memory, data storage, and devices. "The purpose of an operating system is to organize and control hardware and software so that the device it lives in behaves in a flexible but predictable way" (Coustan & Franklin, n.d.). OS examples include Microsoft Windows XP (for stand alone computers) and UNIX (for large networked computers). The OS controls access to all other software installed on the hardware. Other types of software include word processing, database, and spreadsheet programs. Computer users are **customers** (jokingly referred to as "wetware").

There are many types of computers, with power and portability matched to the setting's need. In academic and government settings, supercomputers

CASE SCENARIO 19.1

Mrs. B. is 93 years old and lives by herself in a deteriorating house. A severe kyphosis and arthritis in her hips contribute to her unsteady gait. Rarely using her cane in the house, she steadies herself by holding onto furniture. She has extreme difficulty with homemaking and personal care activities. The student nurse visits on a forty-five-degree day and finds Mrs. B. shivering under a thin blanket. There is no wood for the stove that heats the house. Boxes filled with old papers are stacked within two feet of the stove, and the narrow, two-foot-wide pathway from the bathroom to the living area is crowded with old furniture and grocery bags filled with clothes. A single 40-watt bulb dangling from the ceiling lights the whole house.

The student nurse notes that Mrs. B. has no heat. Mrs. B. states, "I ran out of wood yesterday. I don't know what I'm going to do, but I'm not leaving this house!" Mrs. B. is unsure where she can obtain wood. "People from a church brought me my last load," she states. After taking Mrs. B's vital signs, which are within normal limits, the student asks permission to contact Concerned Neighbors, an organization that can provide Mrs. B. with firewood. Arrangements are made for a small load of split wood to be delivered that day. After preparing Mrs. B a warm cup of tea, the student expresses concern about the boxes of old papers stacked near the wood stove. "Those boxes have been there for years. I like to have paper handy when I light the stove." The student discusses fire safety concerns. "Over the years, I've collected lots of things. Some days I can straighten things up, but I stumble quite a bit. My feet get twisted up real easy. I don't dare go in the bathtub anymore." The student notes that Mrs. B. is wearing a Lifeline necklace and asks about her history of falls. "I fell coming out of the bathroom

last week. I pushed my button and two nice gentlemen from the fire department came and helped me up." The student discusses ways to decrease Mrs. B's risk of falling, and she makes a referral to the Office of Aging for personal care and homemaking services.

Case Considerations

1. List four of Mrs. B's problems. Compare your list with a classmate's. Note that even though you may have identified similar problems, most likely the words you used to describe them differed. This is an example of the inconsistent terminology that standardized languages are designed to address to make sure all users have the same understanding.

2. Look at Figure 19.2. Classify the problems you identified in the first question into the appropriate domains: Environmental, Psychosocial, Physiological, or Health-related Behaviors.

3. Explain the purpose of categorizing problems into domains. See the following Web site for more information: http://omahasystem.org/.

4. Moving from the general to the specific, refer to Figure 19.2 to identify Mrs. B's problems by name.

5. Look at Figure 19.2, Intervention Scheme. Label each of the two interventions the student nurse carried out with one of the categories listed: Teaching, Guidance, and Counseling; Treatments and Procedures; Case Management; and Surveillance. Identify the targets of each intervention.

6. Look at Figure 19.3. Rank Mrs. B's Knowledge (K), Behavior (B), and Status (S) according to the scale given. Describe how this assessment of K, B, and S could be used to assess Mrs. B's outcomes over time.

WRITING EXERCISE 19.1

The text has given one example of the transformation of data to knowledge. (1) Identify at least two different examples of patient data that nurses collect. (2) Give an example of how these data are transformed into information and then knowledge. (3) Describe the persons with whom you would share the information or knowledge once you have created it.

are employed to crunch billions of numbers rapidly. Hospitals were once likely to use very large computers called mainframes, but many now find adequate computing power in newer **minicomputers,** which are smaller versions of mainframes; client-server networks are computers connected through one of them (a **server**). They form a local area network (LAN) that enables individual computers (**clients**) not only to store data locally but also to share data and programs. Larger systems are called wide area networks (WANs). Most hospital nursing stations and other large health care settings have computer terminals by which nurses access the LAN or WAN. Almost everyone is familiar with PCs (personal computers), small but powerful computers; these can be used alone or networked together in a LAN.

Data are stored in **bits** (**B**inary dig**ITs**) and 8-bit collections called **bytes** on a variety of devices. PC users are familiar with compact discs (CDs), DVDs, hard drives, and floppy disks. (The 3.5″ size disk no longer "flops.") Mainframe computers store data on magnetic tape or cartridges. Smaller networks may store data on a series of hard drives wired together.

WIRELESS AND MOBILE COMPUTING

Due to the need to manage information in settings remote from office or nursing station desktops, "laptop" versions of computers were developed to provide portable computing ability. The first portable computer (the Osborne) hit the U.S. market in 1981.

It weighed 25 pounds and had a 5.5″ screen. New "notebook" computers weigh in at about 6 pounds. The **Internet** is a worldwide network of computers that can communicate with one another through specialized programming languages. An **Intranet** is a computer network restricted by password to a particular health care organization or other entity, such as a university. With the advent of wireless Internet and Intranet technology, using telephone or cable wires to connect computers to networks is now optional.

One disadvantage is that wireless devices communicate through electromagnetic spectra, increasing the potential of unauthorized users gaining access. The advantages of ease of use outweigh the risks, though, as long as effective security is built into the wireless network.

Similarly, there are handheld computers, PDAs, Wi-Fi (Wireless Fidelity) badges, and mobile telephones that allow access to electronic information, communication, and e-mail through devices that are small enough to fit into a pocket. The trend is toward merging all functions (communication; data creation, access, and storage; imaging) into a single device. Nurses can carry these devices to the point-of-care (the bedside or other setting).

HEALTH CARE TECHNOLOGY

The **electronic health record** (EHR), sometimes called a computer-based patient record (CPR), is a "secure, real-time, point-of-care, patient-centric information resource for clinicians" (Healthcare

Information and Management Systems Society [HIMSS], 2003, p. 2). "Real-time" refers to instant availability. The EHR is a lifetime record that will document every health care event "using standard terms in computerized systems" (Lunney et al., 2005). Because of the variability in languages used in computer systems, in 2003 the U.S. Department of Health and Human Services formed the EHR collaborative to recommend standards for the EHR. The American Nurses Association was one of eight organizations in the collaborative, which has released its report at *www.ehrcollaborative.org*. The EHR will enable sharing data through an electronic information exchange. In 2005, after the flooding from Hurricane Katrina washed away tons of hospital and medical records in New Orleans, the need for EHRs was writ large. There is no backup system for paper records, but electronic data can be stored compactly in redundant locations.

In 2004 the White House called for an EHR for every American in 10 years. In 2005 a bill was introduced in the U.S. Senate to "help develop a nationwide interoperable health information technology infrastructure that reduces health care costs, improves quality, facilitates health care research and the reporting of public health information, and ensures that patient health information is secure and protected" (U.S. Fed News, 2005). Chief among these laws will be establishing electronic standards. A likely normative standard-setter will be Health Level Seven (HL7), a not-for-profit, American National Standards Institute-accredited Standards Developing Organization. Its mission is

> To provide standards for the exchange, management and integration of data that support clinical patient care and the management, delivery and evaluation of healthcare services. Specifically, to create flexible, cost effective approaches, standards, guidelines, methodologies, and related services for interoperability between healthcare information systems.

The EHR has many advantages, according to the Institute of Medicine (2003):

- Has privacy features incorporated, such as audit trails

- Provides diagnostic decision support
- Improves quality of care
- Enhances patient safety
- Increases productivity
- Contributes to the development of evidence-based health care
- Allows transfer of information among different settings (e.g., hospitals, nursing homes)
- Enables rapid recognition and response to disease outbreaks and bioterrorism

Health care "smart" cards are an emerging technology that will be an integral part of EHSs. These cards resemble plastic credit cards, except that instead of a magnetic strip, they have an embedded microprocessor (computer chip) that stores a person's digitized health records, including insurance information, health history, drug allergies, x-rays, laboratory results, and other data. Smart cards require a special reader to download or upload information, which has been encrypted (coded to make data meaningless if a "hacker" gains access to it). Health smart cards are in widespread use in Europe. In the U.S., a large obstacle to widespread use is the lack of standards for digital data, making data sharing nationally impossible.

The College of American Pathologists (CAP) developed one of the reference terminology systems (SNOMED CT) to be used in EHRs. CAP promotes its system of universal health care terminology with more than 344,000 concepts as one that is "building a seamless infrastructure of worldwide care while integrating an overwhelming amount of clinical data" (SNOMED International, n.d.). SNOMED CT has licensed to the National Library of Medicine its mappings to several nursing terminology systems (e.g., NANDA, NIC, NOC, the Omaha System), ensuring the inclusion of nursing in the EHR.

> SNOMED CT® is one of a suite of designated standards for use in US Federal Government systems for the electronic exchange of clinical health information . . . The NLM, on behalf of the Department of Health and Human Services, entered into an agreement with CAP for

a perpetual license for the core SNOMED CT® (in Spanish and English) and ongoing updates. The terms of this license make SNOMED CT® available to US users at no cost through the UMLS [Unified Medical Language System] Metathesaurus (National Library of Medicine, 2004).

EIIRs are the "gold standard" toward which the world is moving for computerizing health records; however, there is in existence and in use a less comprehensive system: the **electronic medical record** (EMR), although the terms are sometimes used interchangeably. EMRs are computerized versions of paper records with "interoperability within an enterprise (hospital, clinic, practice)" (Waegemann, 2003, p. 44). They contain information regarding the current care episode and may contain free-form text and other noncoded entries, limiting their usefulness. In addition, there is no way (or motivation) to share this information with other health care enterprises due to the lack of uniform standards for EMRs. Nevertheless, Medicare announced in mid-2005 that it would give U.S. physicians free EMR software to computerize their practices with the intent to improve patient care. Each system is expected to cost between $20,000 and $25,000. One clinic in New York was able to expand its waiting room by switching to EMRs, saving 3500 square feet of room previously needed to store paper records (Rogers, 2005).

Hospitals and similar institutions use **healthcare information systems** (HIS). The HIS may be supplied by a vendor or be developed internally ("homegrown"). The HIS is usually divided into a **clinical information system** (CIS) that focuses on patient care and an administrative information system to manage business functions, such as billing, scheduling, and human resources. Just as a hospital is divided into clinical departments, so too are CISs, with separate systems for nursing, radiology, pharmacy, and the laboratory. However, the product (quality patient care) is more than the sum of its parts, which must integrate functions to achieve this aim. The CIS unites all departments and provides additional features beyond data storage to facilitate patient care. "Clinical information systems with applications to support human decision-making and outcomes analysis are slowly being integrated into practice" (Androwich et al., 2003, p. 35).

Nursing information systems (NISs) are part of most CISs. Their purpose is to support nursing practice by providing the information nurses need to practice and the ability to document care. At the end of the last century, although vendors and early adopters predicted many benefits from using NISs (e.g., increased time to spend with patients, better documentation, and increased nursing productivity), a recent Cochrane Review of published research did not find evidence that these systems affected practice (Currell & Urquhart, 2003). In 2003 Androwich and associates, writing for the American Medical Informatics Association and the ANA, called for "a new generation of clinical information systems . . . to support nursing practice" (p. 49), after concluding that "what we have been doing is not working" (p. 47). The next generation of nurses will drive that change by softening the rigid perspective of nursing as a stand-alone component in patient care and adopting a patient-centered approach, working not only with other clinicians but also with CIS vendors to improve electronic information management.

PATIENT SAFETY

When the Institute of Medicine (IOM) released a report in 2000 that 98,000 Americans lost their lives every year due to medical error, the public and health care providers took notice. The IOM pointed out that contrary to the belief of consumers, practitioners, and hospital administrators, the cause of most medical errors was faulty systems, not faulty individuals. In other words, there is a chain of events occurring at the "blunt end" (e.g., inadequate policies, lack of safeguards, staff shortages) that leads up to the final error being made by the nurse, doctor, or other provider at the "sharp end" (the place where the error occurs). The report called for increased use of computers to reduce these adverse events through improved systems management.

The IOM followed this recommendation with another report (2001) calling for more computerization to improve health care quality in the twenty-first century.

> Although growth in clinical knowledge and technology has been profound, many health care settings lack basic computer systems to provide clinical information or support clinical decision making. The development and application of more sophisticated information systems is essential to enhance quality and improve efficiency (p. 15).

As a result of these reports, the U.S. Department of Health and Human Services Agency for Healthcare Research and Quality (AHRQ) became actively involved in the patient safety initiative to reduce medical errors and improve patient safety in federally funded health care programs, and by example and partnership, in the private sector (AHRQ, n.d.). One of its initiatives is the use of information technology to reduce error and prevent adverse medical events. How can technology help meet these goals?

One approach the IOM (2000) recommended was computerizing physicians' orders.

> Having physicians enter and transmit medication orders on-line (computerized physician order entry [CPOE]) is a powerful method for preventing medication errors due to misinterpretation of hand-written orders. It can ensure that the dose, form, and timing are correct and can also check for potential drug-drug or drug-allergy interactions and patient conditions such as renal function (p. 191).

Under the manual system prevalent in most institutions today, physicians write orders by hand or give them verbally, and then a nonphysician transcribes them by keying them into a CIS or other order entry system. This process produces high risk for adverse events from prescribing errors, transcription errors, adverse drug events, and treatment delays. Some studies have shown the CPOE can reduce medication errors, the largest source of medical error, by as much as 81% (Koppel et al., 2005). However, despite the promise of CPOE systems, physicians have been resistant to switching to direct data entry due to their frustrations with many aspects of existing systems and their perception that data entry is clerical work. Once improved systems are designed using human factors engineered to make the process more efficient than handwriting and the different types of errors that CPOE introduces are reduced, clinician acceptance should improve.

Clinical decision support systems (CDSSs) are another potentially powerful information-technology solution for reducing errors in the increasing complex health care environment.

> [CDSSs] are computer-based information systems used to integrate clinical and patient information to provide support for decision-making in patient care. They may be useful in aiding the diagnostic process, the generation of alerts and reminders, therapy critiquing/planning, information retrieval, and image recognition and interpretation (Tan, Dear, & Newell, 2005).

One system under development (N-CODES) is intended to assist novice nurses in making decisions in critical-care environments based on information processing theory (O'Neill, Dluhy, & Chin, 2005). This resource would be very helpful at 3 a.m. to a novice nurse trying to decide what to do after detecting a new symptom in an acutely ill patient.

Smart infusion pumps are another example of technology's potential to reduce adverse events, particularly at the interface between nurse and patient. The Institute for Safe Medication Practices (2002) describes their potential for patient safety.

> These infusion systems allow hospitals to enter various drug infusion protocols into a drug library with pre-defined dose limits. If a dose is programmed outside of established limits or clinical parameters, the pumps halt or provide an alarm, informing the clinician that the dose is outside the recommended range. Some pumps have the capability of integrating patient monitoring and other patient parameters such as age or clinical condition.

WRITING EXERCISE 19.2

Describe a decision-support system intended for student nurses. On what area would it focus? What kinds of questions would it help you answer? With what piece of hardware would you want to access this system? How long do you think it would take to develop the system? Should nursing programs provide your system to students, or would students buy it like a textbook? Name your system and bring details of it to class.

However, as with any technology, nurses have a responsibility to ensure that these high-tech infusion systems are operating as intended. Hardware and software failures have occurred with these automated pumps, putting patients at risk in ways not associated with manual systems. For example, in 2005, the Food and Drug Administration (FDA) required Baxter to recall over 200,000 of its pumps due to flaws that resulted in deadly consequences. One design error was locating the on and off switches side by side, leading some nurses to turn off the pump by mistake instead of activating it.

Information technology assists nurses in performing one of their essential functions: monitoring. Although some of this technology, such as heart monitors, have been in use for about 50 years, the newest generations of these devices are "smarter," in that they can not only directly record their readings in the computer-based patient record but also convert data to information by using computerized arrhythmia analysis to alert nurses to potential deviations from normal. In fact, automated external defibrillators (AEDs) take information processing one step further by not only interpreting the rhythm but also administering an electrical shock to the heart if the machine were to diagnose asystole or ventricular fibrillation. These devices are considered reliable enough to sell for home and public access use.

Other uses of IT to promote patient safety include wireless monitoring devices attached to vulnerable patients to reduce hospital nursery abductions and wandering by Alzheimer's patients, to cite just two examples. A defined perimeter is equipped with sensors that sound an alarm if the monitoring device breaches it. These monitors have quickly become the standard for patient security in facilities and are finding new uses in homes. Newer generation devices contain global positioning devices to pinpoint the location of lost persons, which is the same technology LoJack uses to find stolen cars.

Automated pharmacy systems have also been shown to be effective in reducing medical error. These systems include ones that replace pharmacists' manual review of a patient's record with computerized reviews of clinical information, laboratory results, and other medications prescribed to assess whether new orders are compatible and therapeutic. This type of expert system requires a pre-programmed **database** (information stored in records and fields to allow retrieval by the customer) containing medical knowledge and algorithms (rules). For example, if the physician prescribes a drug that can impair kidney function while the patient has a laboratory result indicating kidney damage, the expert system would flag this conflict for resolution by a clinician. Similarly, if a physician orders a "sound-alike" drug, such as Accupril, the system will issue a warning, questioning the prescriber as to whether this is the actual drug intended or whether it is really Accutane, Accolate, or Aciphex.

Some institutions have installed automated dispensing machines in the pharmacy and on nursing units, reducing (but not eliminating) the errors

CASE SCENARIO 19.2

A 34-year-old woman with AIDS developed a fever and hypotension due to suspected pneumonia. Her past medical history included several AIDS-related complications, but a recent test showed that her viral load was undetectable on a drug regimen of stavudine, lamivudine, and Kaletra (a combination pill containing lopinavir and ritonavir). Given her critical condition, an infectious-disease consultant recommended changing her stavudine, which is associated with lactic acidosis, to abacavir. The intern caring for the patient used a preprinted antiretroviral order template (paper form) to execute the medication orders, requesting a new agent, Trizivir, a combination pill containing abacavir, lamivudine, and zidovudine.

The following morning, a pharmacist noted that the patient's revised orders called for continuation of stavudine, lamivudine, and Kaletra in addition to the new order for Trizivir. The patient was thus set to receive double doses of lamivudine and thymidine analogs, any of which could be terribly toxic in overdose. Apparently, the execution of orders via the template did not automatically cancel the other, free-form orders, a processing issue the intern failed to recognize. Fortunately, the pharmacist caught the error minutes before scheduled administration, and the patient suffered no adverse event because only Trizivir was administered (AHRQ, 2005).

Case Considerations

1. Identify at least two causes of this "near miss" (an error that doesn't result in an adverse medical event).

2. If you were a safety consultant to this hospital, what recommendations for information technology would you make to prevent future occurrences of similar situations?

3. When information technology is introduced, what are some new types of medication errors computerization could produce?

4. If the pharmacist had not discovered the error, what would have been the nurse's responsibility before administering these drugs? How likely is it that the nurse at the sharp end would have caught the error?

5. What would be the consequences to the nurse if she had administered the double dose and it resulted in an adverse drug event?

associated with manually pouring medications according to orders. At the sharp end of pharmacy activities, where up to 30% of errors are made, are bar code medication-dispensing systems. In the optimum version of these systems, the patient wears a bar-coded wristband, the nurse wears a bar-coded badge, and each drug is bar-coded. These systems support the five rights of medication administration: right patient, right time, right drug, right dose, and right route. At the time when a medication is due to be administered to the patient, the nurse goes to the patient's room with the medication cart, a wireless tablet computer, and a bar code scanner. The nurse scans the patient's wristband, after which the medication to be given appears on the screen of the computer. The nurse then scans the medication's bar code. If it is valid for that patient according to the five rights, further information about the medication, along with any alerts, appears on the screen. Otherwise, the system emits a warning. After administering the drug, the nurse scans his or her badge, triggering electronic charting. Several systems sold commercially today automate only part of the process, leaving room for much improvement in work-process convenience and safety.

RESEARCH APPLICATION ARTICLE

Nebeker, J. R., Hoffman, J. M., Weir, C. R., Bennett, C. L, & Hurdle, J. F. (2005). High rates of adverse drug events in a highly computerized hospital. *Archives of Internal Medicine, 165*, 1111–1116.

It should be clear by now that there are powerful consumer, professional, legal, governmental, regulatory, and business forces pressuring health care institutions and practitioners to turn to information technology (IT) to reduce medical error. In light of the hype and the hope associated with this movement, how effective is IT in reducing adverse drug events (ADEs), which are a significant problem in all health care settings? A team of three physicians, a nurse, and a pharmacist (Nebecker, Hoffman, Weir, Bennet, & Hurdle, 2005) asked this question in a study conducted in a Veterans Administration (VA) hospital that had computerized many of its medication processes. Among the IT advances at this facility were "CPOE, bar code-controlled medication delivery, a complete electronic medical record, automated drug-drug interaction checking, and computerized allergy tracking and alerting" (p. 1111). In addition, the facility had full-time patient-safety coordinators, unit dosing (medications packaged singly rather than in bulk), clinical pharmacists who made clinical rounds with the physicians, and resident physicians supervised by senior

doctors. However, the CPOE in use did not have decision-support capabilities. The U.S. government has singled out the VA's "cutting edge" innovations in health care IT as exemplars for medical error reduction.

During a 20-month period in 2000, pharmacists reviewed charts of randomly selected patients admitted during the study time frame and identified ADEs. The researchers defined ADEs as injuries resulting from the use of a drug that started in the hospital. Of 937 charts reviewed, pharmacists found 483 certain or probable clinically significant ADEs. A majority of the ADEs were due to drug interactions. Nine percent of the ADEs were considered serious, the rest moderate. "Errors occurred at the following stages of care: 61% ordering, 0% transcription, 1% dispensing, 13% administration, and 25% monitoring" (p. 1113). The authors concluded that the CPOE had worked as intended to eliminate transcription errors but that an associated clinical decision support system was needed to reduce prescribing errors. They also noted that electronic medical records made ADEs more visible to researchers. It is sobering to consider these troublesome findings of persistent adverse events in light of the VA's position at the "bleeding edge" of health care IT. We are in the infancy of harnessing this technology for patient safety.

TELEHEALTH

In 1998 physician Jerri Nielsen, who was stationed at the South Pole in deepest winter, detected a lump in her breast. Unable to be flown out to treatment due to severe weather, the plucky doctor selected a welder (because of his manual dexterity) to help her perform a breast biopsy. She transmitted pictures over the Internet of the resulting slides to pathologists who confirmed the diagnosis of breast cancer. Planes dropped in chemotherapeutic medications, stopping the spread of cancer until she could be evacuated. That is an extreme example of telehealth, but a memorable one.

According to the Office for the Advancement of Telehealth (n.d.), telehealth "is the use of electronic information and telecommunications technologies to support long-distance clinical health care, patient and professional health-related education, public health and health administration." Telehealth removes time and distance barriers to the delivery of health care.

Certainly the placement of health information on the Internet has resulted in a communication revolution with not only professionals but also the public able to benefit from the easy access to evidence-based information. Unfortunately, this ease of access is both an advantage and a disadvantage, because there is a lot of unreliable, misleading, and false health information available as well. There are no peer reviewers for Internet content. Be sure to refer clients interested in researching health topics to reliable sources, such as government-run Web sites such as Healthfinder (http://www.healthfinder.gov/) or the National Institutes of Health (http://health.nih.gov/).

Telemedicine refers more narrowly to delivering medical consultation and treatment to clients at distant locations. For example, a dermatologist at a university-based medical center could provide services to a geographic area that has no physician trained in that specialty through the use of videoconferencing (real-time two-way transmission of voice and digitized images). However, there continues to be obstacles to delivering medical services this way; among them are the sophistication of the videoconferencing equipment needed at both ends, interstate licensure issues, and lack of reimbursement for this type of remote service. However, pioneers press on with successes such as performing surgery robotically with the surgeon in one country and the patient in another (telesurgery).

One of the most promising uses of telehealth is in home health care for disease management. To successfully manage a chronic disease such as congestive heart failure or diabetes requires a high degree of interaction between the client and the home health nurse or other clinician. Telehealth permits the transmission over the telephone of biometric information (e.g., blood pressure, blood glucose, blood oxygen, cardiac rhythm) collected by a specialized device placed in the home. In addition to the transmission of physiological information, there is also two-way communication of compliance information and education on a more frequent schedule than could be provided by in-person visits, which are more costly. Another application is nurse monitoring of the biometric data for a group of clients. Remote disease management prevents hospital admissions and emergency department visits, so as the U.S. population ages and the burden of chronic disease grows, this use of technology will expand.

RESEARCH WITH IT

It is obvious that health care institutions and providers are collecting massive banks of electronic data. How can nurse researchers convert these data to information and then to knowledge? One approach is to automate the statistical analysis of selected data in large databases to test a hypothesis. In their seminal study in 2002 Aiken and colleagues determined that hospital patient mortality and morbidity were directly related to patient-to-nurse ratios, with high ratios resulting in more deaths and more failures to rescue. To reach these conclusions, the researchers identified and analyzed selected information from the following large databases: the 1999 American Hospital Association (AHA) Annual Survey, the 1999 Pennsylvania Department of Health Hospital Survey, and discharge data for surgical patients from 210 acute-care hospitals. However, they judged hospital administrative databases containing information about registered nurse staffing unreliable, so they collected survey data for this measure instead.

An emerging technique in nursing research is data mining. Like the optimistic child who cheerfully shovels out the manure filling a horse stall because "there's got to be a pony in there somewhere," data miners view large databases as opportunities to use technology such as machine learning, artificial intelligence, pattern recognition, and visualization to discover associations and rules existing in the data. For example, a researcher interested in the work status outcomes of employees who file workers compensation claims could access a state's database of claims and instruct the computer to find patterns. The endeavor might identify previously overlooked factors that are associated with return-to-work success. Data mining unlocks the vast storehouses of already-collected data to allow nurse researchers access to the "gold" within them.

Also useful to nurse researchers are search engines for the databases that contain indexes to scientific journals, such as PubMed or CINHAL. Gone are the days when the researcher had to comb volumes by hand listing articles in print, write down their titles, and then search for hardcopies of them. With more journal articles available electronically (either duplicating the print version or published online only), the nurse researcher can now complete in a matter of hours a literature search that once took days or weeks.

PRIVACY AND SECURITY ISSUES

Just as when patient information is collected on paper, so too must health care organizations (HCOs) protect the privacy of electronically stored health care information. The Health Insurance Portability and Accountability Act (HIPAA) and other federal laws require HCOs to provide physical, technical, and administrative safeguards to ensure the integrity and security of the protected health information (PHI) they collect, store, and transmit.

Every HCO must name a chief privacy officer to keep health information confidential. HCOs also have chief information officers to provide broad oversight of the information system. Because the news is filled with stories of identify theft resulting from unauthorized access to electronic credit-card databases, consumers are concerned that having their PHI stored electronically is riskier than paper records. However, HCOs go to great lengths to prevent illegal intrusions and unauthorized access.

Electronic safeguards include

- Passwords: special codes that customers use to gain access to a network. These provide very limited security due to vulnerability to hacking and the carelessness and forgetfulness of customers.

- User authentication: the following biometric security technologies are already in use: iris recognition, digitized fingerprints, facial recognition, hand geometry, and voice recognition. These provide a high level of security.

- Audit trail: ability to track what electronic information has been accessed, by whom, when, and where. If designed correctly, audit trails can provide HIPAA-required information to consumers about who has accessed their health data. This is a feature not available with paper records.

- Firewalls: hardware or program barriers to prevent security threats from entering through the Internet.

- Encryption (coding) of data. Public-key encryption is a system that uses two keys to transmit information securely over the Internet: a *public key* known to everyone and a *private key* known to only the recipient, who is the only one who can decode the message.

- Virtual private networks (VPNs): enhance security for settings where there are users at remote locations (e.g., a state's public health department headquarters may have numerous regional offices).

With most HCO information stored electronically, a loss of data or service interruption would have a drastic, negative effect on the ability to deliver patient care. HCOs have extensive contingency plans in the event of a disaster to ensure that the system can be restored with data intact. Some of these methods include frequent backup (making copies) of data, storing backed-up data off site, and data mirroring (creation of duplicate data in real time).

Staff education is very important for data integrity and security as well. Before you, as a nursing student, will be allowed to access any HCO's computer system, you will be required to complete institution-specific training. The facility's information technology staff will perform periodic audits to ensure that you are limiting your access to information needed for your assignment only.

PROFESSIONAL NURSE'S ROLE

Nobel prize-winning physicist Max Planck (1858–1947) stated, "An important scientific innovation rarely makes its way by gradually winning over and converting its opponents: What does happen is that the opponents gradually die out." In nursing, those resisting the information revolution are gradually fading away. As the generation that spent their childhoods without computers retires, the Millennium Generation (the e-Generation?) will take their place. They will bring to their practice their expectations that almost all information can be digitized, stored, retrieved upon demand, and harnessed to meet their needs.

Nursing is in the midst of a sea change from a "high touch" profession to a "high tech/high touch" one. IT can assist nurses in spending more time with patients and less time completing tasks. For example, monitoring systems placed on a premature infant collect and record biometric data, giving the nurse time to rub the tiny infant's back, which pleases both of them. However, for this symbiotic system to work, nurses must meet IT at least halfway. Here are some steps to take:

1. *Increase your knowledge.* You may be entering the profession with little IT knowledge or a lot. In this rapidly changing field, yesterday's information may be obsolete tomorrow, so stay connected to groups that can expand and update your knowledge. Join the American Medical Informatics Association Nursing Informatics Working Group (www.amia.org/working/ni/main.html) or the American Nursing Informatics Association (ANIA) (www.ania.org). Once you graduate, take continuing education courses in informatics or attend an informatics conference. You may become so interested that you go on to get a graduate degree in this nursing specialty.

2. *Embrace technology in the workplace.* Speak up to volunteer to try new IT applications, or recommend IT innovations you've read about in other settings. Evaluate how IT can automate repetitive tasks in your work area. It was Kansas nurse Sue Kinnick who first had the idea to use bar coding for medication administration. She had an epiphany as she watched a rental car attendant use a bar-code scanner to check in her vehicle. She championed this idea through her employer, a Veterans' Administration hospital. Perhaps you can be the next Sue Kinnick. Tired of being called through the room intercom to come to the front desk for a telephone call? Ask for a wireless hands-free telephone to wear as you care for patients.

3. *Work with specialists.* If your HCO is considering changing or introducing new technology, it's important for nursing to be at the table during decision making. "If you're not at the table, you're on the menu," is an old political adage. If possible, a certified informatics nurse should represent nursing during the planning phase and assist during the implementation phase. The American Nurses Credentialing Center (ANCC) offers certification to nurses with a minimum of a baccalaureate degree and specified education and experience in informatics. ANCC (2005) describes the specialty:

The Informatics Nurse is involved in activities that focus on the methods and technologies of information handling in nursing. Informatics nursing practice includes the development, support, and evaluation of applications, tools, processes, and structures that help nurses to manage data in direct care of patients/clients. The work of an informatics nurse can involve any and all aspects of information systems including theory formulation, design, development, marketing, selection, testing, implementation, training, maintenance, evaluation, and enhancement. Informatics nurses are engaged in clinical practice, education, consultation, research, administration, and pure informatics.

4. *Work with vendors.* Few nurses have the programming skills to write their own software programs. However, they do have specialized knowledge of how nurses work and how IT can support their practices. If nurses want a better patient-care information system, they must share this knowledge with vendors.

5. *Be vigilant.* No IT "solution" replaces your clinical judgment. The nurse may delegate to machines certain tasks, such as monitoring biometric parameters, but the nurse remains responsible for the accuracy and timeliness of data collection, analysis of data to produce information, and the synthesis of knowledge. Just as humans are fallible, so are machines. Embrace technology, yes, but temper that embrace with critical thinking and common sense.

CHAPTER SUMMARY

Nurses are Information Central in health care. Nurses collect, store, retrieve, analyze, safeguard, and transmit health care client data, information, and knowledge. Information technology has the potential not only to assist nurses in performing their duties but also to improve patient care and reduce adverse events. Because of this potential, there are powerful forces outside of health care demanding the management and processing of information with computers and the adoption of standards to facilitate a lifetime Electronic Health Record for every American. Nursing informatics combines nursing, computer, and information sciences to enhance and support patient care. In the move to computerization of health care information, nursing recognizes several classification systems to standardize terms relating to nursing diagnoses, nursing interventions, and evaluation of outcomes. Most health care organizations

(HCOs) use health care information systems to manage both clinical and administrative information. They must comply with federal laws to safeguard the confidentiality of this information. Advances in information technology include software and hardware systems to reduce adverse events (particularly during medication administration), miniaturization of wire-free hardware to allow exchange of information at point-of-care, biometric data capture systems, wide availability of health information on the Internet, and delivery of health care services without the barriers of time or distance (telehealth). The new generation of nurses will harness technology as a tool to improve patient care. However, evidence-based clinical judgment will remain at the heart of nursing practice.

> *We are drowning in information but starved for knowledge.*
> —John Naisbitt

REFERENCES

Aiken, L. H., Clarke, S. P., Sloane, D. M., Sochalski, J., & Silber, J. H. (2002). Hospital nurse staffing and patient mortality, nurse burnout, and job dissatisfaction. *JAMA, 288*(16), 1987–1993.

AHRQ (n.d.). *Medical errors & patient safety.* Retrieved on July 19, 2005, from http://www.ahrq.gov/qual/errorsix.htm.

AHRQ (2005). *Case and commentary: Two pills, same drug.* Retrieved on July 19, 2005, from http://www.webmm.ahrq.gov/case.aspx?caseID=99.

Androwich, I. M., Bickford, C. J., Button, P. S., Hunter, K. M., Murphy, J., & Sensmeier, J. (2003). *Clinical information systems: A framework for reaching the vision.* Washington, DC: American Medical Informatics Association, American Nurses Association.

ANA (n.d.). *NIDSEC: About NIDSEC.* Retrieved on July 17, 2005, from http://nursingworld.org/nidsec/.

ANCC (2005). Informatics nurse certification exam. Retrieved on July 21, 2005, from http://www.nursingworld.org/ancc/certification/cert/certs/informatics.html.

Currell, R., & Urquhart, C. (2003). Nursing record systems: Effects on nursing practice and health care outcomes. *The Cochrane Database of Systematic Reviews, 3*. Art. No.: CD002099. DOI: 10.1002/ 14651858.CD002099.

Coustan, D., & Franklin, C. (n.d.). *How operating systems work*. Retrieved on July 17, 2005, from http://computer.howstuffworks.com/operating-system.htm.

Hebda, T., Mascara, C., & Czar, P. (2005). *Handbook of informatics for nurses and healthcare professionals* (3rd ed.). New York: Pearson Education.

HIMMS (2003). *HIMSS electronic health record definitional model version 1.0*. Retrieved on July 16, 2005, from http://www.himss.org/content/files/ EHRAttributes.pdf.

HL7 (n.d.) *What is HL7?* Retrieved on July 17, 2005 from http://www.hl7.org/

Institute of Medicine (2000). *To err is human: Building a safer health system*. Washington, DC: National Academies Press.

Institute of Medicine (2001). *Crossing the quality chasm: A new health system for the 21st century*. Washington, DC: National Academies Press.

Institute of Medicine (2003). *Key capabilities of an electronic health record system: Letter report (2003)*. Washington, DC: National Academies Press.

Institute for Safe Medication Practices (2002). "Smart" infusion pumps join CPOE and bar coding as important ways to prevent medication errors. *Medication Safety Alert!* Retrieved on July 19, 2005, from http://www.ismp.org/MSAarticles/Smart.htm.

Koppel, R., Metlay, J. P., Cohen, A., Abaluck, B., Localio, R., Kimmel, S. E., & Strom, B. L. (2005). Role of computerized physician order entry systems in facilitating medication errors. *JAMA, 293*(10), 1197–1203.

Lunney, M., Delaney, C., Duffy, M., Moorhead, S., & Welton, J. (2005). Advocating for standardized nursing languages in electronic health records. *JONA, 35*(1), 1–3.

Martin, K. S. (2005). *The Omaha System: A key to practice, documentation, and information management* (2nd ed.). St. Louis: Elsevier.

National Library of Medicine (2004). *Unified medical language system*. Retrieved on July 18, 2005, from http://www.nlm.nih.gov/research/umls/Snomed/ snomed_main.html.

Nebeker, J. R., Hoffman, J. M., Weir, C. R., Bennett, C. L, & Hurdle, J. F. (2005). High rates of adverse drug events in a highly computerized hospital. *Archives of Internal Medicine, 165*, 1111–1116.

SNOMED International (n.d.). *Welcome*. Retrieved on July 17, 2005, from http://www.snomed.org/.

Office for the Advancement of Telehealth (n.d.). *What is telehealth?* Retrieved on July 19, 2005, from http://telehealth.hrsa.gov/jwgt/jwgt.htm.

O'Neill, E. S., Dluhy, N. M., & Chin, E. (2005). Modelling novice clinical reasoning for a computerized decision support system. *Journal of Advanced Nursing, 49*(1), 68.

Shortliffe, E. H., & Perrault, L. E. (Eds.). (2001). *Medical informatics: Computer applications in health care and biomedicine*. New York: Springer.

Rogers, T. K. (2005, November 20). Square feet: Blueprints; It's a waiting room that keeps patients busy. *New York Times*, Late Edition-Final, Section 3, Page 22.

Tan, K., Dear, P. R., & Newell, S. J. (2005). Clinical decision support systems for neonatal care. *Cochrane Database Systemic Revues*, (2),CD004211.

Thede, L. Q. (2003). *Informatics and nursing*. Philadelphia: Lippincott, Williams & Wilkins.

U.S. Fed News (2005). *Sens. Frist, Clinton introduce Health Technology to Enhance Quality Act of 2005*. HT Media Ltd.

von Bertalanffy, L. (1968). *General system theory*. New York: George Braziller.

Waegemann, C. P. (2003). EHR vs. CPR vs. EMR. *Healthcare Informatics, 20*(5), 40–44.

FOUR

Envisioning the
Future of the Profession

CHAPTER 20

Defining a Professional: Graduate Education

K. Alberta McCaleb

Don't let the fear of the time it will take to accomplish something stand in the way of your doing it. The time will pass anyway; we might just as well put that passing time to the best possible use.

—Earl Nightingale

LEARNING OBJECTIVES

At the completion of the chapter, the learner should be able to do the following:

1. Identify workforce issues in nursing education and practice.
2. Describe the history of nursing education in the United States.
3. Discuss issues in the history of nursing that have assisted with or hindered the progress of nursing as a professional discipline.
4. Discuss the specific application of education level to the roles of nurses in the workplace.
5. Describe current master's preparation in nursing.
6. Describe doctoral preparation in nursing.
7. Identify at least two future trends in graduate nursing education.
8. Discuss issues related to graduate education needed in the practice setting.
9. Discuss issues related to graduate education needed in the academic setting.

KEY TERMS

Associate degree in nursing

Baccalaureate degree

Credentials

Doctoral preparation

Graduate education

Hospital-based diploma programs

Licensed practical nurse

Master's-degree nursing education programs

Nursing education

Professional nursing

The U.S. Department of Labor projects that there will be a need for more than a million new nurses as well as those replacing a retirement-aged workforce by the beginning of the next decade (AACN, 2005a; U.S. Department of Labor, 2003). With the nursing practice shortage at an all time high in the United States and across the globe, nursing education programs are challenged to increase student capacity and meet practice workforce demands. It is a well-known fact that the nursing practice shortage of the twenty-first century is compounded by the national faculty shortage in academic settings. Supply and demand issues for the discipline of nursing can be achieved only with a carefully orchestrated partnership between the nursing education and practice settings. With the demand for new nurses at the bedside and the demand for new faculty who are prepared to educate them comes the challenge of recruiting practicing nurses into graduate nursing education programs. In addition, the supply and demand issues must include creative nursing-career entry programs for individuals with additional educational backgrounds from other disciplines. A clear, specific career trajectory for nurses must be established early in the professional life of a nurse that includes opportunities for educational and career advancement in both the practice and academic settings.

NEED FOR GRADUATE NURSES IN THE WORKFORCE

Since the turn of the century the complexity of a declining professional nursing workforce coupled with an escalation in demand has continued to grow and is expected to reach global crisis by 2020 (USDHHS, 2002). In addition, the National Center for Health Workforce Analysis report (USDHHS, 2003) gives details of both population statistic projections as well as the number of registered nurses needed to serve them. To meet the demands outlined in this report will take a significant increase in the registered-nurse workforce, estimated to be almost

3 million new nurses by 2020. A healthy increase in the licensed practical nurse and nonlicensed nurse assistants is also forecast. The nursing practice shortage is indeed a crisis and is magnified by the need for expanded knowledge among nurses working in the health care industry. Professional nurses at all levels must have knowledge suitable for the information age and competency as a "knowledge worker nurse" who is grounded in practice skills associated with critical thinking, sound clinical judgment, team building, communication skills, who is adaptable and adept in the use of technologies, and leaders with management and delegation capabilities (Gaines, 2001). Thus it is imperative that nursing education and nursing practice work together to achieve the knowledge necessary to fulfill the changing roles of the professional nurse in the health care setting. Nurses must be willing to expand their educational credentials in order to meet the demands not only for increasingly complex caregiver skills, but also for the advanced roles of practitioner, educator, administrator, counselor, researcher, and policymaker (AACN, 1997).

Likewise, nursing education must develop curricula that emulate health care delivery needs. It should not always be the position of nursing programs to respond to practice, but rather to be visionary and shape practice as the health care industry changes. With an aging population before us, it is imperative that graduate programs continue to produce advance-practice nurses who are prepared to provide care to clients across age groups and health care settings (AACN, 1997). Although this push has been evident in master's programs across the country since the 1990s, graduate programs must continue to prepare nurses for role diversity. All graduate nurses will not serve in a primary role of practitioner. Many of them will be managers in primary and secondary health care settings, as well as educators in public health settings, hospitals, and academic settings. Master's-prepared nurses are needed to lead the quality improvement initiatives in health care agencies. Often it is the advanced knowledge of data entry and analysis possessed by graduate nurses that leads them to careers in outcomes assessment, informatics, and clinical research management and utilization. Nursing programs must provide nurses with opportunities to advance their education in these specialty areas in order to sustain professional growth and autonomy in the discipline.

OVERVIEW OF THE HISTORY OF NURSING EDUCATION

Nursing education programs throughout the country offer diverse curricula that lead to some level of entry into practice in the health care delivery arena. Perhaps the profession has experienced interrupted progress and some divisiveness throughout its history because of failure to distinguish the level of knowledge and type of skill acquisition necessary to function in certain health care delivery roles. Throughout nursing history, the focus of education has always been on an identified level of caregiver skill. Nursing is a "practice" discipline, but the role of the nurse is multidimensional. Not only is knowledge of the standards of care and skill sets aimed at quality delivery required, it is deemed the minimum level of knowledge required to function in the caregiver role. However, knowledge and technical skill in delivering care to others is but a minimum requisite for the multifaceted expectation of client- and family-centered care in health care systems today. The profession of nursing must come to terms with issues such as practice and pay differentiation; appropriate economic client-care delivery models utilizing a team of multi- and interdisciplinary team members who function in specific roles based on the knowledge and background of the team members; and an acceptance of upward career mobility for education and credentials obtained by nurses in the profession. To recruit and then retain the number of nurses that will be needed by the health care industry in the next few decades will require change from old paradigms to new, innovative educational programs that attract not only traditional nursing students, but also young adults from other career pathways.

History of Nursing Education

The evolution of educating students for professional nursing practice can be traced back to the late 1800s (Creasia, 2001; Hood & Leddy, 2003). The first nursing program in the United States was established in a hospital setting in Boston, Massachusetts in 1873. The program was a four-month training program that was similar to a model introduced by Florence Nightingale in London, England in the 1860s. Because there was opposition to collegiate education for nurses in the United States, these types of **hospital-based diploma programs** were the predominant models for nursing education for the next century. Diploma education curricula grew to an all-time high in 1958 to near 1000 programs and ranged in length from 2 to 3 years. Since these programs were located primarily in hospital settings, nursing students were used to meet workforce demands in the hospitals rather than solely educational endeavors. Concern over unfair use of nursing students (and other workforce labor issues) became the impetus for new nursing workforce, education, and student life studies, which were implemented by Goldmark in the 1920s and Brown in the 1940s (Creasia, 2001). These important studies marked an educational move for nursing programs from apprentice models that were hospital based to degree-granting, collegiate-based nursing programs. The major decline in diploma education began in the 1960s and has lasted through the turn of the century. However, the few diploma programs that exist today are aligned with academic institutions and grant joint degrees.

The demise of hospital-based diploma programs created a new opportunity to move nursing education programs into academic institutions of higher learning. The University of Texas was the first to recognize nursing education in the university setting in the early 1890s (Hood & Leddy, 2003). However, the University of Minnesota was the first to offer nursing as a college major within the School of Medicine in 1909 (Creasia, 2001). It was 1923 before the first university offered an independent nursing program and awarded the **baccalaureate degree** in nursing at Yale University. Other universities, such as Case Western Reserve University, the University of Chicago, and Vanderbilt University, followed this academic initiative. It should be noted that the first programs were implemented at the university level, but it was not until the 1970s that the number of graduates from these types of programs began to increase. Issues related to involvement in World War II, attitudes toward the education of women, women in the workforce, and physician opinion about the knowledge needed by nurses to perform their roles were all hindrances to increasing numbers of programs and graduates of baccalaureate education in nursing. Other important deterrents to the proliferation of baccalaureate nursing programs were the lack of qualified faculty to teach at the university level and the length of programs. Today, baccalaureate programs in nursing are approximately four years in length, organized with nursing at the upper division of the curriculum, and prepare a nurse generalist who is educated to obtain registered nurse licensure. The number of baccalaureate-prepared nurses has grown from approximately 3700 per year between 1975 and 1999 to over 12,000 per year in 2000 (AACN, 1996). Further, the baccalaureate degree in nursing was designated in 1965 by the American Nurses Association as the point of entry into professional nursing practice (Creasia, 2001). Likewise, the American Association of Colleges of Nursing Board of Directors published a position statement in 1996 recognizing the Bachelor of Science degree in nursing as the minimum educational requirement for professional nursing practice (AACN, 1996). The National Advisory Council on Nurse Education and Practice (1996) recommended more educational preparation of nurses in the workforce and that the baccalaureate- or higher-degrees in nursing constitute at least two-thirds of the registered-nurse workforce by 2010. Both of these declarations came on the heels of the infamous Pew Health Professions Commission report (1995), which directed nursing programs to produce more bachelors- and higher-degree nursing graduates. Within the last year the American Organization of Nurse Executives (AONE) has joined these

professional groups in support of the baccalaureate degree in nursing as the educational level required for registered nurses (AACN, 2005b). In 2005 there were over 700 baccalaureate- and higher-degree programs available to nursing students in the United States.

Historically, the next nursing education program type to be developed was for a technical/vocational nurse in 1942 (Creasia, 2001). This type program led to a new licensure category for nurses or the licensed practical nurse/licensed vocational nurse (LPN/LVN). The 9- to 15-month LPN program was developed in response to the workforce shortage created by World War II. Because many of the registered nurses were deployed to work during the war, this phenomenon left many hospitals understaffed. During this time unlicensed personnel, such as nurse aides and volunteers, provided much of the care delivered in the local hospitals. The need for another skilled worker who would be licensed was obvious. Since the 1950s licensed practical nursing programs have increased to over 1,000 (Creasia, 2001).

For nurses who wanted to enroll in a shorter educational program and still work as a registered nurse, nursing education programs in community colleges began to offer an **associate degree in nursing** (ADN). These registered-nurse programs prepare a nurse to provide direct care using a problem-solving approach and specific technical skill set that has an average program length of two years. Graduates of ADN programs are eligible to sit for registered-nurse licensure examination. Perhaps no other nursing program type has grown as much as the associate degree in nursing programs. In 2000 there were approximately 900 associate-degree programs in the United States, which graduated about two-thirds of the entering registered-nurse workforce (Creasia, 2001). Today associate-degree RNs make up 34% of the total nursing workforce compared with 43% of all nurses who possess a baccalaureate or higher degree in nursing (AACN, 2005a).

It should not be surprising that while baccalaureate- and associate-degree programs began to grow on college campuses throughout the country, so did the establishment of **master's-degree nursing**

education programs in university settings. If registered nurses were to be taught in institutions of higher learning, nurses must prepare themselves to teach and supervise in academic settings as well as clinical practice settings. Master's education in nursing began in 1899 at the Teachers College of New York to prepare nurses with knowledge of nursing management and education (Creasia, 2001). However, it wasn't until the late 1950s that master's degree education in nursing became more visible nationally due to its strength in preparing nursing for role function in a particular clinical area or client-focused population. It would be approximately 40 more years (1990s) before graduate education at the master's level focused predominately on the role of the advanced-practice nurse. Traditionally, master's programs in nursing are built on the baccalaureate-degree foundation and are 1.5 to 2 years in length. By 2005 there were over 350 master's-degree programs in nursing throughout all states and territories of the United States.

In the relatively short history of nursing education in the United States, doctoral education for nurses was essential, but slow to proliferate. With the first undergraduate nursing education programs beginning at the university level in the early 1900s and master's-level graduate programs established in the 1950s, it is to be expected that there was a tremendous need for doctoral education in nursing. The first doctoral programs in nursing were recorded in the 1930s at Teachers College Columbia University and New York University (Fisher & Haberman, 2001). Colleges and universities were in need of nurses educated beyond the master's level to assume faculty leadership roles in the academy relative to teaching, service, and research. These first two doctoral programs offered a Doctor of Education in Nursing degree. Prior to the 1970s there were fewer than 12 doctoral programs in nursing to serve all of the nursing programs in academic institutions. By the turn of the century there were more than 75 doctoral programs across 35 states offering doctorates in nursing, such as Doctor of Science in Nursing (DSN), Doctor of Nursing Science (DNSc), and Doctor of Philosophy in Nursing (PhD) (Creasia, 2001). The traditional doctorate in nursing varies in length from three to five years of full-time study and requires advanced content in concept and theoretical formulations, testing, and analysis; issues and trends in the discipline of nursing; and in-depth study, problem solving, statistical analysis, and research dissemination in a concentrated area of study.

The evolution of nursing education programs in the United States predominantly spans the twentieth century. The need to address issues of educational entry into practice; role differentiation at the various educational levels; and strategies to address both an increasing nursing practice and the nursing faculty shortage, which is estimated to continue well into the twenty-first century, are essential. Nurses must take charge of the educational milieu and develop nursing curricula at all levels of education that will serve the changing health care delivery environment. There is room in the nursing workforce for nurses with different degrees and skill sets to function in the multifaceted roles needed on behalf of the client and family. Resolution of the educational entry into practice would be a giant step in moving the profession toward a new paradigm of educational models as well as nursing-care delivery models in the practice setting.

GRADUATE PROGRAMS IN NURSING

In order to attract the most qualified applicants to a graduate program in nursing, potential students must see the cost/benefit ratio for expending energy over and beyond that which is necessary to carry out the day-to-day work as a professional nurse. The work environment for the nurse is a challenge and in some instances serves as a barrier for educational mobility. Many nurses entered the nursing profession with the goal of obtaining advanced degree(s) after a few years of concentrated clinical practice; however, the demands of the work setting and the typical workload of the bedside nurse pose

WRITING EXERCISE 20.1

The text has presented an overview of the history of nursing education in the United States. (1) Identify one nurse that you know from the clinical area or from your own experience who has been affected by the history of education in nursing; (2) Describe how this nurse functions in her or his role and what educational level is appropriate for that professional nursing role; (3) Describe issues in the history of professional nursing education that have positively and/or adversely affected the overall nursing profession; (4) Identify solutions to any problems you mentioned in item #3. Write up a short essay for each of the questions, and be prepared to discuss this in class.

a question of whether or not there is time and energy to complete the graduate nursing degree. Many are looking for creative, flexible approaches to graduate education that will still allow time for work, school, family, and the community.

Masters of Science in Nursing (MSN) Preparation

Graduate education in nursing provides an opportunity for nurses and entering second-professional-degree students to acquire advanced knowledge and specialized skill beyond the nurse-generalist level. The master's degree in nursing is awarded by universities after approximately 30 to 50 semester credits have been achieved in content areas, such as core concepts for advance practice, issues and trends in professional role behaviors, evidenced-based-practice analysis, and intense clinical practice in a focused client-population area. These program types usually prepare a nurse for specialty practice, such as clinical nurse-specialist or nurse practitioner. Master's degrees in nursing that prepare nurses for advanced-specialty practice are typically 1.5 to 2 years in length; however, other clinical-practice specialties, such as nurse midwifery and nurse anesthetist are also prepared at the master's level. The nurse anesthetist programs were historically postbaccalaureate in nature, but now require a master's educational level as the outcome. A master's program preparing the nurse anesthetist is laden with theory, science, and clinical-practice hours.

These programs are usually 24 to 36 months in length and require 50 to over 100 credit hours to complete. The goal of a master's curriculum in nursing is to prepare the nurse to assume a selected advanced-practice role, such as practitioner, clinical specialist, administrator, teacher, clinical researcher, or other specialty roles including nurse midwife or nurse anesthetists in a dynamic, changing health care delivery system (Blais, Hayes, Kozier, & Erb, 2006). As master's programs strive to remain competitive and flexible in the educational approach, standards of care for the advance-practice nurse who will be required not only to obtain a degree but also achieve national certification in a specialty area must be maintained. Graduate programs are continuing to modify curricular models to incorporate advanced study for indirect client-care roles, such as nursing leadership and management; outcomes and quality evaluators; informatics and technology experts; and academic- and clinical-setting educators.

In an effort to attract traditional nursing students as well as nontraditional students from other career paths, many master's programs have developed accelerated master's programs. As of March 2005 there are approximately 50 accelerated programs at the master's level, with an estimated increase of 20 more by the end of the year (AACN, 2005a). Accelerated programs at the graduate level build on previous knowledge in nursing and include essential knowledge from the generalist to advanced-practice level of nursing all in one curriculum plan. If students have not completed the first professional degree at the baccalaureate level, they will be required to take the registered-nurse licensure exam prior to clinical practice as a professional nurse. The accelerated master's degree is typically designed for students who have proven their ability to be successful in a university environment (AACN, 2005a). Many successful students in accelerated graduate programs are encouraged to pursue advanced roles as nurse educators in an effort to grow nurse faculty for the future.

Another model for graduate education at the master's level is the dual-degree option. The graduate student can complete two master's degrees in one curriculum plan and be awarded two degrees upon graduation. In some cases the dual curriculum plan includes two separate programs of study taken simultaneously, with a degree in two separate majors as the outcome. In other curriculum plans, the coursework is a blending of courses from two separate majors with a total number of credits for graduation in each major sufficient to award two degrees. Popular dual majors include Master's in Nursing Administration and Master's in Business Administration; Master's in Nursing Administration and Master's in Hospital Administration; Master's in Nursing and Master's in Public Health.

Some graduate nursing programs have been flexible in allowing students to design an individualized program option tailored to incorporate advanced-practice knowledge with a particular skill set required for a specific role. In this type of curriculum plan, courses are designed to complete the core knowledge needed for an advanced degree. Research and statistical requirements are included as well as a set of courses designed to gain knowledge in a specific specialty, role function, or field. These advanced-practice-program plans may include a curricular design for indirect care roles such as clinical research associate, information systems manager, or clinical nurse educator.

Doctoral Preparation

According to Fisher and Habermann (2001), the goal of doctoral programs in nursing is twofold. First, doctoral programs should prepare nurse scientists who can develop scientific knowledge for the discipline

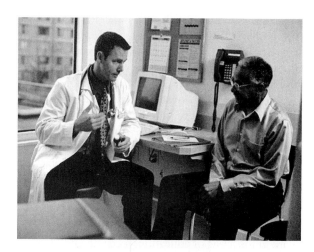

Figure 20.1 **Nurse practitioners' roles include health screenings for the chronically ill client.** Photo courtesy of Photodisc.

through research and scholarship productivity. Second, doctoral programs must meet the increasing demand for doctorally prepared educators who are credentialed to teach in university-based nursing programs. Both goals are absolutely essential for the discipline. Doctoral degrees awarded in nursing include the Doctor of Philosophy in Nursing (PhD), Doctorate of Science in Nursing (DSN), and Doctorate of Nursing Science (DNSc). However, since the degree most awarded in nursing is a doctor of philosophy (PhD) with a major in nursing, it is common that new PhD faculty are prepared to assume the research and scholarship role but have not been educationally or experientially prepared to teach in academic institutions. Nurses interested in pursuing a doctoral degree should examine program philosophy, goals, and curricular emphasis that match their professional career goals (Blais, Hayes, Kozier, & Erb, 2006). If the career goal of the doctoral student is to teach in an academic setting upon completion of the degree, the student should enroll in additional courses that emphasize topics such as teaching principles, curriculum development, educational processes, and classroom and clinical evaluation processes.

Doctoral programs are typically three to five years in length and include content relative to the profession of nursing: health care policy; societal and global health care delivery issues; and scientific knowledge and process necessary to create, test, and analyze theory relative to the discipline. Research and statistical knowledge for scientific discovery is integrated into all doctoral programs, and a doctoral dissertation is required as a culminating educational requirement. Because nursing is grounded in clinical practice, many doctoral programs emphasize clinically relevant research and scholarship activities. Traditional doctoral programs in nursing, such as the PhD, DSN, and DNSc, share common elements within the educational program of studies, but more emphasis must be placed on support coursework in the areas of education, teaching and learning principles, and educational research if nurse faculty are to exhibit beginning competency in the tripartite role of teaching as they enter university settings.

In an effort to grow young faculty in the nursing profession, some nursing programs have developed accelerated PhD programs, which link the first professional degree (the baccalaureate degree or Bachelor of Science in Nursing—BSN) with PhD coursework. Students accelerate past many of the credit hours required in the master's program into a carefully designed BSN to PhD program of study. Coursework required at the master's level often includes only advanced-practice role development, basic statistics, and evidenced-based inquiry or research process. The PhD coursework then builds on foundational advanced-nursing content acquired from the master's-degree program. However, students can elect the option of completing a master's degree in an individualized program of study, such as teaching of nursing, policy analyst, consultation, or administration. The accelerated PhD track is an exciting, innovative opportunity for nurses who have either a strong experiential base or a successful academic track record in order to bypass some of the clinically intense coursework required in a clinical advanced-practice master's program. Students who excel in research and scholarship and who have exhibited a desire to grow as nurse educators can benefit from a fast-track educational plan with a doctoral degree outcome.

Another model for nursing education at the doctoral level is the nursing doctorate program (ND). This curricular design builds on a baccalaureate degree in another field. The model is similar to that used by other professional health care delivery disciplines, such as medicine, dentistry, and optometry. The first ND was established at Case Western Reserve University in 1979 (Creasia, 2001). The nurse doctorate degree prepares a nurse generalist who is eligible for the registered-nurse licensure examination at the completion of the generalist component of the four-year program. Although the program emphasizes research utilization, the main focus is on building expertise in clinical practice. It should be noted that the ND, much like the degree in medicine (MD), does not replace the need for an advance-practice degree or an academic doctoral degree in order to focus on research generation as a scientist or to serve as a faculty member at a major university. In 2004 the AACN recommended that all ND programs convert to the new Doctorate of Nursing Practice (DNP) terminal degree, and by the end of 2005 all ND programs in the United States had made commitments to become DNP programs (AACN, 2004b; AACN, 2005e).

Future Trends in Graduate Education

Transforming nursing education to allow for flexibility and innovation without sacrificing quality and the essential knowledge necessary for the practice of professional nursing will be a challenge that educational programs face for decades to come. Careful monitoring and planning for workforce supply-and-demand issues are required for both the health care delivery system as well as resources in nursing programs located in academic institutions. A response to the nursing-practice shortage and the need for nurses educated to fulfill various advanced roles in the practice setting has recently been publicized by the American Association of Colleges of Nursing. The Clinical Nurse Leader (CNL) is a master's-prepared, highly skilled clinician who focuses on outcome-based practice and quality improvement

(AACN, 2004a). In addition, an AACN task force developed a position statement and curriculum plan for the Practice Doctorate in Nursing (DNP, DrNP) (AACN, 2004b). If adopted by nursing programs across the country, both initiatives will affect the curricular outcomes of graduate nursing programs.

Unlike the Nurse Doctorate, the Clinical Nurse Leader, approved by the AACN Board of Directors in 2003, supports the role of a nurse generalist prepared at the master's level (AACN, 2003b; AACN 2004a; AACN 2005c). The CNL fulfills a role in the practice setting for an expert clinician who can provide leadership in coordinating care, evaluating patient outcomes, directing evidenced-based care delivery, and implementing and evaluating quality improvement measures. "Clinical nurse leaders will direct the care team, consulting with clinical nurse specialists and other disciplines to ensure better outcomes for patients with complex needs. These nurses will integrate evidence-base nursing practice into daily care and help to more effectively provide quality, cost-effective services" (Wood, 2005).

In October of 2005 the American Nurses Association (ANA) acknowledged the need for careful deliberation of the development of the new CNL role, which must address issues in nursing practice (ANA, 2005). Likewise, the ANA leaders agreed to join the AACN's CNL initiative in both the implementation and evaluation of outcomes phases in order to assist with shaping the future role of the CNL in the practice setting.

In an effort to support a more consistent approach to the new CNL role, the AACN initiated a national pilot project, beginning in the Spring and Fall academic terms of 2005, that included education and practice partnerships in nearly 90 institutions across 35 states and Puerto Rico (AACN, 2005d). Curriculum models for the new CNL program vary by school and practice setting, but most of the pilot programs across the country include 12 to 15 months of full-time coursework including a residency phase during or after coursework is completed and the eligibility for certification upon completion of the program (Steefel, 2005). The AACN task forces acknowledge that the role needs to remain flexible

so that institutions can adapt the CNL role to the needs of their agency. It is acknowledged that the new CNL will be a master's-prepared generalist who is educated to work collaboratively with other clinical nurse specialists and as a member of the interdisciplinary health care team in planning, implementing, and evaluating comprehensive patient care and the outcomes of that care (AACN, 2004a). An example of variation in program was described as a 15-month, 36-semester credit program developed for the postbaccalaureate nurse (Wood, 2005). In addition, a second-degree program was developed at one university that integrates bachelor's and master's degree coursework over a 24-month period. In this program type, graduates will be prepared in a curriculum that uses the competencies outlined in the AACN (1998) Essentials of Baccalaureate Education for Professional Nursing Practice as well as the AACN Working Paper on the Role of the Clinical Nurse Leader (AACN, 1998; AACN 2003b). Graduates of the CNL master's programs will be eligible to sit for a certification exam developed under the supervision of AACN.

Another trend in graduate nursing education is the development of a practice-focused doctoral degree program (DNP). Created by a task force of nurse leaders in education and practice from AACN in 2002, the concept of the DNP is closely aligned with the research-focused degrees such as PhD and DNSc, DSN, or DNS (AACN, 2004b). The doctorate of nursing practice degree (DNP) is proposed to be different from the research-focused doctorate (PhD) in that the DNP will include (1) less focus on theory and meta-analysis; (2) less research methodology with a focus on evaluation of research rather than knowledge generation through the conduct of research; (3) different requirements for the capstone project of the program ranging from no dissertation requirement to clinical-focused theses or dissertation; (4) completion of a practicum or residency requirement; and (5) emphasis on scholarly practice, practice improvement, evaluation of health care outcomes, and expertise in shaping clinical practice excellence through leadership and health policy reform (AACN, 2004b). In an effort to provide

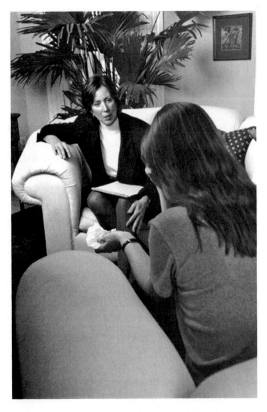

Figure 20.2 **The DNP-prepared psychiatric nurse practitioner often sees clients in crisis.** Photo courtesy of Photodisc.

continuity in terms and distinguish the DNP as the terminal degree for a practice-focused role, the AACN task force recommended that the ND degree, which prepares a nurse generalist, be phased out.

The practice doctorate is proposed as the minimum graduate degree for at least four advanced-practice nurse roles: clinical nurse specialist, nurse anesthetist, nurse midwife, and nurse practitioner. In addition, the AACN membership voted to accept all of the recommendations of the DNP task force including the evolution of master's curricula that prepare advanced-practice nurses for the doctorate of nursing practice (DNP) by the year 2015 (AACN, 2004b). Further, the Commission on Collegiate Nursing Education (CCNE) accrediting body for

baccalaureate- and higher-degree nursing programs has agreed to develop a process to begin accrediting practice doctorate programs (AACN, 2005e). Beginning in the fall of 2005 the AACN appointed two task forces to (1) describe DNP program development, transition from the master's education curriculum to the DNP curriculum plan, examine regulation and licensure issues, and explore any advanced-practice reimbursement issues; and (2) develop a set of standards and competencies to guide curriculum development and outcome assessment to be entitled "Essentials of the Doctorate of Nursing Practice" (AACN, 2005b). Regional meetings to promote stakeholder support as well as refine the essentials document are projected for final completion in 2006. This essentials document will be a guiding force in the accreditation process for the newly developed DNP programs as well. It is anticipated that DNP program development will continue to increase throughout the next decade, with educational pathways such as the post-master's DNP option, BSN to DNP option, and a generic DNP educational model being developed by many nursing programs across the country.

Many specialty organizations have begun to assess the feasibility of the transition to a DNP degree for their advanced-practice nurses (AACN, 2005c; Marion et al., 2005; National Association of Clinical Nurse Specialists, 2005). Although it is anticipated that the DNP initiative will not be accepted by all stakeholders, many nursing programs and practice-setting leaders agree that the current system for health care delivery does not work, and that a new role for the nurse is absolutely necessary for today and in the future. This role requires a focus on comprehensive evaluation and use of evidence in making decisions and implementing clinical innovations, application of research, a theoretical understanding in the patient-care setting, and an overall change in practice models (AACN, 2005e). Such a change in the methods by which the nursing discipline educates its academicians and clinicians will obviously bring concern and doubt to the forefront of the discipline. Organizations that support advanced-practice nurses and faculty who teach them have documented concern

WRITING EXERCISE 20.2

The text has provided an overview of degree-granting programs offered by nursing education programs at the graduate level. Using the program descriptions, (1) create a table contrasting different role preparation at the master's level, including the newly proposed CNL model, and (2) create a table describing the various approaches to doctoral education in nursing. Be prepared to discuss the strengths and weaknesses of each educational option.

over the outcomes of such a dynamic shift in the educational model for advanced-practice nurses (Dracup, Cronenwett, Meleis, & Benner, 2005; Marion et al., 2005). Regardless of support or opposition, it is expected that a transition period will be necessary to (1) allow master's-prepared advanced-practice nurses who are currently in practice to earn credits to complete the practice doctoral degree; (2) allow doctoral-granting institutions the opportunity to transition and develop new doctoral program curricula and procedures; (3) allow practice settings to carve a new role for advanced-practice nurses within the institution; and (4) allow for time to plan, implement, and evaluate educational outcomes for accreditation processes. These new program initiatives will take time, but it is clear that the decades of the 2000s and 2010s will experience a shift in educational

paradigms that prepare nurses with generalist knowledge for expert clinical practice as well as preparation of specialized, advance-practice nurses.

GRADUATE EDUCATION AS A CAREER DECISION

It is without question that entry into a career in nursing can be somewhat confusing to the individual. Multiple entry pathways have hindered professional progress in the discipline by promoting the societal notion that a nurse is a nurse is a nurse. Often consumers are left bewildered by the many different health care workers who parade before them,

CASE SCENARIO 20.1

Joe has been a Director of Nursing of the surgical division for five years. He is debating the merits of returning to graduate school to obtain a doctoral degree in nursing. His strength has always been related to his clinical expertise in surgical care of the adult as well as his organization and leadership abilities in working with the interdisciplinary team. Joe is considering the new DNP as compared to the more traditional PhD. Considering Joe's

dilemma, answer the following questions: (1) What knowledge and skill will Joe obtain by enrolling in a DNP program? (2) What knowledge and skill will Joe obtain by enrolling in a PhD program? (3) What professional nursing role will Joe be best prepared for upon completion of the DNP versus the PhD program? (4) Discuss the merits of enrollment in a PhD program in either hospital administration or business administration.

all claiming to be a "nurse." The media has done little to change this image of the practicing nurse. In addition, members of the interdisciplinary health care delivery team are often confused or lack knowledge about the educational preparation and outcome competency expected of the professional nurse. As we continue to push for more registered nurses to enter the workforce throughout the next decade, an opportunity arises for the nursing profession to address entry-level issues, clarify differentiation of nursing-practice roles, and resolve confusion about career pathways in the discipline of nursing.

Advancement in the Practice Setting

Nurses of the future have an excellent opportunity to provide leadership in the entire health care delivery system. It is the nurse who provides the majority of patient care in hospitals, long-term care facilities, and ambulatory and community-based health care settings. Often it is the nurse who leads the health care delivery team with regard to patient- and family-focused care decisions; practice changes based on sound empirical evidence; and educational agendas for patients, families, and other health care delivery personnel. The work environments of the twenty-first century are among the most demanding of all types of work settings for the contemporary professional nurse (AACN, 2002). Exacerbating the challenge to create a work environment where nurses can deliver the best quality care possible for clients who exhibit the most complex, high acuity illness condition is the increasing demand for more qualified nursing personnel. These work environments are laden with workload issues for the sickest of clients, increased overtime demands, and the stress of burnout in the profession of nursing.

Practice environments where nurses are allowed to function in roles compatible with their education and competency are the most satisfying. Prominent among the environments that support professional nursing practice and career advancement are those that promote the highest level of nursing achievement through recognition of excellence in quality

nursing care services (AACN, 2002). Today one of the highest honors for excellence in nursing services in health care organizations is the Magnet Nursing Services Designation, awarded under the auspices of the American Nurses Credentialing Center of the American Nurses Association (ANCC, 2004). Magnet Hospital Designation is achieved only in organizational environments where a high level of integration of professional nursing-practice standards is consistently documented at all levels of nursing practice throughout the institution. Organizations that promote professional nursing-practice advancements also recognize that the work environment of today requires mentoring and professional development. In these institutions, professional nurses with baccalaureate and higher degrees serve as preceptors for new nurses as well as nursing students who are transitioning from the classroom to the clinical practice environment. In many facilities, these nurses serve as facilitators of learning for clinical practice for nurses who are employed and working in internship and residency programs. In addition, professional nurses new to the organization need assistance with learning policies and procedures as well as the variances in nursing practice among different practice levels. The preceptor can assist the nurse in recognizing practice models, such as interdisciplinary team collaboration, that are specific for that unit or exhibited throughout the agency. A hallmark of the practice environment is an atmosphere in which professional nurses can grow and advance in their expertise not only clinically, but also through mobility in obtaining advanced nursing degrees.

Academic Careers

Professional nurses must take on the responsibility of furthering the discipline through career advancement. The nursing shortage cannot be solved without qualified faculty resources. The education of professional nurse graduates entering the workforce is a complex issue. In 2002 a survey of baccalaureate, master's, and doctoral programs by the AACN revealed that over 5,000 qualified applicants were turned away from nursing programs, due in large part to an insufficient number of faculty to teach them (Berlin, Stennett, & Bednash, 2003). Compounding issues related to the faculty shortage are faculty age and retirement timelines, a decline in the number of nurses who wish to stay in the academic setting, salary differentials between education and practice settings, diminishing applicant pools for graduate school, the burden of the nursing practice shortage, demands of graduate study, faculty workloads and role expectations, the increasing age of doctorally prepared faculty, and attractive alternative career pathways for nurses with advanced education (AACN, 2003a; Berlin & Sechrist, 2002).

Strategies to expand the nursing faculty workforce must be actualized.

- Nursing students in their bachelors' programs who are adept at teaching and show promise of future graduate study must be identified early.
- Academic climates must be fostered that offer professional development to master's-prepared nurse faculty and practitioners and encourage progression toward the doctoral degree.
- Nursing-education theory, principles, and evaluation must be integrated into all nursing doctoral programs.
- Potential nurse faculty must be recruited from among those nurses in the practice setting who are serving in preceptor and educator roles.

The nursing education setting must develop an attitude of ongoing nurturing and mentoring of its young in order to sustain the growth in faculty supply that will be needed in the future.

FUTURE PLANNING FOR THE DISCIPLINE OF NURSING

The profession of nursing is at an important stage in its 100-year development. In the next few years nursing has a chance to grow and develop in both the practice and educational settings. Further differentiation of nursing roles and educational outcomes

that must be exhibited to function in those roles will be a challenge. Perhaps the most important challenge that nursing faces is to take control of its own destiny. Nursing must provide the leadership for necessary changes and become proactive rather than reactive in leading health care delivery now and in the future. The opportunities that exist for a career in professional nursing are more numerous than ever. Likewise, advancement in nursing through experience and expansion of educational credentials is very rewarding. There is a place in the health care delivery system and higher education arena for every nurse who has the courage to step forward and continue on the professional career path.

Future Nursing Population Projections

Let us not be discouraged by the projections of the need for future nurses. As a profession, we must embrace them and be empowered in solving our own professional issues. The shortage of nurses in both the practice and academic settings is a challenge that is affected by a plethora of societal issues. Heller, Oros, and Durney-Crowley (2000) identified trends that will affect the advancement of the nursing profession, which include socioeconomic and population demographic changes; an increase in the diversity of nursing-student populations to include ethnic and underrepresented populations; technological and information explosions; globalization of the world's economy and society; consumer-driven expectations of the profession of nursing; the economics of the health care industry; the impact of changing health policy and regulation; an increased need for interdisciplinary education to promote collaborative nursing practice models; advances in nursing science, research, and technology; and the dynamics of the nursing shortage. These trends will affect both nursing education and the health care delivery system. As the health care industry continues to see an older population needing health care services, nurses will experience a more educated consumer. Alternative treatments and therapies as well as traditional treatment

RESEARCH APPLICATION ARTICLE

Berlin, L. E. & Sechrist, K. R. (2002). The shortage of doctorally prepared nursing faculty: A dire situation. *Nursing Outlook, 50*(2), 50–56.

It is a well-known fact that the nursing shortage in the practice setting is currently severe and will be with us for several decades to come. However, the accompanying faculty shortage is a growing problem. In fact, it has a reciprocal effect on the overall nursing shortage in the practice sector. This study by Berlin and Sechrist (2002) describes an evaluation of the impact of faculty age and retirement projections on the availability of doctorally prepared faculty for the future.

This descriptive study examines the American Association of Colleges of Nursing data from the survey of 4,451 full-time doctorally prepared faculty in schools granting baccalaureate and higher degrees in 2001. The overall mean age was 53.2 years; with a mean age of 56.2, 53.8, and 50.4 years for professors, associate, and assistant professors, respectively. On average, nursing faculty retire at age 62.5, with faculty 65 years or older accounting for only 3% or less of the population. Regression analysis of faculty age revealed that between 1993 and 2001 the mean age changed significantly from 49.7 to 53.3 (Beta = .437; $F = 3319.79$; $df = 1,7$; $P < .0001$). Conversely, regression analysis of years to faculty retirement significantly decreased from 13 years in 1993

to <10 years in 2001 (Beta = .593; $F = 4102.54$; $df = 1,7$; $P = < .0001$). Data in the survey revealed that the proportion of faculty in the age group of 50 years and older increased from 50.7% to 70.3% from 1999 to 2001. Of concern is the decrease in number of faculty who are 35 years and younger: 49.3% to 29.7% from 1999 to 2001. Another alarming statistic related to faculty loss is the number of doctorally prepared nurses who leave the academic setting for nursing services or private-sector clinical or executive positions (approximately 17.7% in 1993 and similar statistics in 1994).

If nursing faculty are to make an impact on the shortage of nurses in the practice setting, there must be an increase in the number of nurses at the master's and doctoral levels who are prepared to teach. Nursing education must engage in creative, innovative strategies that will increase the number of doctorally prepared faculty among its ranks at an earlier age. Career pathways that are positively embraced by the entire academic community are essential. Exploring opportunities for young nurses with master's degrees to continue the educational pathway to doctoral completion is imperative. The research confirms that the gap between master's education and doctoral study must be closed from the current mean time of 15.9 years to a shorter, more reasonable timeframe.

regimens will be the "business" of nurses. Educational programs must continue not only to strive and improve supply and demand issues for the health care system, but also to produce a knowledge worker who is on the cutting edge of the business of health care delivery issues. Nurses of the

future must be aware of the impact of globalization on the economy as well as on the methods used to deliver health care.

It has been well documented that the future will find the profession of nursing challenged to fill important nursing positions, both in the practice

WRITING EXERCISE 20.3

Given the content in the previous sections, write a short essay discussing the impact that globalization has on the profession of nursing. Be prepared to lead this discussion in the next class/seminar.

and education sectors. A goal of increased supply nearing 2.5 million by 2020 is somewhat overwhelming. However, the nursing profession has been challenged in the past, accomplishing many advances through creative and innovative transitions. Many of the issues concerning supply and demand will need to be addressed through decisions related to the basic level of preparation for nurses, the advanced role function of nurses with different levels of educational preparation, and the transition to new ways of teaching and delivering nursing care.

CHAPTER SUMMARY

The challenge of supply and demand for the profession of nursing in the United States is a twofold problem, touching both the nursing practice and nursing education enterprises. Historically, this is not the first supply-and-demand issue for the profession. What may be new, though, are the strategies that nursing will need to employee to solve it. Questions of the educational preparation of the nursing workforce must be addressed. Educational preparation needed for entry into practice as a professional nurse has been debated for over half a century. Support for the baccalaureate degree as the minimum level of education necessary for the professional nurse has been provided by various professional organizations since the 1960s; however, the need for nurses with advanced knowledge beyond the basic entry education preparation is a growing concern. Nurses must be willing to advance their educational credentials beyond the bachelor's level and move into master's and doctoral programs in graduate nursing programs. Because the current work environment requires a more knowledgeable professional nurse, proposals for a master's-prepared clinical nurse leader and a clinically focused, doctorally prepared nurse have been explicated through work by both practice and education nurse leaders under the auspices of the American Association of Colleges of Nursing. The next few decades hold numerous challenges for professional nurses in both practice and educational settings. Nurses must make an effort to solve some of their own professional issues and move forward toward a clearer, specific plan for educational advancement and career trajectories within the discipline. There are many challenges, but nurses must move from old to new paradigms of professional nursing, even in the midst of uncertainty. What is certain is that change will occur, and more nurses will be needed to address the health care delivery issues well into the twenty-first century. What is also certain is that if nursing doesn't take charge of its own destiny and find resolutions to professional issues, some other discipline will do it for us!

Keep away from people who try to belittle your ambitions. Small people always do that, but the really great make you feel that you, too, can become great.

—Mark Twain

REFERENCES

American Association of Colleges of Nursing (1996). The baccalaureate degree in nursing as minimal preparation for professional practice. Updated December 12, 2000. Retrieved July 1, 2005, from http://www.aacn.nche.edu/Publications/positions/baccmin.htm.

American Association of Colleges of Nursing (1997). A vision of baccalaureate and graduate nursing education: The next decade. Updated March 1, 2005. Retrieved July 1, 2005, from http://www.aacn.nche.edu/Publications/positions/vision.htm.

American Association of Colleges of Nursing (1998). *The essentials of baccalaureate education for professional nursing practice.* Washington, DC: Author.

American Association of Colleges of Nursing (2002). *Hallmarks of the professional nursing practice environment: A white paper.* Washington, DC: Author.

American Association of Colleges of Nursing (2003a). *Faculty shortages in baccalaureate and graduate nursing programs: Scope of the problem and strategies for expanding the supply.* Washington, DC: Author.

American Association of Colleges of Nursing (2003b). *Working paper on the role of the clinical nurse leader (updated June, 2004).* Washington, DC: Author.

American Association of Colleges of Nursing (2004a). *Working statement comparing the clinical nurse leader and clinical nurse specialist roles: Similarities, differences, and complementarities.* Washington, DC: Author.

American Association of Colleges of Nursing (2004b). *AACN position statement on the practice doctorate in nursing.* Washington, DC: Author.

American Association of Colleges of Nursing (2005a). *Accelerated baccalaureate and master's degrees in nursing fact sheet.* Washington, DC: Author.

American Association of Colleges of Nursing (2005b). AACN applauds decision of the AONE to move registered nursing education to the baccalaureate level. Retrieved July 1, 2005, from http://www.aacn.nche.edu/Media/NewsReleases/2005/AONE505.htm.

American Association of Colleges of Nursing (2005c). *AACN applauds the National Academy of Sciences' report which supports the practice doctorate in nursing and calls for more nurse scientists (September 12, 2005).* Washington, DC: Author.

American Association of Colleges of Nursing (2005d). Fact sheet: The clinical nurse leader (updated June 15, 2005). Retrieved July 1, 2005, from http://www.aacn.nche.edu.

American Association of Colleges of Nursing (2005e). *Frequently asked questions: Doctor of Nursing Practice (DNP) programs.* Washington, DC: Author.

American Nurses Association (2005). ANA joins the AACN clinical nurse leader implementation and evaluation task forces. Retrieved November 10, 2005, from http://www.nursingworld.org/pressnl/2005/pr1013.htm

American Nurses Credentialing Center (2004) *Magnet recognition program: Recognizing excellence in nursing services, 2005.* Silver Springs, MD: Author.

Berlin, L. E., & Sechrist, K. R. (2002). The shortage of doctorally prepared nursing faculty: A dire situation. *Nursing Outlook, 50*(2), 50–56.

Berlin, L. E., Stennett, J., & Bednash, G. D. (2003). *2002–2003 enrollment and graduations in baccalaureate and graduate programs in nursing.* Washington, DC: American Association of Colleges of Nursing.

Creasia, J. L. (2001). Pathways of nursing education. In Creasia, J. L. & Parker, B. (Eds.) (2001), *Conceptual foundations: The bridge to professional nursing Practice* (3rd ed., Chapter 2, pp. 26–35). St. Louis: Mosby.

Dracup, K., Cronenwett, L., Meleis, A. I., & Benner, P. E. (2005). Reflections on the doctorate of nursing practice. *Nursing Outlook, 53*: 177–182.

Fisher, A., & Habermann, B. (2001). Transitions: From doctoral preparation to academic career. In N. L. Chaska (Ed.), *The nursing profession: Tomorrow and beyond* (Chapter 21, p. 252). Thousand Oaks, CA: Sage Publications, Inc.

Gaines, B. C. (2001). From revolution to transformation: Curriculum development in a new millennium. In N. L. Chaska (Ed.), *The Nursing profession: Tomorrow and beyond* (Chapter 12, p. 144). Thousand Oaks, CA: Sage Publications, Inc.

Heller, B., Oros, M. T., & Durney-Crowley, J (2000). The future of nursing education: 10 trends to watch. *Nursing and Health Care Perspectives, 21*(1), 8–13.

Hood, L. J., & Leddy, S. K. (2003). The professional nurse. In Hood, L. J. & Leddy, S.K. *Conceptual bases of professional nursing* (5th ed., Chapter 1, pp. 2–40). Philadelphia: Lippincott Williams & Wilkins.

Marion, L. N., O'Sullivan, A. L., Crabtree, M. K., Price, M., & Fontana, S. A. (2005). Curriculum models for the practice doctorate in nursing. *Topics in Advanced Practice Nursing eJournal, 5*(1): 1–5.

National Advisory Council on Nurses Education and Practice (1996). *Report from the National Sample Survey of Registered Nurses.* Washington, DC: Division of Nursing, Health Resources and Services Administration.

National Association of Clinical Nurse Specialists (2005). White paper on the nursing practice doctorate. *Clinical Nurse Specialist, 19*(4), 215–217.

PEW Health Professions Commission (1995). *Critical challenges: Revitalizing the health professions for the twenty-first century.* San Francisco, CA: University of California Center for the Health Professions.

Steefel, L. (2005). Partnerships pilot CNL program. Retrieved July 1, 2005, from http://www2. Nurseweek.com.

United States Department of Health and Human Services. (2002). *Projected supply, demand, and shortage of registered nurses: 2000–2020.* Health Resources and Services Administration, Bureau of Health Professions, National Center for Health Workforce Analysis. Washington, DC: Author.

United States Department of Health and Human Services, The National Center for Health Workforce Analysis. (2003). *Changing demographics: Implications for physicians, nurses, and other health workers.* Washington, DC: Author.

United States Department of Labor (2003). May 2003 Occupational employment and wage estimates. Retrieved December 2003, from http://stats.bls.gov/oes/2003/may.htm.

Wood, D. (2005). Nursing schools launch CNL master's programs. Retrieved July 1, 2005, from http://www.nursezone.com.

CHAPTER 21

Mentoring and the Profession

Sheryl Curtis

So never lose an opportunity of urging a practical beginning, however small,
for it is wonderful how often in such matters the mustard-seed
germinates and roots itself.

—Florence Nightingale

LEARNING OBJECTIVES

At the completion of the chapter, the learner should be able to do the following:

1. Describe current trends in health care in relation to nursing shortages.
2. Identify characteristics of an effective mentor.
3. Analyze factors that affect the mentoring relationship.
4. Apply Benner's theory of the five levels of nursing skill development to the role and function of a mentor.
5. Describe effective mentoring strategies.
6. Identify stages of the mentoring relationship.
7. Compare and contrast mentoring strategies for the new graduate nurse, minority nurses, nurse managers, and nursing faculty.
8. Discuss the benefits of developing mentoring relationships to both individual nurses and the health care system as a whole.

KEY TERMS

Coach

Mentor

Mentoring

Mentoring culture

Preceptee

Preceptor

Protégé/Mentee

Teacher

It is a scenario played out all across the country, familiar to many who have worked in health care for any length of time: new graduate nurses and those nurses just returning to the workforce for varied reasons, including personal, financial, or professional needs, enter into the profession with fresh ideas and high expectations, only to find themselves confronted with self-doubt, difficult and demanding workloads, and often little, if any, support from other members of the staff. These staff members may also resent the fact that these new nurses have been hired at starting salaries equal to or greater than their own. It is little wonder that, over time, many of these new nurses become discouraged, burnt-out, and eventually leave the profession entirely.

Nursing has historically been a profession accused of "eating its own"—and for good reason. A March 2000 survey by the U.S. Department of Health and Human Services found that of the 2,696,540 currently licensed registered nurses in the United States, 494,727 (18.3%) were not practicing. Over half of these individuals (263,856) had been employed as nurses within the five years preceding the survey (Spately, Johnson, Sachalski, Fritz, & Spencer, 2000). A survey of employed staff nurses found that only 65% reported job satisfaction in the hospital setting (Spatley et. al., 2000).

There have been many changes in the delivery of health care that have directly affected all nurses and the facilities within which they work. The patient population has become much more ethnically and culturally diverse, requiring nurses to be more sensitive to these differences and, in some instances, to become fluent in a second language. The patient population has become older and more medically complex, creating increased workloads for many nurses. Increased use of technology and immediate access to information, both accurate and inaccurate, for both patients and medical personnel has also added responsibilities to the nursing workforce. There have been many changes in medical funding in the past decade, especially from the government sector, leading to institutional budgetary constraints and fierce competition for patients among health care institutions. The patient is now seen as a "consumer" of health care, and many have high expectations of what that care should be.

In this age of higher demand for nurses and increasing complexity of care, coupled with decreasing numbers of nurses entering the workforce, many health care facilities are evaluating the reasons why nurses leave the profession and are beginning to implement strategies to improve retention and job satisfaction of nurses. One such strategy, **mentoring**, is beginning to gain popularity in nursing (see Figure 21.1). Mentoring is seen as a method of giving novice nurses the consistent support and guidance that they will need in order to be successful in the multifaceted and ever-changing landscape of health care today.

HISTORICAL PERSPECTIVES ON MENTORING

Mentoring is not a new concept. It has been used in the business world successfully for many years. In fact the first mention of the word "mentor" dates back to Greek mythology in Homer's *The Odyssey*. Mentor was a very old friend of King Odysseus, and he entrusted his household, including his son Telemachus, to him when Odysseus was required to sail to Troy to fight in the Trojan War. The goddess of wisdom, Athena, wanting to help young Telemachus, would often disguise herself as Mentor so that she could give guidance and wise council to Telemachus, helping him in his journey to find his father. Through time, the word "mentor" has come to mean a wise, experienced, and trusted advisor to someone wanting to develop as a professional (Thorpe & Kalischuk, 2003; Cameron-Jones & O'Hara, 1996).

Mentoring is well documented in historical accounts, literature, and media. Roman generals fought beside mentors who advised them in battle. Medieval guild masters were responsible for not only the development of the skills of their apprentices, but also the guiding of their values and beliefs.

More recently we have had the mentoring relationships of Sherlock Holmes to Watson, Yoda to Luke Skywalker in the *Star Wars* movies, and of course Professor Albus Dumbledore to the young Harry Potter in the series of books popularized by J.K. Rowling.

It has also been well documented that Florence Nightingale had many mentoring relationships with her former students (Lorentzon & Brown, 2003). One such relationship was with Rachel Williams, the reforming matron of St. Mary's Hospital, Paddington. Nightingale had a very active correspondence with her, and in 1876, prior to her being appointed as matron of St. Mary's, was advised by Nightingale to proceed with caution and "not frighten doctors by starting at once any proposal to reform the nursing system or to have a training school" (Lorrentzon & Brown, 2003, p. 269); and she was also counseled in reference to her relationship with Dr. Sievking, an influential medical member of the Board of Governors: "St. Mary's is his primary object—the proposition of the training school would have to come from him" (Lorentzon & Brown, 2003, p. 269). Nightingale gave Rachel Williams emotional support, advice, and inspiration while preparing her for the role of matronship during their longstanding correspondence with each other.

DEFINITION OF TERMS

The words "coach," "preceptor," "teacher," "instructor," and "mentor" have all been use interchangeably at times, but there are some basic differences predicated on their contexts. A **preceptor** is usually an assigned, experienced person who helps the **"preceptee"** or novice "learn the ropes" of the job, so to speak. It is usually a formal relationship, very job specific, and of a much-defined duration (Hom, 2003). Horton describes a preceptor as "an individual, such as a clinical instructor, who has responsibility for facilitating a student's application of theory to practice and for assessing a student's progress" (2003, p. 191). A **coach,** in the opinion

of Carolyn Hope Smeltzer (2002), is someone who "provides an objective analysis and professional advice." Again this is usually a formal relationship, although there is not always a limit to the time involved in the relationship. A **teacher** or instructor involves a predominately formal relationship with a student or pupil, with the teacher/instructor having knowledge or information needed by the student/pupil and the ability to share that information, and necessarily the ability to influence them.

The mentoring relationship is most often informal, chosen mutually by both the **mentor** and **mentee,** and with the mentor more experienced and able to assist the mentee with personal, career, and professional development (Horton, 2003). It is a "role that an individual takes in order to assist someone to grow and learn through transference of expertise" (Hom, 2003, p. 39).

CHARACTERISTICS OF MENTORS

What is it that draws one person to another for mentoring? What qualities do they possess that sets them apart from others? The first and most prominent characteristic of a mentor is the ability to inspire. Mentors are usually, but not always, older and have a sense of self-confidence, knowledge, and expertise that attracts the novice to them. They are comfortable in their roles, their advice is sought after, and they are at a point of strength in their careers. They embody everything that someone just beginning a career would aspire to, becoming a much-respected role model worthy of observation and emulation (Owens & Patton, 2003).

Mentors can possess the means to advance the career of their **protégé.** They are able to give career counseling and advice while also integrating the novice into the social culture of the profession. They freely share their dreams; help instill a sense of vision; encourage and promote independent thinking; often have high, but achievable

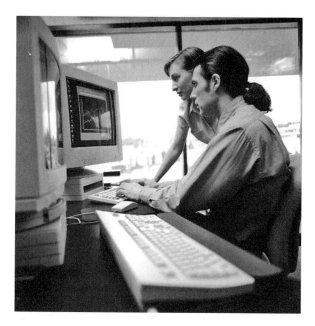

Figure 21.1 Mentors can offer much needed emotional support to the novice during technology training. Photo courtesy of Photodisc.

expectations; and provide opportunities for the protégé to excel. They challenge and mentally stretch the novice; they are the "eye opener, door opener, idea bouncer, and problem solver" (Horton, 2003, p. 191).

Mentors can also be available to offer much-needed emotional support to the novice. They are usually accepting, nonjudgmental, patient, empathetic listeners, and possess good communication skills. They can provide an atmosphere of trust that allows the novice to test boundaries and grow; they are there to nurture an often-fragile sense of self-esteem. They demonstrate both professional and personal values, acting as a gauge against which novices measure their own personal development. More often than not, mentors have a sense of connection or personal chemistry with their mentee, which makes them willing to invest the time and energy required for a mentoring relationship (Roberts, 2003).

CHARACTERISTICS OF MENTEES

Why do nurses want and even seek out mentoring relationships? What would they stand to gain by having a mentor? The predominant answer to this question is that many nurses feel that mentoring aids them in skill development, career advancement, and growth as a professional (Horton, 2003). As nurses begin to seek out peers to mentor them, they also need to be aware that certain characteristics, personality traits, and attitudes enhance their ability to be mentored and increase their appeal to potential mentors.

Motivation, a passion for work, professionalism, strong self-identity, willingness to take initiative, and a commitment to career are all characteristics that aid in the mentoring process. Mentees need to be open to receiving assistance, constructive criticism, and unafraid to ask for help or guidance (Sherwen, 2003). Those who are active and assertive learners, displaying confidence and the ability to share opinions, ideas, and thoughts, are the nurses who tend to benefit more from the mentoring process (Grindel, 2003).

For a mentoring relationship to be effective, mentees must be able to adequately assess their own needs, know their unique strengths and talents, determine and articulate their specific goals, and understand the limits of the relationship. Nurses who have good listening and observation skills are able to utilize feedback, open to different learning processes, not afraid to take risks, and able make good use of the opportunities provided by their mentor will most likely thrive and grow professionally under the guidance and support of a mentor. It is also beneficial for the mentee to develop and demonstrate trust-building behaviors such as consistency, confidence, speaking firmly and frankly, asking appropriate questions, treating others as unique individuals, and not being overly critical or judgmental.

The mentoring process is a very dynamic and individual phenomenon, with many different factors

RESEARCH APPLICATION ARTICLE

Meno, K. M., Keaveny, B. M., & O'Donnell, J. M. (2003). Mentoring in the operating room: A student perspective. *American Association of Nurse Anesthetists Journal, 71*(5), 337–341.

It was determined by the American Association of Nurse Anesthetists (AANA) Education Committee that a need exists to examine student nurse anesthetists' (SNA) perceptions of the concept of mentoring as it pertained to the nurse anesthesia-education programs. A previous study involving Certified Registered Nurse Anesthetists (CRNA) showed that many members of the profession believed that didactic educators should serve as the primary mentors to the SNAs. The purpose of this descriptive research study was to solicit the opinions of SNAs on mentoring in the clinical setting and to have them identify characteristics that set clinical mentors apart from educators. In the survey, 56% of the SNAs indicated that

they believed a mentor should be assigned to them, and 98% felt that this mentor should be a CRNA and not an educator. There were 1,251 students (65% response rate) who completed and returned this survey. The SNAs who responded also identified three of their most important (perceived) adjectives to describe a clinical mentor: knowledgeable (93.8%), approachable (88.9%), and encouraging (74.2%). They also listed three of the most important adjectives to describe an educator: knowledgeable (95.4%), resourceful (64.5%), and approachable (58.9%). These did not differ greatly from those selected for a clinical mentor. The researchers involved in this study felt the results revealed that there should be greater assistance initiated to help match students with clinical mentors while in the anesthesia program, and that the concept of a mentor role is highly valued.

affecting the development of mentoring relationships, but it is important for potential mentees to understand that mentoring is a two-way street: they should play an active role in the relationship, committed to developing and changing themselves—partnering with their mentors to take full advantage of all that can be offered through their relationship.

MENTORING RELATIONSHIPS AND THE FACTORS THAT AFFECT THEM

Strong, effective mentoring relationships can be very powerful and transforming for both the mentor and the protégé. Vance and Olsen (1998) describe the

mentoring relationship as "a developmental, empowering, nurturing relationship that occurs over time with mutual sharing, learning and growth promotion in an environment of respect, collegiality, and affirmation." Bell (2002) uses the SAGE model for describing the mentoring relationship. In this model, SAGE stands for "Surrendering, Accepting, Giving, and Extending." Surrendering is the leveling of the playing field by means of the dissolution of power and authority and the encouragement of creativity and critical reflection. Accepting is inclusion without evaluation or judging—the provision of a safe, nurturing environment. Giving is the giving of oneself by advising, offering feedback, direction, and focus. Finally, Extending is the challenging, pushing, and mental stretching of the mentee.

Glass and Walter (2000), in their research on student-nurse peer mentoring, determined that some of the characteristics of the mentoring process were shared learning and caring, reciprocity, friendship, and a commitment to each other's personal and professional growth. Kochan and Trimble (2000) discussed how mentoring/comentoring relationships provide the tools to succeed both professionally and personally in the workplace. They identified some themes from their research and personal mentoring/comentoring relationship. The first theme was that of mutual benefit for both the mentor and comentor from initiating these mentoring relationships. The second theme was that of the development of the mentoring/comentoring relationship in cyclical and overlapping phases, in which certain actions can be taken to further the development and effectiveness of these relationships. The third theme they described was that of open and trusting relationships that encourage the personal and professional development of both members. Finally, they found that the consistent discussion of the status of the relationship by those involved could facilitate the maintenance of, provide the necessary changes to, and initiate the resolution of the relationship.

Young and Perrewe (2000) developed a model that examines the relationships of formally assigned mentors and their mentees in a corporate setting. They described five factors that affect the development and maintenance of a mentoring relationship: individual characteristics, relationship factors, environmental factors, career factors, and relationship type.

In looking at individual characteristics that can affect a mentoring relationship, consideration should be given to learning styles and mentoring skills. As a general rule, most mentors tend to present material in a manner that reflects the learning style they are most comfortable with; but they need to be aware that their mentee's learning style may be different than their own. Adult learners generally fall into a combination of three styles: auditory learners, kinesthetic and/or tactile learners, and visual learners (Hom, 2003). Auditory learners make up 20%–30% of adults who learn best by material presented in a lecture format or with audio situations discussed. Kinesthetic/tactile learners comprise 30%–50% of adults who learn best when they involve their whole

bodies in the process through role-playing, hands-on, and return demonstration. Finally, visual learners are the 30%–40% of adults who learn best with visual stimulation such as videos, flip charts, handouts, and pictures (Hom, 2003).

Mentoring skills can greatly affect a relationship; an inexperienced or insecure mentor can have profound effects on its success. Poor mentors break promises, lack structure in their teaching, change their minds often, and are either overprotective or have unrealistic expectations of their mentees abilities. They may even possibly be products of poor mentoring themselves. Good mentors have well-developed skills in facilitating, guiding, encouraging, coaching, managing conflict, problem solving, providing and receiving feedback, reflecting, building and maintaining relationships, and goal setting (Zachary, 2000). Other characteristics that can affect the relationship are an individual's locus of control, self-esteem, need for power and control, need for achievement, altruism, and ability to communicate (Young & Perrewe, 2000).

Relationship factors include backgrounds and past experiences of individuals, attraction, commitment to the relationship, personal and professional interests, and the presence of generational differences or a mentoring gap. Usually older, more experienced nurses fall into a different generational category than younger, newer nurses. Understanding and demonstrating sensitivity to generational differences can be a key factor in the success of a mentoring relationship. Nurses from different generations have varying values and career expectations that may determine how they react or respond to various work-related situations (Kupperschmidt, 2000). Traditional or veteran nurses who grew up in the aftermath of the Great Depression typically respect authority, are conformers, and value logic. These nurses usually possess qualities of "hard work, frugality and loyalty to organizations and managers" (Kupperschmidt, 2000, p. 68). Nurses of the Baby-Boomer generation may value strong work ethics and commitment to an organization. They are frequently idealists and workaholics, who value challenge and self-fulfillment in their careers and who have a distrust of authority figures (Kupperschmidt, 2000). On the other hand, younger, Generation-X or "millennial" nurses seek to strike a balance between work and play, placing value on time off and flexible scheduling. They are often more committed to skills acquisition and marketability than to loyalty to an organization. They tend to have a preference for "teamwork, experiential activities, and more involvement in their learning" (Billings, Skiba, & Connors, 2005, p. 130). These younger nurses are usually multitaskers who are comfortable using technology and view it as a necessary part of everyday life.

Older nurses who may have had to work a substantial number of years and "do their time" before being able to work schedules of their choosing might also feel a sense of resentment toward younger nurses who may be able to demand equal or greater wages and ask for and receive a more preferential work schedules of their preference, while at the same time the older nurses had to work a substantial number of years and "do their time" before they were able to work schedules of their choosing. McKinley (2004) describes a phenomenon called a "mentoring gap," wherein more-experienced nurses have a "seen it all, done it all" attitude toward younger nurses and may even label those who speak up as cocky and arrogant; neither of these attitudes fosters creativity and new ideas. Identifying and being knowledgeable about these generational differences can help mentors keep the lines of communication open and bridge the "generation gap."

Environmental factors, such as the amount of organizational support, the presence of adequate resources, and whether there is some form of reward structure, can play a substantial role in the mentoring process. In looking at how an organization supports mentoring, Zachary (2000) discussed indicators of an organization's **"mentoring culture."** Some of the indicators described were the accountability of the organization toward mentoring; infrastructure in place to support mentoring programs; demand for mentoring; a common mentoring vocabulary; multiple venues for mentoring; role modeling; the presence of safety nets, including expectations of

confidentiality in the relationship; and adequate training and education programs for potential mentors. Zachary (2000) also looked at how the alignment of mentoring within the culture of an organization was reflected by the organization's goals and mission statement and whether mentoring was valued by the organization.

Time and effort are the primary resources needed for effective, meaningful mentoring. Other resources needed include opportunities for education and training to aid in the acquisition of needed skills. Mentoring relationships in and of themselves can be very rewarding, but having an organizational system of rewards, whether by financial incentive or recognition, can go a long way toward encouraging and fostering mentoring in the workplace.

Career factors to be considered in the mentoring relationship concern both the potential mentees and mentors. Whether mentees see mentoring as essential for career development or increased access to opportunities, protection and support determines the amount of effort they put into finding a mentor. The intrinsic value that potential mentors place on the need for mentoring itself, increased respect from peers, and the fresh perspective that comes from keeping up with new information all determine whether or not they are willing to engage in a mentoring relationship.

Finally, the structure of the relationship as well as the methods of communication are important factors. Mentoring relationships can be either formal or informal. Formal relationships are usually structured, with one mentor assigned to a specific mentee. Informal relationships can form spontaneously, are usually voluntary in nature, and typically more effective and meaningful; but there are no guarantees that they will occur in the average work setting. Communication is another important factor in how successful a relationship will be. It needs to occur on a regular basis and be focused on the learning needs of the mentee, with adequate support for career growth and development, but can be effectively maintained via telephone, e-mail, or correspondence if a face-to-face relationship is not always possible (Grindel, 2003).

WRITING EXERCISE 21.1

Different factors affecting the mentoring relationship have been discussed. Think of a mentoring relationship that you have been in, witnessed, or perhaps a historical mentoring relationship. Describe the factors that either helped that relationship develop or hindered its success. Write up your description of these factors, and be prepared to discuss it in class.

MENTORING FUNCTIONS AND STRATEGIES

The concept of mentoring has been gaining popularity in all areas of nursing, from hospital organizations to nursing colleges, all of which are trying to find newer, creative ways of effectively training and retaining new members, while at the same time improving their productivity through job satisfaction and skills acquisition. In the evaluation of the relevance of mentoring, it is important to determine some of the functions of a mentoring relationship and to examine strategies used to facilitate the success of the relationship.

Pinkerton (2003) stated that there are two components of a mentoring relationship: the career function and the psychosocial function. The career function involves coaching, challenging, protection, sponsorship, exposure and visibility, skills acquisition, and an ongoing belief on the part of the mentor that the mentee will be successful. The psychosocial function involves promoting competence, counseling, nonjudgmental acceptance, clarification of identity, role modeling, role development, and friendship. Darling (1985) conducted a two-year research study to define what nurses wanted from a mentor. Study participants cited the need for mentors to be inspirers, inventors, and supporters.

One of the main goals of mentoring is to develop mentees' careers, smoothing the path, encouraging them, and facilitating their personal and professional growth, thus expediting the mentees' ability to function in their new role. The mentor should be able to recognize protégés' future potential and strive to help them discover and fully utilize their strengths, while finding ways to overcome and compensate for their weaknesses.

Another important function of mentoring is that of the socialization of the mentee into the organizational culture. By their mentor's reflected power and guidance, mentees are able to navigate the challenges and barriers to their acceptance as a peer into the organization. Mentors can also introduce mentees to influential colleagues and help establish a networking system for them. Good mentoring relationships can affect all aspects of a mentee's career, and through role modeling, the mentor can demonstrate a sense of pride and respect for the nursing profession (Greene & Puetzer, 2002).

Awareness of mentoring strategies can help determine the success of a relationship. The first strategy is to develop defined goals and periodically reevaluate them as the relationship evolves. It should also be understood that there is a shared responsibility for goal achievement. Time for the relationship should be considered a priority, and steps should be taken to allow for frequent contact, utilizing communication methods that are convenient and accessible to both individuals. The mentor should be well versed in the principles of adult learning and concepts of a process-oriented relationship, which include knowledge acquisition, application, and critical evaluation (Grindel, 2003). Finally, it is essential for a successful relationship to maintain an atmosphere of trust and confidentiality.

CASE SCENARIO 21.1

You are the manager of a busy Medical/Surgical Unit at Pleasantville Hospital. The CEO of the hospital has been made aware that there has been a hospitalwide shortage of nursing staff for some time, which seems to be worsening, and he has created a task force to examine the problem. After hiring a consultant and examining the issue extensively, the task force found numerous areas of concern. One such concern was that after one year the retention rate of new hires was only fifty-five percent, decreasing to forty percent after three years. The consultant has recommended forming a hospitalwide mentoring program. The task force has given you the job of working with them to develop the program and implementing it on your unit, which will be the model unit for the hospital.

Case Considerations

1. What are some of the factors, unique to your unit, that you will consider while developing this mentoring program?

2. Discuss whether you feel that the program should formally assign mentors to new staff or provide an environment that encourages the formation of mentoring relationships and how you would implement this on your unit.

3. List ways that you would work with the hospital to foster a mentoring culture on your unit and ultimately hospitalwide. What kind of incentives would be provided to encourage senior staff members to become mentors?

4. In what way will you present this program to your staff? Discuss how your approach might differ if you had been managing the unit for less than one year and for ten years or more.

MENTORING STAGES/PHASES

Many aspects of our lives have defined patterns of progression. The changing of the seasons, the growth of a child, the attainment of a goal, even the nursing process itself all demonstrate different stages of change in the world around us. As a dynamic relationship between two individuals, the mentoring process has also been shown, by various authors in the literature, to have progressive stages or phases of development.

Kram (1991) postulated that the mentoring relationship has four distinct stages. The first stage is initiation, when the relationship begins, by either formal or informal means; then comes the cultivation stage, when the relationship grows and develops; then the separation stage, as the mentee becomes more independent; and then the stage of redefinition, when the relationship is either terminated or develops into a new type of relationship.

Gordon (1998) defined three distinct phases of mentoring. Initially there is the phase of "recognition and development," then "emerging independence," and finally "letting go." Owens, Herrick, and Kelley (1998) determined that there are four phases of mentoring, beginning with the "initiation and acquaintance" phase, then progressing to "passage," then to "integration and accomplishment," and finally to "evaluation and termination."

Kochan and Trimble (2000), in their examination of mentoring relationships, concluded that mentoring occurs in four stages. The first stage is that of "laying the groundwork." In this stage individuals decide that they would like to engage in the mentoring process and then begin to assess their needs and define their goals. Next is the "warm-up" stage, when mentees begin to approach potential mentors and select the person whom they feel would best meet their needs and help them accomplish their goals. The two of them then begin to define the terms of their relationship. They then enter the "working" stage of the relationship, which involves the ongoing process of mentoring. The final stage is "long-term status," when an assessment of the relationship is made to determine whether the goals have been achieved and whether the relationship should be continued or terminated. This involves a reevaluation and redefining of the relationship.

All of these authors seem to agree that mentoring relationships have a defined progression, and that the goal of the relationship should be the development of the mentee into an independent, successfully functioning member of an organization. It is at that point that many of those involved in these relationships go on to become colleagues, friends, and even develop comentoring relationships.

MENTORING A NEW GENERATION

In a lifetime, nurses may experience many different phases and changes in their career path. They most likely will begin as a student and then progress to the position of a nurse working within an organizational structure. As time goes on they may decide to become a manager or administrator, to return to school, to become an educator, or to develop the skills and obtain the education necessary to work as a specialist or nurse practitioner. Or they may even decide to change to an altogether different profession. Through each of these transitions, a strong mentoring relationship can help make the process of developing a new role much easier and more rewarding. Mentoring for each of these roles have similarities, but also some unique differences. Mentoring strategies for new graduate nurses, minority

nurses, nurse managers, and nursing faculty will be examined in the following paragraphs.

Mentoring New Graduates

The first year working as a novice can be one of the most challenging of a nurse's career (Greggs-McQuilkin, 2004). Orientations are not always well planned, may be limited in scope, and can be quite short in length. This time of transition can be extremely mentally, physically, and emotionally taxing. The novice nurse can feel overwhelmed, physically exhausted, and confused when the concepts and absolutes that were learned in nursing school suddenly seem inadequate and unrealistic in the day-to-day struggle to cope with the myriad challenges encountered in providing nursing care to patients.

There also may be generational differences encountered by the novice while relating to the older, more experienced nursing staff (Green & Puetzer, 2002). New nursing graduates are generally computer literate; self-assured; and willing to voice their beliefs, concerns, or dissatisfactions. They are typically visual learners and strive for a balance between career and personal life. These characteristics can often be at odds with the views and work ethics of senior nurses, who may view the novice as arrogant, self-absorbed, not a team player, and having a poor work ethic (Hom, 2003).

Patricia Benner (2001) identified a continuum of five levels of nursing skill development: novice, advanced beginner, competent, proficient, and expert. Novices initially begin as very task-oriented, linear thinkers and develop through these levels until they become an expert. Expert nurses are able to "identify meaningful patterns, organize them, and use their skill base to apply the needed action" (Hom, 2003, p. 38).

Often new graduate nurses, shocked by the reality of actual bedside nursing, may feel that they have no one to turn to or confide in for fear of appearing incompetent (Hwang, 2004). New graduate nurses require guidance and nurturing to begin progressing in skill level from novice to the more advanced levels

CASE SCENARIO 21.2

You have been working as a staff nurse on a pediatric floor for the past ten years. Finally last year, two years after you requested the scheduling change, you have been able to move to a day-shift schedule of forty hours per week. You have greatly enjoyed working a "normal" schedule and being able to spend time with your family, although lately it seems that you have been constantly asked to work overtime to compensate for staffing shortages.

The previous manager recently retired, and a new nurse manager has begun running your floor. At a recent staff meeting she stated that in order to aid in the recruitment of new nursing staff, everyone would be expected to rotate schedules to accommodate the staffing needs of the floor, and that there would no longer be any permanent shifts with absolutely no exceptions. This information has greatly angered you because you feel that you have paid your dues by having to work odd schedules, and it is unfair to change the scheduling system to accommodate the desires of new nursing staff members. You have also seen recent recruiting advertisements for your hospital in the local paper

offering substantial sign-on bonuses, compensation for moving and educational expenses, and starting salaries that are equal to your own. Yesterday you were approached by the nurse manager to participate in a new nurse mentoring program, pairing you with a recent nursing graduate. You are flattered to be chosen by your manager and with some hesitation agree to be a mentor.

Case Considerations

1. Describe actions that you could take to help you deal with any negative emotions that could potentially affect your mentoring relationship adversely.

2. Discuss how the learning needs of a new graduate might differ from those of a newly hired, more experienced nurse.

3. List some strategies that would be appropriate for mentoring a new graduate nurse.

4. Develop some creative ideas and strategies that could be implemented to help this floor achieve a mentoring culture.

of practice. They need role models to teach prioritizing, the performance of both basic and more advanced nursing skills, and how to interact effectively with other members of the health care team (Hom, 2003). They must learn not only the policies, procedures, and skills necessary to function in an organization, but also the more subtle language, rules, methods of communication, taboos, and power structure of the organizational culture in which they find themselves. Effective mentoring of these new graduate nurses has been found to greatly decrease costs to health care organizations by increasing retention of new nurses and thus lowering the costs attributed to the orientation process (Greggs-McQuilkin, 2004).

Active, respectful listening is critical when mentoring new graduate nurses. Interruptions, physical distractions, and anticipation of a reply all act as barriers to listening and should be limited whenever possible. Good eye contact should be maintained, and mentors should acknowledge and respond to their mentees by paraphrasing and summarizing their thoughts and ideas. It is essential that mentors evaluate and confront any of their own negative emotions and then work to control them. Mentors must also drop any authoritative, superior attitudes, be open-minded, and gain knowledge themselves from the relationship (McKinley, 2004).

Mentoring Minority Nurses

The United States has seen a tremendous increase in the cultural and ethnic diversity of its population in the last few decades (Washington, Erickson, & Ditomassi, 2004). Yet at the same time, minority groups continue to be underrepresented in nursing. Organizations are struggling to find ways to increase diversity and cultural sensitivity in their staff members and to recruit and retain minorities. Increasingly, these organizations are looking at mentoring programs as a way of accomplishing this.

Mentoring is "a key component in building a diverse workplace focused on the development of multicultural leaders" (Washington et al., 2004, p. 167). Mentors can help assist minority nurses in navigating the cultural landscape of an organization, teaching them networking skills and helping them maintain their sense of self-worth and personal identity. To effectively mentor minorities, individuals must possess good communication and coping skills. They need to have the ability to help minority nurses understand the intricacies of an organization's culture, while at the same time having a perspective on how nurses' particular cultures and ethnic backgrounds might influence their reactions to situations.

Washington, Erickson, & Ditomassi (2004) discuss their "Five Cs" of effective mentoring strategies for minority nurses. They are "Candor, Compromise, Confidence, Complexity, and Champion" (p. 168). Candor is the ability to be frank about issues such as bias or concerns related to the loss of ethnic identity while maintaining an atmosphere of trust and inclusion. Compromise is teaching minority nurses not to "win the battle while losing the war" and teaching them effective problem solving and negotiation skills. Confidence is the concept of preserving minority nurses' ethnic and cultural individuality while at the same time encouraging them to function as valued members of the team. Complexity is the acknowledgment that cultural and diversity issues have strong historical roots and can be highly emotional. It is critical that the mentor establish a trusting relationship so that these issues can be worked through and dealt with in a constructive manner.

Finally, Champion represents the idea that the mentor will become the minority nurse's advocate and supporter, providing opportunities for personal growth and career advancement.

Some of the goals for the minority nurse include learning to be assertive in confronting issues rather than demonstrating avoidance or passive/aggressive behaviors, the ability to determine if there are "hidden agendas" in feedback that is received, becoming skilled at negotiation, learning to develop crosscultural relationships, and learning effective strategies for dealing with intracultural conflicts.

Mentoring Nursing Faculty

The ever-growing shortage of nurses affects not only hospitals and health care organizations, but also nursing colleges across the country. Thus a vicious cycle ensues: colleges must limit enrollment due to fewer faculty resources, and this in turn contributes to the inadequate number of available qualified nurses. Nursing colleges are also examining how the mentoring of junior faculty can help with retention and foster excellence in teaching. Wocial (1995) stated that mentoring was critical in promoting integrity among developing nurse scientists and could also prevent incidences of scientific misconduct during research activities.

New faculty are often overwhelmed with the stresses of meeting the needs of students, the education system, work expectations, and meeting obligations to professional organizations in which they are involved. Mentoring by senior faculty members can help junior faculty members prioritize activities, learn organizational skills, and assess their own learning needs. Senior faculty can also provide opportunities for junior faculty to gain new knowledge and participate in activities that can strengthen their curriculum vitae. They can help promote team building and socialize newer faculty into the culture of the college organization (Horton, 2003).

To be successful mentors, senior faculty members should be aware of the policies and procedures of their particular educational organization. They should expect and be prepared to deal with mistakes that will be made by junior faculty, offering support, guidance, and modeling appropriate responses to situations. Senior faculty need to provide ongoing, constructive feedback and help junior faculty develop teaching strategies, discover methods to improve their subject knowledge, and help them in identifying available resources.

Mentoring Nurse Managers/Leaders

Historically, nurses who excel in the clinical setting are the ones who are encouraged to transition to leadership and management positions. Very often these same nurses, who possess such excellent clinical skills, have little if any management training or skills. They find that they have gone from a position of expert knowledge in their clinical area to one of being a virtual novice at the skills required for effective management (Gershenson, Moravick, Sellman, & Somerville, 2004). They usually do not have any formal orientation to the role and many times find themselves feeling overwhelmed, frustrated, and inadequate, and ultimately experience failure in this role.

New managers need to devise new paradigms to help them thrive in this role. They must move from a task-oriented to a skill-oriented pathway of career development. They need to look at not only short-term goals, but also at the long-term view or the big picture, and they will have to begin to consider the needs of the whole unit at the possible expense of individual needs and desires. Being able to function in this role requires much planning because there are constant interruptions. The new nurse manager must develop skills in conflict resolution, budget management, staff motivation, and effective communication.

Mentoring can be critical to the development of a nurse manager/leader, and organizations have much to gain by having mentors for these novice leaders, which can ultimately decrease costs by minimizing management turnover, increasing staff satisfaction, and improving unit efficiency through effective management. Organizations can groom new leaders by identifying appropriate learning opportunities, serving as resources, and guiding them through many of the multiple challenges of management. Mentors need to be aware that these new managers, as adult learners, have the ability to diagnose, plan, implement, and evaluate their own learning. They are usually self-motivated and self-directed, but need guidance on how to achieve their goals.

New nurse managers can have several different mentors, each to facilitate growth in different areas of their role. New managers should seek out mentors who have similar philosophies and goals; having a mentor both inside and outside of the organization can also be advantageous (Grindel, 2003). An effective mentor can help a novice manager acquire the skills and qualities necessary for good leadership, such as integrity, political sensitivity and candor, management, team building, the ability to network and work collaboratively, as well as communication and organizational skills (Gershenson et al., 2004).

BENEFITS OF MENTORING

The benefits of mentoring relationships are numerous, from organizational, professional, and personal perspectives. From an organizational standpoint, mentoring can decrease attrition, which has been shown to increase costs and decrease the morale of remaining members. Mentoring can enhance the quality, creativity, and productivity of members while at the same time decreasing boredom and stagnation (Grindel, 2003). An organization that fosters a work environment based on a mentoring culture increases the job satisfaction of its members and has been shown to improve retention rates (Grindel, 2003).

From a professional level, nurses who have been mentored have higher earnings, increased confidence and self-esteem, increased opportunities for promotion, and are generally more prepared for leadership roles (Grindel, 2003). They do not have to "reinvent the wheel" because they can learn from mistakes that mentors have made in the past and made their mentees aware of. Mentoring also strengthens the nursing profession by developing new leaders and building a professional culture among nurses. Nurses who are mentored tend to mentor others. It has been documented that Rachel Williams, who was mentored by Florence Nightingale, went on to mentor several protégés (Lorentzon & Brown, 2003).

Lastly, mentoring can have very profound rewards for both the mentee and the mentor. There can be personal and professional growth for both individuals from the stimulation and challenge of the relationship. Mentors can also gain insights into their own goals and experience career revitalization and satisfaction from peer and organizational recognition of their efforts.

CHAPTER SUMMARY

As today's health care environment becomes more complex, diverse, and ever-changing, nurses need experienced, reliable mentors more than ever to guide them into productive and satisfying roles. Mentoring is an ongoing, dynamic process that not only prepares individuals for their career paths, but also instills in them the desire to return the favor by mentoring others. Developing good mentoring skills and strategies can do much to stop nursing from "eating its young" and help organizations begin to deal with and correct some of the issues that have led to the current nursing shortage. The nursing profession and individual nurses can experience many benefits from involvement in mentoring relationships and programs.

> *We do not grow in a vacuum; the caring, mentoring, and support of others form our career trajectories as well as our professional and personal experiences.*
> —Carolyn L. Murdaugh

REFERENCES

Bell, C. R. (2002). *Managers as mentors: Building partnerships for learning*. San Francisco: Berrett-Koehler Publishing, Inc.

Benner, P. (2001). *From novice to expert: Excellence and power in clinical nursing practice (commerative edition)*. Upper Saddle River, NJ: Prentice Hall Health.

Billings, D. M., Skiba, D. J., & Connors, H. R. (2005). Best practices in Web-based courses: Generational differences across undergraduate and graduate nursing students. *Journal of Professional Nursing, 21*(2), 126–133.

Cameron-Jones, M., & O'Hara, P. (1996). Three decisions about nurse mentoring. *Journal of Nursing Management, 4*, 225–230.

Darling, L. W. (1985). So, you've never had a mentor. *Journal of Nursing Administration, 13*(12), 38–39.

Department of Health and Human Services. Retrieved August 8, 2005, from http://bhpr.hrsa.gov/healthworkforce/reports/rnsurvey/rnss.1.htm.

Gershenson, T. A., Moravick, D. A., Sellman, E., & Somerville, S. (2004). Expert to novice: A nurse leader's evolution. *Nursing Management, 35*(6), 49–52.

Glass, N., & Walter, R. (2000). An experience of peer mentoring with student nurses: Enhancement of personal and professional growth. *Journal of Nursing Education, 39*(4), 155–160.

Gordon, F. A. (1998). The road to success with a mentor. *Journal of Vascular Nursing, 18*(1), 30–33.

Greggs-McQuilkin, D. (2004). Mentoring really matters: Motivate and mentor a colleague. *Medsurg Nursing, 13*(4), 209, 266.

Greene, T. M., & Puetzer, M. (2002). The value of mentoring: A strategic approach to retention and recruitment. *Journal of nursing care quality, 17*(1), 63–70.

Grindel, C. G. (2003). Mentoring managers. *Nephrology Nursing Journal, 30*(5), 517–522.

Hom, E. M. (2003). Coaching and mentoring new graduates entering perinatal nursing practice. *Journal of Perinatal and Neonatal Nursing, 17*(1), 35–49.

Horton, B. J. (2003). The importance of mentoring in recruiting and retaining junior faculty. *AANA Journal, 71*(3), 189–195.

Hwang, L. (2004). Sounding board. *California Nurse, 100*(6), 12–13.

Kram, K. E. (1991). *Mentoring at work: Developing relationships in organizational life.* Glenview, IL: Scott Foresman.

Kochan, F. K., & Trimble, S. B. (2000). From mentoring to co-mentoring: Establishing collaborative relationships. *Theory into Practice, 39*(1), 20–28.

Kupperschmidt, B. (2000). Multigeneration employees: Strategies for effective management. *Health Care Manager, 19*(1), 65–76.

Lorentzon, M., & Brown, K. (2003). Florence Nightingale as 'mentor of matrons': Correspondence with Rachel Williams at St. Mary's Hospital. *Journal of Nursing Management, 11,* 266–274.

McKinley, M. G. (2004). A mentor gap in nursing? *Critical Care Nurse, 24*(2), 8–11.

Meno, K. M., Keaveny, B. M., & O'Donnell, J. M. (2003). Mentoring in the operating room: A student perspective. *American Association of Nurse Anesthetists Journal, 71*(5), 337–341.

Murdaugh, C. L. (1998). The value of mentors and facillitatiors in the pursuit of excellence. *Journal of Cardiovascular Nursing, 12*(2), 65–72.

Owens, B. H., Herrick, C. A., & Kelley, J. A. (1998). A prearranged mentorship program: Can it work long distance? *Journal of Professional Nursing, 14,* 78–84.

Owens, J. K., & Patton, J. G. (2003). Take a chance on nursing mentorships: Enhance leadership with this win-win strategy. *Nursing Education Perspectives, 24*(4), 19–204.

Pinkerton, S. E. (2003). Mentoring new graduates. *Nursing Economics, 21*(4), 202–203.

Roberts, D. (2003). Mentoring: The future of nursing. *MedSurg Nursing, 12*(3), 143.

Sherwen, L. N. (2003). Finding a mentor: What every nursing student should know. *Nursing News, 27*(3).

Smeltzer, C. H. (2002). The benefits of executive coaching. *Journal of Nursing Administration, 32*(10), 501–502.

Spatley, E., Johnson, A., Sochalski, J., Fritz, M., & Spencer, W. (2000). March 2000: Findings from the national sample survey of registered nurses. Washington, DC: U.S.

Thorpe, K. & Kalischuk, R. G. (2003). A collegial mentoring model for nurse educators. *Nursing Forum, 38*(1), 5–15.

Vance, C., & Olson, R. K. (1998). *The mentor connection in nursing.* New York: Springer Publishing Company.

Washington, D., Erickson, J. I., & Ditomassi, M. (2004). Mentoring the minority nurse leader of tomorrow. *Nursing Administration Quarterly, 28*(3), 165–169.

Wocial, L. D. (1995). The role of mentors in promoting integrity and preventing scientific misconduct in nursing research. *Journal of Professional Nursing, 11*(5), 276–280.

Young, A. M., & Perrewe, P. L. (2000). The exchange relationship between mentors and protégés: The development of a framework. *Human Resource Management Review, 10*(2), 177–209.

Zachary, I. J. (2000). *The mentor's guide.* San Francisco: Jossey-Bass.

CHAPTER 22

Responsibilities of the Profession

Mary Jo Regan-Kubinski and Karin A. Polifko

Talent only gives you the opportunity to win.
—Chad Brown, NFL Linebacker

LEARNING OBJECTIVES

At the completion of the chapter, the learner should be able to do the following:

1. Describe the characteristics of a profession.
2. Identify the ways in which nursing can be characterized as a profession and ways in which it cannot.
3. Discuss the role of nursing organizations in the promotion of the profession, improving practice, and influencing health.
4. Analyze the interplay of the image, role, and behavior of nurses in defining the nursing as a profession.
5. Identify specific actions that individual nurses can take to strengthen the voice, influence, and effectiveness of the nursing profession.
6. Discuss the implications of future trends on the profession of nursing.

KEY TERMS

Characteristics of a profession	Profession	Professional responsibilities
Political activity	Professional organizations	Voice of nursing

The **profession** of nursing has had a long and proud history. However, throughout that history, nursing has struggled with both defining and actualizing itself as a profession. The work of the nurse, in particular the bedside care of patients, is not viewed as the work of a professional. The personal and social background of many nurses, mostly women, was such that they entered nursing as a means to secure a job; the thought of a career in nursing was not the norm. The lack of autonomy and the handmaiden-to-the-physician image hardly illustrates the image of a professional person. And even today people enter nursing through various educational routes, giving rise to the question of whether nurses can be considered professionals. Thus, history, attitude, and education work together to create a current image of nursing that is incongruent with that of a profession. Yet, at the very same time, nursing is perceived by the public as being the most trusted and most ethical among the professions (Sigma Theta Tau International, 1999).

DEFINING A PROFESSION

The definition of a profession in American culture arose as workers sought to move from heavy labor, menial work, or lack of control over the conditions of work. Indeed, even medicine, today considered the prototype of a profession, was a part of the movement to define its work as professional.

The classic **characteristics of a profession** are generally accepted to be autonomy, a defined body of knowledge, independent standards for practice, accountability, responsibility to society, a code of ethics, and self-governance (Flexner, 1910). In addition, a profession needs to have a strong internal organization that is learned through a rigorous process, generally obtained at the college or university level. These standards address issues of independence in thinking and in practice, a body of knowledge that continues to develop, integrity of the practitioner, and a responsibility beyond individual needs and concerns. Also implied is self-organization and self-governance, so that the profession regulates its practice and its practitioners.

THE NURSING PROFESSION: ISSUES AND IMPLICATIONS

Using the widely accepted criteria of a profession, there is historical and current debate about whether nursing meets those criteria. Against the backdrop of medicine's journey to the status of a profession, nursing separated from medicine and attempted to become recognized as a profession. Even today, nursing appears to meet some, but not all, of the criteria of a profession.

Nursing has a specified body of knowledge, premised on the requisite to deliver holistic care to individuals, groups, and populations. Nurse researchers pursue answers to problems that concern the delivery of care as well as add to the theoretical base of nursing practice. There is a National Institute for Nursing Research, a strong indication that the government considers the development of nursing knowledge worthy of funding as a separate entity. Today's nursing practice requires the use of sophisticated technology, so that what were once simple tasks now include an element of functioning beyond routine. The hallmark of independent nursing judgment and assessment is a highly developed knowledge base. Yet the nature of nursing knowledge and research is not entirely independent of the knowledge base of other disciplines. Nursing knowledge builds on the foundations of psychology, sociology, anthropology, pharmacology, biology, and medicine. The unique combination and application of the knowledge of the various other disciplines together with nursing's own knowledge is holistic patient-centered care.

A traditional image of the nurse, that of a handmaiden to the physician, has diminished, even if it has not entirely disappeared. But do nurses have the autonomy that is characteristic of professional status? Most nurses practice in a hospital setting, where there are structured units and expectations for hours of work. The workweek may be flexible and may even be spread over more than one 7-day period, but most nurses do not have control over the hours or the schedule that they work. The questions of control over working conditions as well as the education needed for nursing have been addressed by nursing leaders for years. And although advanced-practice nurses and others in independent roles do have higher degrees of autonomy, the interdependent nature of nursing practice remains a reality.

The characteristics of a code of ethics and acceptance of a commitment to society are well met by nursing. The Code of Ethics for Nurses (ANA, 2001) was first published in 1971 and is accepted as the standard for nursing in the United States; other countries have developed their own codes. The intent of a code of ethics is to serve as a guideline and general principles. These codes cannot give answers to specific problems, but they do summarize the guiding principles that premise professional practice. It is also important to note that the ANA has revised and updated its Code of Ethics. Nursing as a profession is attentive to changes in the delivery of health care, changes that are reflected in the revised document and that serve as evidence of professional behavior.

The commitment of nursing to the health and well-being of society, having accepted a contract to provide for societal needs, is another indication that nursing is a profession. Attending to client and societal needs is a defining characteristic of nursing practice, one that is acknowledged by consumers and prized by nurses. "Helping others" is the driving force behind many a decision to enter nursing.

However, given the parameters of the core competencies of health care professions as stated by the Institute of Medicine (2003), individual nurses will need to move beyond the initial conception of helping that primarily focuses on working directly with individuals and families (see Table 22.1). Nursing as a profession, and nurses as professionals, will need to move to interdisciplinary, evidence-based

Table 22.1 The Core Competencies Needed for Health Care Professionals

- Provide patient-centered care
- Work in interdisciplinary teams
- Employ evidence-based practice
- Apply quality improvement
- Utilize informatics

SOURCE: Institute of Medicine (2003). *Health professions education: A bridge to quality.* Washington, DC: National Academies Press.

patient care using technology as a means of both communication and improvement of that care. The challenge rests with both the individual and the profession more broadly: to move beyond the bedside image of the nurse even though the primary site of care delivery may be at the bedside.

Even though nursing might not demonstrate all of the characteristics of a profession, it is in the best interest of nurses to act as if they have attained professional status. On the collective level, nursing has the responsibility to support and maintain professional organizations, nursing's research agenda, and to fulfill nursing's social contract. On an individual level, there are also important contributions that each and every practicing nurse can be engaged in. With collective and individual action, nursing will further its own agenda and become increasingly autonomous.

WRITING EXERCISE 22.1

Are you satisfied with the image of nursing? Is it what you expected when you entered into your nursing education program? Is the fact that nursing does not meet all of the criteria of a profession a hindrance to you as a nurse? Do you think it is an issue for the profession of nursing or society in general?

THE COLLECTIVE RESPONSIBILITIES OF THE PROFESSION

Strong **professional organizations** are a hallmark of a profession. Organization confers a strength that individual members cannot attain on their own. A variety of organizations have emerged to represent nurses, nursing practice, and to promote specialty-nursing practice. Nursing's reach and interests are many and varied, and these factors have lead to the establishment of organizations to represent the many facets of nursing.

The American Nurses Association (ANA) emerged from the recognition of a need to promote and oversee the quality of nursing care. As a direct result, the main concern of the ANA is the maintenance and improvement of the standards for nursing care. The ANA accomplishes its goals through setting standards and through services that assist nurses to grow and develop. It is engaged in a continual process of review and revision of the standards of practice, which have become the benchmark for legal and ethical decision making. The ANA is likewise concerned with the working conditions of nurses and their financial well-being. In some states, the ANA provides collective bargaining representation for nurses; and it has been a constant voice in the discussions about the educational preparation of nurses and the debate about requirements for entry into practice. An arm of the ANA, the American Nurses Credentialing Center (ANCC), offers testing and certification for specialty-nursing practice. As the largest U.S. nursing organization, the ANA has the potential to represent the voice of nursing on the national level, playing an important role in political action and lobbying efforts. However, the ANA has not attained the power or the stature of other professional organizations, in particular, the American Medical Association.

The role of the National League for Nursing (NLN) is more focused than that of the ANA. The NLN's purpose is to oversee the standards and accreditation of nursing education; however, the NLN is also an organized voice for nursing in the areas of health policy and promotion of public health. One of the major activities of the NLN is the accreditation of schools of nursing through the National League for Nursing Accrediting Commission (NLNAC), which has developed criteria and standards for nursing education with which schools of nursing must demonstrate compliance. The NLNAC is the only nursing-accreditation-granting body that deals with all levels of nursing education—diploma, associate degree, baccalaureate degree, and master's degree. (Historically, doctoral programs in nursing have not been accredited.) The NLN also offers testing and evaluation services for new graduates, continuing education for the faculty of schools of nursing, literature pertaining to nursing issues, and publishes comparative data about nursing education programs.

Sigma Theta Tau International (STTI), as its name indicates, represents nursing globally. In addition, STTI has membership criteria intended to honor nurses who have attained or who are expected to attain leadership roles in nursing. Influence within the profession and development of leadership skills in nursing are the specific concerns of STTI. Knowledge development, support for research, and leadership development of members are indirect means to influence the delivery of nursing care. An international platform encourages learning across cultures and sharing of best practices around the world. Support for nurses in poorer and developing nations is central to the mission to improve health worldwide.

Groups representing specific nursing entities have emerged, such as the American Association of Colleges of Nursing (AACN), which represents baccalaureate- and higher-degree nursing-education programs. The vast majority of baccalaureate and graduate programs are members exclusively of the AACN. Data collection, research, and governmental advocacy are some of the areas the AACN engages in; they also produce educational programs and publications as well as set standards for bachelor's- and graduate-degree nursing programs. The AACN has established the Commission on Collegiate Nursing

Education (CCNE), which accredits baccalaureate- and master's-level nursing programs, ensuring implementation of quality standards. The AACN greatly influences nursing education, practice, and research endeavors, and promotes public support for the profession of nursing.

Nurses have found it either necessary or desirable to join forces in seeking representation for special interests in order to establish forums for discussion or platforms for actions. International organizations seek to establish communication and share concerns across national borders. Groups representing groups have emerged, such as the American Association of Colleges of Nursing or the National Federation for Specialty Nursing Organizations.

Broad representation of nurses or the nursing profession is attained through the very large national and international organizations. Other nursing organizations represent much more narrowly defined aspects of nursing. For example, the American Organization of Operating Room Nurses (AORN) promotes standards and quality and represents the interests of operating-room nurses. The American Association of Critical Care Nurses, the American Holistic Nurses Association, the National Association of Neonatal Nurses, the Emergency Nurses Association and the Society of Urologic Nurses illustrate the range of specialty interests represented by a professional nursing organization. Indeed, there is a nursing specialty organization for almost every kind of nursing practice and interest. The American Association for the History of Nursing and the American Association of Legal Nurse Consultants illustrate further the range of available opportunities for nurses to find collegiality and share common interests and concerns.

Many varieties and levels of nursing organizations indicate that, on the whole, the profession has developed the means to represent nursing and nurses. The existence of these many professional nursing organizations gives the individual nurse the opportunity for involvement on many levels. Despite the plentiful options, it is not yet the norm for nurses to join and actively participate in professional organizations. As a result, organizations may not develop their full potential—whether their focus is improved patient care or support for the nursing profession.

Nurses can initiate involvement in professional organizations at the local level. National organizations are typically organized into their regional or local chapters, facilitating individual involvement. Often regionally based organizations will rotate meeting sites, making it more convenient for members to attend at a local site. Nurses are very busy people, and local leaders know and understand that. They may schedule meetings in restaurants, providing opportunities for socialization as well as business. There may even be opportunities to meet with chapter members in one's place of employment. For example, a local chapter of the American Association of Critical Care Nurses may meet in a conference room within a hospital.

It is true that national leaders of professional organizations have the greatest visibility, and so it is easy to overlook that there are numerous opportunities to be effective on smaller stages. Participation at a local level offers both the means and the opportunity for broader action, such as on the regional, state, and national levels. Holding office at the local level often leads to the need to represent the local group on a regional or state board. Similarly, involvement at the state level offers networking at the national level at conferences, workshops, and meetings. Taking first steps is much easier to think about and to do at the local level. Opportunities for wider involvement will present themselves with continued participation, networking, and a willingness to step into leadership roles. But taking those first steps is crucial!

Students of nursing have an opportunity to participate in their own professional organization, the National Student Nurses Association (NSNA). Chapters exist at many schools of nursing, sometimes with support from the college or university student government. There are state and national conferences, and opportunities for students to be groomed for leadership roles with the support of faculty mentors. Student nurses can try out organizational leadership, support for a cause, political involvement on campus, and participation in national forums through involvement in the NSNA. If the school chapter is relatively inactive, the potential for leadership abounds, and opportunities for action are extensive. Participation in the NSNA is a wonderful bridge to continued and sustained involvement as a professional nurse.

Time and motivation are constant issues that influence and impact nurses' participation in professional organizations; but if one has a vision for improvement or for instituting change, the realization that one is not alone can be a powerful factor in joining forces to work together on issues. Nurses must move beyond the walls of their places of employment to affect the wider arena of health care and its delivery. Nursing organizations offer ready-made venues to begin participation beyond the bedside.

PROFESSIONAL RESPONSIBILITIES OF THE INDIVIDUAL NURSE

The plight of nursing in its journey to find professional status is dependent upon the actions of individual nurses. The mentality of many who enter nursing is that it is a job, rather than a career to be developed. Instead of merely putting in time, nurses need to have an attitude of growth and development. The prevailing attitudes and self-images of nurses are not congruent with those of professionals who believe that they have power to effect change in either their own working lives or in the broader delivery of health care. Yet the very fact that nursing possesses most of the characteristics of a profession offers hope and provides opportunity to individual nurses.

For nursing to attain professional stature and power, individual nurses must accept the invitation to accountability and **responsibility** inherent in professional practice. First and foremost, each and every nurse must be dedicated to continued education. Lifelong learning is not merely a slogan; it is a fact of life in the rapidly evolving health care system. It is no longer adequate to be educated at the associate-degree level in nursing; instead, the baccalaureate should be the minimal preparation, with the expectation that regardless of position, further education is necessary in order to advance. Nurses need to update practice skills and their knowledge of the technology that is used in the delivery of care. Information systems will alter the systems of care delivery, and nurses must be at the forefront of the design as well as the implementation of these new systems. Practicing nurses must ask and answer whether they are performing at the highest level and pursue certification or advanced-practice status to make the most of their talents. Nurses must seek the right fit between their talents and the many options available to them in clinical practice, administration, research, or educational settings. These responsibilities and accompanying actions might sound familiar—and they should. These are the core competencies outlined by the Institute of Medicine (2003).

A first step for many nurses might be joining and becoming active in a local professional organization. Local groups offer stepping stones to regional and national organizations. Collective action will increase the power and the influence of nursing and give the individual nurse a new source of motivation and sense of identity. The profession of nursing should not be looked upon as merely a job in which the same techniques and skills learned in school will maintain the person for her entire work life without returning to school. By joining a professional organization, the nursing professional takes the initiative for supporting policy surrounding a specialized practice area through effective lobbying efforts, through increased visibility of certain issues, or through various political action committees.

POLITICAL ACTION

Nurses must also consider individual political action. Professional organizations represent nursing and provide a voice for nursing's interests, but each and every

CASE SCENARIO 22.1

As an almost-graduated nurse with a BSN, you have been encouraged by your faculty members to join your professional organization. After school, you will have many expenses: you are moving to a new state, your family will have to buy a new house, and you will be paying off your school loans.

1. As an AD nurse graduate, you never joined any professional organizations. Why should you now, especially since you are about to graduate with your BSN?

2. Or as a second-degree student, the whole notion of the nursing profession is fairly new to you. Why should you join your professional organization now?

3. What organizations(s) are you thinking of joining and why?

4. What are some reasons that others would not consider joining their professional organization? How would you respond to them as a challenge to their thinking?

5. Identify at least three benefits to joining a professional organization. What do some organizations do for their new graduate applicants?

individual nurse can also effectively influence the political decision-making process on a smaller scale.

What is "political"? Broadly viewed, politics is the use of influence to effect the distribution of resources (Leavitt & Mason, 2006). Applying this perspective may help nurses recognize that since resources are not infinite, it is in the best interest of their patients if they use their professional influence in the decision- making process related to the allocation of those resources. Nurses must also develop an attitude that they have knowledge that is needed in that decision-making process. Nurses publicly promoting nursing knowledge, coupled with a vision of improved health outcomes, can make powerful statements in support of the use of resources to maximize health on local, state, and national levels. Nurses think of themselves as patient advocates; political involvement offers the opportunity to advocate for those patients on a broader stage, with greater effect. Keeping in mind that professions have a social responsibility may help nurses understand that they need to add their knowledge and perspective when issues regarding their profession, patient care, or the delivery of health care are concerned.

Similar to participation in professional organizations, opportunities for political involvement begin at the local level. Regional and state politicians are eager to represent the interests of their constituencies, and nurses are well poised to raise issues and concerns regarding health, health policies, and nursing practice. Individual nurses, representatives of a well-respected profession, add to the power of their statements by identifying that profession when weighing in on or calling attention to issues. At times, legislators may not have the information or the knowledge regarding matters of importance to nurses, and it is up to nurses to inform them of how those issues could affect their constituents. Groups of nurses may also join together, to both hear from and speak to the legislators representing their geographic area. For example, the local chapter of a state's nursing organization might invite legislators from all parties to attend a "nursing forum," attended by nurses who listen and speak to their own legislators.

It is not difficult to keep the names of one's senators and representatives nearby one's computer, ready for an e-mail contact with one's legislators. Given present-day concerns about security, e-mail is the preferred method of communication with legislators. An e-mail message does not have to be sent for inspection, and congressional aides are astute in identifying timely and well-presented input. With the contact information readily available, one can easily send messages to the legislature when issues related to nursing and health care arise. One might become identified as a trusted expert on nursing and be invited to contribute thoughts and opinions as well as to offer them as they arise.

If nurses continue to think narrowly of political action, confining it to legislative sessions or campaigns, they will continue to miss chances to make changes in health care and in nursing. Broadening the perspective of nurses to include political action as a tool to improve patient care is a task that the professional cannot afford to overlook. The collective voice of the largest group of health care professionals can be very powerful, but the voice of nursing does not represent the power of those numbers.

MEDIA AND THE VOICE OF NURSING

Similar to the reticence that characterizes nurses' involvement in political forums, nurses generally are not prominent in media reports. Their thoughts and opinions are not typically sought out, unless there is an issue focused on nursing, such as the nursing shortage or the possibility of nurses striking for better working conditions. It is much less likely that journalists or reporters will seek the thoughts and opinions of nurses regarding health care. It is also not likely, dissimilar to the case for medical research, that the results of nursing research are reported. For too long nurses and nursing have not made the most of opportunities for improved professional stature, to bring attention to nursing, nurses, and the factors that influence providing patient care, with the result that nurses are silent members of the health care

team (Buresh & Gordon, 2006). It is not difficult to see that nurses, collectively, have not made it a priority to ensure that the public hears, knows, and understands the nursing profession's stance on a wide variety of health-related topics. The knowledge base that nurses have acquired through education and practice, although recognized in the abstract, is not concretely identified and sought as a source of information. Yet nurses can develop (and some have developed) the requisite skills to influence the media and thereby the public (Sullivan, 2004).

Nurses must take the responsibility to move from a silent position to one of public attention. Just as the initial learning of nursing skills takes time and practice, so does the learning of the skills that will move nursing to the forefront of media attention and public awareness. Nurses need to move past the role that they learned and practiced while in school, recognizing that their own professional development requires them to move beyond the bedside.

LOOKING TO THE FUTURE: BEYOND THE BEDSIDE

The present nursing shortage has greatly increased public awareness of nursing and has generated interest in nursing as a career. Or has it increased interest in nursing as merely a secure, dependable job? At a time when the average age of nurses indicates that many will be ready to retire in the next decade, there is a pressing need to ensure an adequate supply of nurses to meet the needs of the public. But what will those nurses look like, who will they be, and what will they do? Students of nursing are poised to make changes, going boldly into the future with a new vision for nursing. But what exactly does this vision look like? What are some of the issues that are being actively discussed at this point in nursing education?

RESEARCH APPLICATION ARTICLE

Swearington, S. & Liberman, A. (2004). Nursing generations: An expanded look at the emergence of conflict and its resolution. *Health Care Manager, 23*(1), 54–64.

Currently in the health care system there are at least three generations of nurses who are working together—with many a misunderstanding and intergenerational conflict. The three generations are known as the Veteran Nurses, the Baby Boomers, and Generation X. The authors believe that one of the reasons that there are nursing shortages—and that there will continue to be so—is that the youngest generation, Generation X, has little desire to seek or maintain a career in nursing for a variety of reasons. The conceptual frameworks of conflict and cohort theories were theoretically applied to the three abovementioned cohorts in an attempt to distinguish—and hopefully plan for—some of the discrepancies among the groups, particularly among Generation X. Although the article does not clearly describe the application of the two theories, it does mention that a shortcoming to the cohort theory application is that it fails to show the importance of the intergenerational differences that need to be appreciated for the diversity that the three intergenerational groups of nurses can bring to the workplace.

Future Trends of the Profession

As this book has discussed, there are multiple tenets in the profession of nursing that are at its core: bedside skills; leadership and management capabilities; and the ability to act in the roles of delegator, mediator, mentor, teacher, and change agent while ensuring that the patient and his family receive the best care to achieve optimal outcomes. But can the profession maintain itself in the same way it has for the past fifty years? Can it afford to? What are the current and future trends that will alter the way in which we deliver care?

WRITING EXERCISE 22.2

Many people have commented on the image of popular nursing as seen in the movies or on television—and it isn't all viewed in a positive, professional light (how many female nurses do you know wear 4-inch heels to work a 12-hour shift?). Further, men who have chosen the nursing profession have not always been portrayed in the best possible way either.

If you were given the opportunity by a public relations firm with unlimited resources, what kind of media campaign would you develop to promote the profession of nursing? What are some of the highlights that you would want to make sure are viewed by the public? What are some of the images that you would work hard to dispel? What are your ideas for a campaign name?

WRITING ASSIGNMENT 22.3

What does the future of nursing hold? Some say that the profession has had several discussions in the last 20 to 30 years that really haven't been resolved, such as the entry-into-practice debate. Why does a profession such as nursing still have several entry points: the associate degree, the hospital-based diploma, the baccalaureate degree, and the generic master's degree? How have these multiple entry points helped or hindered the profession? Will this discussion ever reach consensus?

There are at least twelve significant trends that we suggest will alter the landscape of both nursing education and the resultant nursing delivery system in the United States.

- The aging of the American population, including the nursing workforce. Not only are we as a nation getting older and living longer, but we are existing with more chronic diseases that would have decreased our survival rates years ago. Concurrently, the nursing workforce is aging, causing hospital systems to rethink how they expect older nurses to continue work that is as physically demanding as it is mentally challenging.

- Changing demographics including increasing cultural diversity, increased immigration, and increasing poverty rates. What was once a majority race may be the minority race in many areas throughout America, bringing new challenges and barriers to effective health care delivery.

- Continued increases in the level of the uninsured in the United States and in the cost of health care both to the individual and to the employer at a rate that is increasing faster than inflation. Managed care has not altered the landscape for providing care for all, and with the struggle with unemployment or in the challenges of the working poor, families are finding it increasingly more difficult to pay for health care, because care is sought only when the illness is debilitating. Preventative care is generally

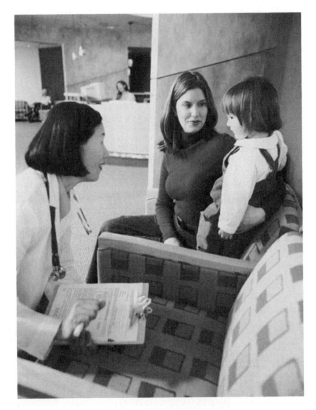

Figure 22.1 The registered nurse is at the forefront of the health care delivery team, often being the one provider who can influence people's health care decisions directly through education, understanding and compassion. Photo courtesy of Photodisc.

unheard-of in certain populations—and not because of lack of desire, but lack of finances and priorities.

- Continual changes to the technology landscape as it relates to patient care: documentation, delivery, and maintenance of data. Hopefully, one day soon patient charts will be computerized, with information following a patient from facility to facility and episode to episode.

- Emergence of health care issues that continue to affect large populations of people, including more drug-resistant strains of disease and responses to major disasters, such as the health issues related to hurricane Katrina in 2005. What will the next epidemic be?

- Enhanced consumer education resulting in expectations for informed and collaborative health care decisions, rather than being told what to do by health care providers. No longer do the majority of health consumers do what the physician wants them to do merely because he is the physician; patients and their families are information-hungry, seeking answers to their questions on the Internet and then validating with their health care provider.

- Demands for more ethical and involved end-of-life care through the use of advanced directives, palliative care, and active participation in decision making. Families will become increasingly more participatory as they help guide health care providers in end-of-life care.

- The continued focus on care outcomes and the achievement of patient goals as health care settings and providers will continue to be evaluated on their ability to achieve preestablished results.

- A sustained regulation effort by state and federal governments as health care costs continue to rise, resulting in more people needing services due to their uninsured or underinsured status. The maintenance of the health care system will continue to be shifted to managed care because the states remain challenged in meeting specific population needs as compared with economic

limitations. Priorities will be reshuffled, resulting in significant policy action, to which nurses and other health care leaders must be prepared to contribute meaningful discussion.

- A need for a more educated nursing workforce. Already there is a movement afoot that addresses the enhanced bedside nurse's skills through the Clinical Nurse Leader (CNL) position and the increased clinical knowledge necessary to provide care through the Doctorate in Nursing Practice (DNP) role. But how will these roles be effectively implemented within the health care system?

- A continued nursing shortage in both clinicians and nursing faculty. Unless there are some significant changes in the ability for nursing colleges to produce more faculty, the next decade will sorely challenge them to educate the increasing numbers of prospective nursing students, many of whom, at least in the early 2000s, were turned away for lack of qualified faculty (AACN, 2003).

- Due to the shortage of nurses, hospitals will continue to be challenged by the way they utilize their current and future staff; but regardless of the perspective, the time spent with the patient and family will need to be more meaningful, because many other tasks that are time-consuming (tray delivery, documentation, and other pieces of patient data) will (hopefully) be enhanced by bedside technology. Registered nurses should finally be allowed to "reconnect" with their patients, providing the human touch and putting the care back in health care.

When individual nurses internalize and accept responsibility for their own professional growth and development, the by-product will be an actualization of the Institute of Medicine's core competencies. In the future, with the rapid technological changes and the knowledge explosion, nurses will not be able to keep pace without constant effort and involvement. Similarly, nursing as a profession is dependent upon engaged and active nurses influencing the direction of the profession—and the ability to attract others to the profession in order to carry on its goals, its vision, and its dreams.

CHAPTER SUMMARY

Nursing's past has created an image and expectations for the practice of nursing that at times have resulted in a variety of impressions. However, changes in the delivery of health care, a knowledge explosion, and the rapid evolution of technology, coupled with globalization and expectations for cultural sensitivity, have greatly altered the conditions in which nursing is practiced. Nursing as a profession does not meet all of the generally accepted criteria of a profession, but it is still the responsibility of the individual nurse to strive to meet the core competencies for professional practice. Collectively, nurses who can successfully meet the challenges of the rapidly changing health care delivery system will gain recognition and develop further influence for themselves and their profession, while providing optimal care for their patients. Nursing must continue to address its internal issues in order to emerge with unquestioned professional status, reshaping its image and ensuring its legacy.

> *Be bold, be bold, and everywhere be bold.*
> —Edmund Spenser

REFERENCES

American Association of Colleges of Nursing (2003). *White paper: Faculty shortages in baccalaureate and graduate nursing programs: Scope of the problem and strategies for expanding the supply.* Washington, DC: Author. Available from http://www.aacn.nche.edu/Publications/positions/whitepaper.htm.

American Nurses Association (2001). *A code for nurses.* Washington, DC: Author.

Buresh, B., & Gordon, S. (2006). *From silence to voice. What nurses need to know and must communicate to the public* (2nd ed.). Ottawa, Ontario: The Canadian Nurses Association.

Catalano, J. T. (2003). The development of a profession. In J. T. Catalano, *Nursing now! Today's issues, tomorrow's trends* (3rd ed.). Philadelphia, PA: F. A. Davis Company.

Institute of Medicine. (2003). *Health professions education: A bridge to quality.* Washington, DC: Author.

Mason, D. J., Leavitt, J. K., & Chaffee, M. W. (2006). *Policy and politics in nursing and health care* (5th ed.). Philadelphia, PA: W.B. Saunders.

Sigma Theta Tau International (1999). *Harris poll on consumer attitudes about nursing.* Conducted by Louis Harris & Associates, commissioned by Sigma Theta Tau International and NurseWeek Publishing, Inc.

Sullivan, E. J. (2004). *Becoming influential. A guide for nurses.* Upper Saddle River, NJ: Pearson Education Inc.

Swearington, S., & Liberman, A. (2004). Nursing generations: An expanded look at the emergence of conflict and its resolution. *Health Care Manager, 23*(1), 54–64.

INDEX

A

AACN. *See* American Association of Colleges of Nursing

Academic Center for Evidence-based Nursing (ACE) Star model of knowledge transformation, 103, 105, 105f

Accommodation, coping strategies, in conflict, 302, 303t

Accountability, 280

Acculturation, 180–181

ACE. *See* Academic Center for Evidence-based Nursing Star model of knowledge transformation

Adult-learning theory, 244, 244t

Advance directive, 203, 205f

Advanced-practice nurses, 119–120

Advanced-practice registered nurse (APRN), 144

Agency Healthcare Research and Quality (AHRQ), 102

AHRQ. *See* Agency Healthcare Research and Quality

Aiken, Linda, 139

AIN. *See* Associate degree in nursing

ALLHAT. *See* Antihypertensive and Lipid Lowering Treatment to Prevent Heart Attack Trial

Allied health practitioners, 120–121

Allocative health policy, 161

Ambiguity era, in nursing, 5–6

American Association of Colleges of Nursing (AACN), 380–381

American Nurses Association (ANA), 139, 380
first position paper, 39–40

American Nurses Credentialing Center (ANCC), 149, 150–151t, 151

American Psychological Association (APA), baccalaureate-degree program and, 47

ANA. *See* American Nurses Association

ANCC. *See* American Nurses Credentialing Center

Andragogy, 49

Antihypertensive and Lipid Lowering Treatment to Prevent Heart Attack Trial (ALLHAT), 101

Antiquity, nursing in, 17–18
Greece, 17–18
primitive societies, 17
Rome, 17–18

APA. *See* American Psychological Association

APRN. *See* Advanced-practice registered nurse

Army Nurse Corps, 25, 38

Asclepius, 17, 18

Associate degree in nursing (AIN), 248

Associate-degree program, in nursing education, 38–39, 40

Authority, 280

Autonomy, 218

B

Baby boomers, 127, 190

Baccalaureate-degree program, 47–48
adult learners, 47, 48
concepts of, 49–50
uniqueness of, 49
American Psychological Association, 47
in nursing education, 39, 40
professional student responsibilities and, 46–47
returning to school for, 46–47

Barton, Clara, 23–24

Behavioral learning theory, 234–235, 234f

Beliefs, in health care environment, 216

Beneficence, 219

Bits, 330

Black nursing program, development of, 36–38

Boolean logic, 68f
BPI. *See* Brain preference indicator
Brain preference indicator (BPI), 249t
Brewster, Mary, professional accountability and, 138
Britain training evolution, Florence Nightingale and, 31–32
Bruner, Jerome, 237
Bytes, 330

C

Cadet Nurse Corps, 25–26
Carnegie, Mary Elizabeth, 37
CCNE. *See* Commission on Collegiate Nursing Education
CDSSs. *See* Clinical decision support systems
Certification, in nursing, 148–152
Certified Nurse Midwife (CNM), 120
Certified Registered Nurse Anesthetist (CRNA), 120
CE. *See* Continuing education (CE), mandatory
Change agent, 270
Change theory, 269–270, 269f
    contemporary, 270–272
        first-order, 271
        second-order, 271
    of families, 275
    of individuals, 275
    of staff, 274–275
    traditional, 270, 270t
Chaos and complexity, 272
Christian era, early, nursing in, 18
CINAHL, 72
CIS. *See* Clinical information systems
Civil War, nursing and, 21–24, 23f
    confederate, 24, 24f
    union, 22–24
Clients, 330
Clinical decision support systems (CDSSs), 333
Clinical information systems (CIS), 332
Clinical nurse leader (CNL), 352–353, 387
Clinical nurse specialists (CNS), 119, 179
Clinical practice guideline (CPG), 97, 98f
CNL. *See* Clinical nurse leader
CNM. *See* Certified Nurse Midwife
CNS. *See* Clinical nurse specialists
Coach, mentoring and, 354
Coercive power, conflict and, 299, 300t
Cognitive learning theory, 235–238, 237f, 238t
Collaboration, 11–12
    conflict and, 308–310
    coping strategies, in conflict, 303, 303t
    elements of, 310

Commission on Collegiate Nursing Education (CCNE), 141, 381–382
Communication
    delegation and, 289–291
    technology and, 5–6
Community-based care, 116
Competency, 280
Competition, coping strategies, in conflict, 303, 303t
Complexity/chaos theory, 272–273
Compromise, coping strategies, in conflict, 303, 303t
Computer-based patient record (CPR), 325. *See also* Electronic health record (EHR)
Confederate nursing, 24, 24f
Conflict
    addressing of, 305–310
        collaboration, 308–310
        negotiation, 305–307
        negotiation, principled, 307–308
    coping strategies in, 302–303, 303t
        accommodation, 302, 303t
        collaboration, 303, 303t
        competition, 303, 303t
        compromise, 303, 303t
        confrontation, 303, 303t
        force, 302, 303t
        withdrawing, 302, 303t
    definition of, 295
    dysfunctional, 295–296
    emotional response to, 303–304, 304f
    functional, 295–296
    leadership during, 310
    potential for, 296–298
    power and, 298–299, 300t
        coercive, 299, 300t
        expert, 299, 300t
        information, 299, 300t
        legitimate, 299, 300t
        referent, 299, 300t
        reward, 299, 300t
    results of, 301–302
    staging of, 301
    types of, 289–301, 301t
        intergroup, 300–301, 301t
        interpersonal, 300, 301t
        intragroup, 300, 301t
        intrapersonal, 289–300, 301t
        role, 301, 301t
    work/family, 53

Confrontation, coping strategies, in
    conflict, 303, 303t
Consent form, 202f
Continuing education (CE), mandatory, nursing, trends
    in, 146–148, 147t
Continuous Quality Improvement (CQI), 126
Coping strategies, in conflict, 302–303, 303t
    accommodation, 302, 303t
    collaboration, 303, 303t
    competition, 303, 303t
    compromise, 303, 303t
    confrontation, 303, 303t
    force, 302, 303t
    withdrawing, 302, 303t
Core competencies, health professionals overlap
    of, 12f
Court decisions, health policies and, 162
CPG. See Clinical practice guideline
CPR. See Computer-based Patient Record
CQI. See Continuous Quality Improvement
Credentialing, in nursing, 148–152
Crimean War, Florence Nightingale and, 31
CRNA. See Certified Registered Nurse Anesthetist
Cultural Heritage Model, 183
Customers, hardware, access/management of
    electronic information, 328

D

Data, 323
    capture, 325
    integrity, 325
Databases
    in health care information, 72–74
        CINAHL, 72
        MEDLINE (PubMed), 72–74, 73f
        PsycInfo, 72
    health care information and, 67–68
Deep change, 271
Delegated care, evaluation of, personnel
    providing care, 318
Delegation
    accountability and, 280
    authority and, 280
    barriers of, 286–287
    communication and, 289–291
    competency and, 280
    considerations in, 282f
    definition of, 280–281
    dumping or, 289
    effectiveness of, 285–286

evolution of, 281–282
    feedback and, 289–291, 291f
    five rights of, 283–285, 284t
    high-context communication and, 290
    liability and, 287–289
    low-context communication and, 290
    overdelegation in, 286
    right circumstance and, 284t
    right direction/communication and, 284t
    right person and, 284t
    right supervision and, 284t
    right task and, 284t
    underdelegation in, 286
DePree, Max, 267
Diagnostic Related Groupings (DRGs), 5, 121
    urbanization and, 27
Dimock, Susan, 6, 32–33
Diploma program, in nursing education, 39
Discrimination, in health care environment, 201–202
Diversity
    aging nurses, 190–192, 191f
    definition of, 180–181, 181f
    management of, 193–194
    nursing, 185–188, 187f, 188f
    sexual orientation and, 192–193
Dix, Dorothea, 22–23
DNP. See Doctorate of Nursing Practice
DNR. See Do Not Resuscitate
DNSc. See Doctorate of Nursing Science
Doctoral, preparation for, graduate programs,
    351–352, 351f
Doctorate of Nursing Practice (DNP),
    352–354, 354f
Doctorate of Nursing Science (DNSc), 351
Doctorate of Science in Nursing (DSN), 351
Doctor of Philosophy in Nursing (PhD), 351
Do Not Resuscitate (DNR), 219
Dreyfus Model, 233
DRGs. See Diagnostic Related Groupings
DSN. See Doctorate of Science in Nursing
Dunn and Dunn Learning Style Inventory, 249t
Durable Power of Attorney, 203, 204f
Dysfunctional conflict, 295–296

E

EBP. See Evidence-based practice
EFT. See Embedded figures test
EHR. See Electronic health record
Electronic health record (EHR), 330–331
Electronic medical record (EMR), 332

Embedded figures test (EFT), 249t
Emergency care, 116
Emergency medical technicians (EMTs), 116
Emergency Medical Treatment and Active Labor
        Act (EMTALA), 161
Employment, issues of, 198–199
Employment trends, 179–180
EMR. *See* Electronic medical record
EMTALA. *See* Emergency Medical Treatment
        and Active Labor Act
EMTs. *See* Emergency medical technicians
End-of-life care, 224–226, 225f
Ethics, in health care environment, 216
    beliefs, 216
    decision making, 222
    development of, 216–217
    end-of-life care, 224–226, 225f
    moral behavior, 216
    morals, 216, 217–220, 220f
    religions, 216
    resolving dilemmas in, 220–222
    United States applications to health
        care, 223–226
    values, 216
Euthanasia, 219
Evaluation
    definition of, 312–313
    of delegated care, 318
    formative, 315
    nursing-sensitive patient outcomes, 319–320
    in patient care, 313–314, 314f, 314t
    of patient care process, 314–315, 314t
    of peers, 317–318
    of personnel providing care, 314t, 316–318
    of policies, 316
    of programs, 316
    of protocols, 316
    of self, 316–317
    standards of, 318–319
    summative, 315
    types of, 314f
Evidence-based practice (EBP)
    clinical practice guideline, 97, 98f
    concerns regarding, 100
    definition of, 97–98
    historical perspective of, 98–100
        economics, 98–99
        heath care, 99
        nursing, 99–100

implementation of, 105–107
    education, 107
    populations, 107
    practice, 105–107
literature synthesis, 100–103
    evaluating research, 102–103
    finding evidence, 100–101
    research designs, 101–102
model of implementation for, 103–105
    ACE Star model of knowledge transformation,
        103, 105, 105f
outcomes of, 98
in patient care process evaluation, 315
resources, 75
Expert power, conflict and, 299, 300t

F

Fabiola, 18
Families, change theory of, 275
Family interferes with work (FIW), 54
Family/work conflict, 53–55
    imbalance, 54
Feedback, delegation and, 289–291, 291f
Feminization, 24
FIW. *See* Family interferes with work
Flexner Report, 35
Flexnex, Abraham, 35
Force, coping strategies, in conflict, 302, 303t
4MAT System, 249t
Functional conflict, 295–296

G

Gender issues, nursing and, 188–190
Goldmark, Josephine, 35
Goldmark Report, 35–36
Good Samaritan statutes, 212–213
Graduate nurses
    as career decision, 355–357
        academic careers, 356–357
        practice setting advancement, 356
    workforce and, 346–347
Graduate programs, 349–255
    doctoral, preparation for, 351–352, 351f
    future trends in, 352–355, 354f
    Masters of Science in Nursing, preparation
        for, 350–351
Great Depression, nursing and, 25
Greenleaf, Robert, 267
Gregorc Style Delineator, 249t

H

Hampton-Robb, Isabel, 33–34, 34f
Hardware, access/management of electronic
  information, 328–330
  bits, 330
  bytes, 330
  clients, 330
  customers, 328
  minicomputers, 330
  operating system, 328
  server, 330
  software, 328
Harmony
  coping strategies for, 59–60
  work/family, 53
HCOs. *See* Health care organizations
Health care, demands of, 126–134
  baby boomers, 127, 190
  changing trends in, 126–134
  demographic changes, 127–128, 127t
  genetics, 128–129
  information technology, 128
  natural disasters, 128–129
  primary care, 134
  technological innovations, 128–129
  technology, 128
  terrorism, 128–129
  unhealthy lifestyle, 130–133, 132f, 133f, 134f
Health care environment
  assignment rejection in, 199–201
  discrimination, 201–202
  employment issues in, 198–199
  ethics in, 216
    beliefs, 216
    decision making, 221
    development of, 216–217
    end-of-life care, 224–226, 225f
    moral behavior, 216
    morals, 216, 217–220, 220f
    religions, 216
    resolving dilemmas in, 220–222
    United States applications to health care, 223–226
    values, 216
  Good Samaritan statutes, 212–213
  Health Insurance Portability and Accountability
    Act and, 205–206
  informed consent, 207–211
  legal instruments in, 202–205
    advance directive, 203, 205f

    consent form, 202f
    durable Power of Attorney, 203, 204f
    living will, 205f
    Power of Attorney, 202–203
  liability risk, decrease, 207t
  negligence, 206–207
  Nurse Practice Act and, 211–212
  protected health information, 205–206
Health care finance, 121–124
  health policy and, 165–168
    Medicaid, 167
    Medicare, 165–167
    military insurance, 167–168
    private-sector financing, 168
    public-sector financing, 165–168
    social security, 168
    State Children's Health Insurance Plan, 167
  Medicaid, 122
  medical expenditures, 124f
  Medicare, 121–122, 123t
  private health insurance, 122, 124
  worker's compensation, 122
Health care information
  databases, 72–74
    CINAHL, 72
    MEDLINE (PubMed), 72–74, 73f
    PsycInfo, 72
  evidence-based practice resources, 75
  Internet searching tips, 68, 68f
  lifelong learning, 76
  literature types, 65–66
    peer-reviewed publications, 66
    refereed publications, 66
  locating information, 66–68
    databases, 67–68
    search engines, 67–68
  needs of, 70–71
  retrieval of, 71–72
  search statement development, 70–71
  trends in, 65–74
  web site evaluation, 68, 69f
  web site recommendations, 68–70
    keywords, 69–70
    subject headings, 69–70
  writing resources, 75–76
Healthcare information systems (HIS), 332
Health care organizations (HCOs), 338–339
  accrediting bodies for, 152–154
Health care professionals, core competencies for, 379t

Health care settings
    inpatient, 114–115
        hospice care, 115
        long-term care, 115
    outpatient, 114, 116–117
        community-based care, 116
        emergency care, 116
        primary care, 117
        secondary care, 117
        tertiary care, 117
Health care team, 117–121
    advanced-practice nurses, 119–120
    allied health practitioners, 120–121
    employment of, 118t
    pharmacists, 120
    physician assistants, 120
    physicians, 120
    registered nurses, 119
    social workers, 120
Health care technology, 330–332
    clinical information systems, 332
    electronic health record, 330–331
    electronic medical record, 332
    healthcare information systems, 332
    privacy issues and, 336–337
    security issues and, 336–337
Health insurance
    Health Maintenance Organizations, 125–126
    military, 167–168
    no coverage, 125f
    preferred provider organizations, 126
Health Insurance Portability and Accountability Act
        (HIPAA), 205–206, 236
Health Maintenance Organizations (HMOs), 125–126
Health policy, 180–181
    health and, 162
    health care finance and, 165–168
        Medicaid, 167
        Medicare, 165–167
        military insurance, 167–168
        private-sector financing, 168
        public-sector financing, 165–168
        social security, 168
        State Children's Health Insurance Plan, 167
    issues of, 168–174
        access, 169
        community, 174
        cost, 169
        global, 172–173
        government, 173–174
        health professions and, 172–174
        healthy people 2010, 169–172, 170t,
            171f, 172t
        quality, 169
        workplace, 174
    social policy and, 160–161
    types of, 161–162
        allocative, 161
        court decisions, 162
        laws, 161
        regulatory, 161–162
High-context communication, delegation and, 290
High school students, health care, demands of
        drinking and driving, 135f
        physical activity and, 134f
        seatbelt use, 135f
Hill-Burton Act, 27
HIPAA. See Health Insurance Portability and
        Accountability Act
Hippocrates, 17–18
HIS. See Healthcare information systems
HMOs. See Health Maintenance Organizations
Hospice care, 115
Hospital-based diploma programs, 247
Human Genoma Project, 224
Humanistic learning theory, 243–244

Incremantalism, 163
Industrial revolution, nursing in, 19, 20f
Informatics, 323
    data, 323
    information, 323
    information technology, 323
    nursing, 323
Information management, trends in, 323–324
Information manager, nurse as, 324–328, 324t
    computer-based patient record, 325
    data capture, 325
    data integrity, 325
    data transformation to knowledge, 324f
    nursing classifications systems, 325
    Nursing Information Systems, 325
    Omaha System, 326–328f
    standardized nursing languages, 325
Information power, conflict and, 299, 300t
Information technology (IT), 323, 324
    health care, demands of, 128

Informed consent, 207–211
Inpatient health care settings, 114–115
    hospice care, 115
    long-term care, 115
Integration, work/family, 53
Interest bargaining, 305
Intergroup conflict, 300–301, 301t
Internet, 330
    libraries and, 74–75
Internet searching tips, health care information
        and, 68, 68f
Interpersonal conflict, 300, 301t
Intragroup conflict, 300, 301t
Intranet, 330
Intrapersonal conflict, 289–300, 301t

J

JCAHO. *See* Joint Commission on Accreditation of
        Healthcare Organizations
Joint Commission on Accreditation of Healthcare
        Organizations (JCAHO)
    body accreditation and, 152–154
    teaching/learning and, 232
Justice, 219–220

K

Kolb's Learning Style Inventory, 249t

L

Labor, in American, 50–51
    of females, 50f, 51f
LaTourette, Steven, 199
Learner, in teaching/learning, 244–252, 245f
    characteristics of, 240–242t, 246–247
    findings of, 245–246, 246f
    literacy of, 250–252, 252t
    motivation of, 249, 250t, 251t
    overview of, 245
    purpose of, 245
    research design of, 245
    research focus of, 244
    styles of, 247–249, 248t, 249t
Learning organization, 269
Learning-style instruments, 249t
Legal instruments, in health care environment, 202–205
    advance directive, 203, 205f
    consent form, 202f
    durable Power of Attorney, 203, 204f
    living will, 205f
    Power of Attorney, 202–203

Legitimate power, conflict and, 299, 300t
Leininger, Madeline, 181
Liability, delegation and, 287–289
Libraries, Internet and, 74–75
Licensure, of nurses, 143–144
    mutual recognition model of, 144–146, 145t
Lifelong learning, 76
Life satisfaction, 58–59
Literature synthesis, 100–103
    evaluating research, 102–103
    finding evidence, 100–101
    research designs, 101–102
Living will, 205f
Lomas Model, 163, 164f
Longest Model, 164–165, 165f
Long-term care (LTC), 115, 172–173
Low-context communication, delegation and, 290
LTC. *See* Long-term care

M

Mahoney, Mary Eliza, 36–37, 37f
Managed care, 124–126, 125f
Mandatory continuing education (MCE), nursing,
        trends in, 146–148, 147t
Marcella, 18
Master's-degree nursing education programs,
        248–249
Masters of Science in Nursing (MSN), preparation for,
        graduate programs, 350–351
MCE. *See* Mandatory continuing education
Medicaid, 122
    public-sector financing, 167
Medical expenditures, 124f
Medicare, 121–122, 123t
    public-sector financing, 165–167
MEDLINE (PubMed), 72–74, 73f
Men, nursing and, 38
Mentees
    characteristics of, 365–366
    mentoring and, 354
Mentoring. *See also* Mentors
    benefits of, 374–375
    coach and, 354
    culture, 368
    historical perspectives on, 353–354
    mentee and, 354
    mentor and, 354
    new generation of, 371–374
        graduates, 371–372
        minority nurses, 373

Mentoring (*continued*)
    nurse managers/leaders, 374
    nursing faculty, 373–374
  preceptee and, 354
  preceptor and, 354
  relationships, factors affecting, 366–368
  stages/phases, 370–371
  strategies, 369
  teacher and, 354
Mentors
  characteristics of, 364–365
  mentoring and, 354
Metaparadigm, 80
Middle ages, nursing in, 19
Military insurance, public-sector financing, 167–168
Minicomputers, 330
Mobile computing, 330
Moral behavior, in health care environment, 216,
        217–220, 220f
  autonomy, 218
  beneficence, 219
  justice, 219–220
  nonmaleficence, 218–219
Motivation theory, 273–274, 274t
MSN. *See* Masters of Science in Nursing,
        preparation for
Mutual recognition model of nurse licensure,
        144–146, 145t
Myers-Briggs Type Indicator, 249t

N

National Association of Nursing Superintendents,
        33–34
National Bioethics Advisory Commission
        (NBAC), 223
National Black Nurses Association, 37–38
National Council Licensure Examination
        (NCLEX), 144
National Council of State Boards of Nursing (NCSBN),
        141–142
National League for Nursing (NLN), 380
National League for Nursing Accreditation Commission
        (NLNAC), 140–141, 380
National Student Nurses Association (NSNA),
        381–382
Natural disasters, health care, demands
        of, 129–130
NBAC. *See* National Bioethics Advisory Commission
NCLEX. *See* National Council Licensure Examination

N-CODES, 333
NCSBN. *See* National Council of State Boards of
        Nursing
Negligence, in health care environment, 206–207
Negotiation
  conflict and, 305–307
    interest bargaining, 306
    positional bargaining, 306
  principled, 307–308
  process of, 306–307
Nielsen, Jerri, 336
Nightingale, Florence, 6, 7, 19–21, 80, 81, 90, 91b
  nursing licensure requirements and, 143
  nursing theory and, 82–84, 87t
  professional accountability and, 138
  tradition of, 31–32
    Britain training evolution, 31–32
    Crimean War, 31
Nightingale Training School for Nurses, 31, 33
NIS. *See* Nursing Information Systems
NLC. *See* Nurse Licensure Compact
NLNAC. *See* National League for Nursing Accreditation
        Commission
NLN. *See* National League for Nursing
Nonmaleficence, 218–219
NP. *See* Nurse practitioners
NSNA. *See* National Student Nurses Association
N-STAT. *See* Nurses Strategic Action Team
Nurse Licensure Compact (NLC), 144, 145t
Nurse Practice Act, 211–212
Nurse practitioners (NP), 119
Nurses. *See also* Nursing
  advanced-practice, 119–120
  graduate, workforce and, 346–347
  licensure of, 143–144
  minority, mentoring and, 373
  political action of, 382–384
  politics and, 162–163
  professional responsibilities of, 382
  professional role of, 339–340
  registered, 119
Nurses Strategic Action Team (N-STAT), 9
Nurse Training Act, 26
Nursing. *See also* Nurses
  21st century and, 27
  1950s through 1970s, 26–27
  accreditation of certification programs in, 151
  advanced practice certification in, 149
  aging workforce, 190–192, 191f

ambiguity era in, 5–6
American Nurses Credentialing Center, 149, 150–151t, 151
in antiquity, 17–18
    Greece, 17–18
    primitive societies, 17
    Rome, 17–18
certification in, 148–152
in changing times, 4–5
Civil War and, 21–24, 23f
    confederate nursing, 24, 24f
    union nursing, 22–24
concepts of, 79
    environment, 79
    health, 79
    nursing, 79
    person, 79
confederate, 24, 24f
continuing education, mandatory, trends in, 146–148, 147t
credentialing in, 148–152
cultural assessment interview guide and, 184f
discipline of, future planning for, 357–359
diversity of, 36–38, 185–188, 187f, 188f
    black nursing program development, 36–38
    men and, 38
early American health care and, 31
in early Christian era, 18
faculty, mentoring and, 373–374
futures of, 286f, 384–387
gender, issues of, 188–190
graduate programs in, 349–355
    doctoral, preparation for, 351–352, 351f
    future trends in, 352–355, 354f
    Masters of Science in Nursing, preparation for, 350–351
Great Depression and, 25
historical events influencing evolution of, 42–43t
in industrial revolution, 19, 20f
in middle ages, 19
opportunity era in, 5–6
population projections of, 357–359
as profession, 79
professional identity of, 7–8
in Protestant Reformation, 19
race and, 183–185, 185f
society and, 183–185
Spanish-American War and, 25
transcultural, 181–183

union, 22–24
voice of, media and, 384
World War I and, 25
World War II and, 25–26
Nursing classifications systems, 325
Nursing education, 30–31
    accreditation in, 140–142
    approval in, 140–142
    associate-degree program in, 38–39, 40
    baccalaureate-degree program in, 39, 40
    diploma program in, 39
    history overview of, 247–249
        associate degree, 248
        baccalaureate degree, 247–248
        doctoral, preparation for, 351–352, 351f
        hospital-based diploma programs, 247
        master's-degree, 248–249
    models for, 24, 38
    practical nurse training, 38
    specialty nursing certification in, 41
    standards for, 35
        Flexner Report, 35
        regulatory board institution, 35
Nursing informatics, 323
Nursing Information Systems (NIS), 325
Nursing practice
    licensure requirements in, 143–144
    theory and, 89–91
Nursing-sensitive patient, outcomes of, 319–320
Nursing theory, 79–80
    controversy and, 93
    element of, 82b
    grand, 81–82
    historical overview of, 80–81
    levels of, 81–82
    middle-range, 81–82
    Nightingale, Florence, and, 82–84, 87t
    Pepula, Hildegard, and, 84–85, 87t
    practice and, 81–82, 89–91
    Rogers, Martha, and, 85, 87–88t
    Roy, Sister Callista, and, 85–86, 87t
    structural hierarchy, 85f
    types of, 81–82
Nursing world force, 4

O

Obesity, health care, demands of, 132f
Olympias, 18
Omaha System, 326–328f
Operant Conditioning Model, 234

Operating system (OS), 328
Opportunity era, in nursing, 5–6
OS. *See* Operating system
Outpatient health care settings, 114, 116–117
  community-based care, 116
  emergency care, 116
  primary care, 117
  secondary care, 117
  tertiary care, 117
Overdelegation, 286
Overtime, mandatory, 198
Overweight, health care, demands of, 132f

P

PA. *See* Physician assistants
Patient care, evaluation in, 313–314, 314f, 314t
Patient care process, evaluation of, 314–315, 314t
  evidence-based practice, 315
Patient-centered care, 4
Patient education materials (PEM), 252
Patient safety, 332–335
PDAs. *See* Personal digital assistants
Pedagogy, 49
Peer-reviewed publications, health care information
    and, 66
Peers, evaluation of, in personnel providing care,
    317–318
Pember, Phoebe, 24
PEM. *See* Patient education materials
Peplau, Hildegard, 81, 91b
  nursing theory and, 84–85, 87t
Peplau's Theory of Interpersonal Relationships, 81
Personal digital assistants (PDAs), 328, 330
Personnel providing care, evaluation
    of, 314t, 316–318
  delegated care, 318
  peers, 317–318
  self, 316–317
Pharmacists, 120
PhD. *See* Doctor of Philosophy in Nursing
PHI. *See* Protected health information
Phoebe, 18
Physician assistants (PA), 120
Physicians, 120
Piaget, Jean, 237
Planck, Max, 339
Planned change, 270
POA. *See* Power of Attorney
Policies

evaluation of, 316
  health, 180–181
    allocative, 161
    court decisions, 162
    health and, 162
    laws, 161
    regulatory, 161–162
    social policy and, 160–161
    types of, 161–162
  making of, 162–165, 164f, 165f
  social, health policy and, 160–161
Political action, of nurses, 382–384
Politics, nurses and, 162–163
Positional bargaining, 305
Power, conflict and, 298–299, 300t
  coercive, 299, 300t
  expert, 299, 300t
  information, 299, 300t
  legitimate, 299, 300t
  referent, 299, 300t
  reward, 299, 300t
Power of Attorney (POA), 202–203
  durable, 203, 204f
PPC. *See* Progressive Patient Care
PPOs. *See* Preferred provider organizations
Preceptor, mentoring and, 354
Preferred provider organizations (PPOs), 126
President Clinton, 114
Principled negotiation, conflict and, 307–308
Private health insurance, 122, 124
Profession
  definition of, 378
  nursing, 377–378
    collective responsibilities of, 380–382
    health care professionals core competencies, 379
    implications of, 378–379
    issues of, 378–379
Professional accountability, 137–138
  in nursing, 138–140, 139f
Professional identity, of nurses, 7–8
Professionalism, 7
Professional nurse's role, 339–340
Professional organizations, 380
Professional roots, 6–7
Professional workforce, of 21st century,
    11–13, 12f
Programs, evaluation of, 316
Progressive Patient Care (PPC), 4
Protected health information (PHI), 205–206

Protégé, 364–365
Protestant Reformation, nursing in, 19
Protocols, evaluation of, 316
Psychodynamic theory, 239, 240–242t, 243
PsycInfo, 72
Public identity, of nurses, 9, 11
Public-sector financing, 165–168
    Medicaid, 167
    Medicare, 165–167
    military insurance, 167–168
    social security, 168
    State Children's Health Insurance Plan, 167
PubMed (MEDLINE), 72–74, 73f

Q

Quality improvement, 5

R

Race, nursing and, 183–185, 185f
RAM. See Roy's Adaptation Model
Randomized clinical trials (RCTs), 99, 100, 101, 102
RCTs. See Randomized clinical trials
Refereed publications, health care information and, 66
Referent power, conflict and, 299, 300t
Registered nurse (RN), 119
    as change agent, overview of, 267–269, 268f
    as leader, overview of, 267–269, 268f
Regulation, 139
Regulatory health policy, 161–162
Religions, in health care environment, 216
Reorganizing care era, 4, 5
Research utilization. See Evidence-based practice (EBP)
Responsibility, 382
Reward power, conflict and, 299, 300t
Richards, Linda, 6
Right circumstance, delegation and, 284t
Right direction/communication, delegation and, 284t
Right person, delegation and, 284t
Right supervision, delegation and, 284t
Right task, delegation and, 284t
Rogers, Martha, 81, 91b
    nursing theory and, 85, 87–88t
Role, 50
Role conflict, 301, 301t
Role overload, 50
Role set, 50
Role stress, 50
Roy's Adaptation Model (RAM), 50, 85–86
Roy, Sister Callista, 81, 91b
    nursing theory and, 85–86, 87t

S

Sackett, David, 97
SCHIP. See State Children's Health Insurance Plan
Science of Unitary Human Beings (SUHB), 85
Search engines, health care information and, 67–68
Self-awareness, 316–317
Self-evaluation, in personnel providing care, 316–317
Servant leadership, 267
Server, 330
Sexual orientation, 192–193
Sigma Theta Tau International (STTI), 380
Skinner, B. F., 234
SNOMED CT, 331–332
Social learning theory, 238–239, 239f
Social policy, health policy and, 160–161
Social Role Theory, 51–52
Social security, public-sector financing, 168
Social workers, 120
Software, 328
Spanish-American War, nursing and, 25
Specialty nursing certification, in nursing
    education, 41
Spillover, 55–56
Staff, change theory of, 274–275
Standardized nursing languages, 325
Stark, Pete, 199
State Children's Health Insurance Plan (SCHIP),
    public-sector financing, 167
Staupers, Mabel Keaton, 36–37
STI. See Sigma Theta Tau International
Styles, Margretta, 139
SUHB. See Science of Unitary Human Beings

T

Teacher
    mentoring and, 354
    in teaching/learning, 260, 260t, 261t
Teaching/learning, 232–233
    instructional materials in, 256–258, 257t
    instructional methods in, 252–256
        definitions, 252t
        select nursing educational intervention
            studies, 256t
        teaching tips and, 254t
        terms, 252t
    instructional strategy planning, 258–259, 258t
    learner, 244–252, 245f
        characteristics of, 240–242t, 246–247
        findings of, 245–246, 246f
        literacy of, 250–252, 252t

Teaching/learning (*continued*)
    motivation of, 249, 250t, 251t
    overview of, 245
    purpose of, 245
    research design of, 245
    research focus of, 244
    retention of, 258t
    styles of, 247–249, 248t, 249t
  models, 233, 233f, 233t
  nursing process *versus* education process, 233t
  teacher, 260, 260t, 261t
  theories of, 234–244, 234t
    adult-learning, 244, 244t
    behavioral learning, 234–235, 234f
    cognitive learning, 235–238, 237f, 238t
    humanistic learning, 243–244
    psychodynamic, 239, 240–242t, 243
    social learning, 238–239, 239f
Telehealth, 336–337
Telemedicine, 337
Terrorism, health care, demands of, 129–130
Theory(ies)
  change, 269–270, 269f
    contemporary, 270–272
      first-order, 271
      second-order, 271
    traditional, 270, 270t
  complexity/chaos, 272–273
  definition of, 79
  derivation of, 79
  motivation, 273–274, 274t
  of teaching/learning, 234–244, 234t
    adult-learning, 244, 244t
    behavioral learning, 234–235, 234f
    cognitive learning, 235–238, 237f, 238t
    humanistic learning, 243–244
    psychodynamic, 239, 240–242t, 243
    social learning, 238–239, 239f
Thompkins, Sallie, 24
Transcultural Assessment Model, 181–182, 182f
Transcultural Nursing Theory, 181–183
Transformational leadership, 267
21st century
  nursing in, 27
  professional workforce of, 11

U
UAP. *See* Unlicensed assistive personnel
Underdelegation, 286
Union nursing, 22–24
Unlicensed assistive personnel (UAP), 179, 279–280
U.S. Preventative Services Task Force (USP-STF),
    102–103, 103t
  rating scale for evidence quality, 103t
  strength of recommendation guidelines, 103t
USP-STP. *See* U.S. Preventative Services Task Force
U.S. Training Schools of Nursing, 32–35
  first, 33
  foundation of hospital training, 33–35
  National Association of Nursing Superintendents, 33–34

V
Values, in health care environment, 216
Virtual private networks (VPNs), 338
VPNs. *See* Virtual private networks

W
Wald, Lillian, 6–7
  professional accountability and, 138
Web sites
  evaluation of, 68, 69f
  recommendations, 68–70
    keywords, 69–70
    subject headings, 69–70
WIF. *See* Work interferes with family
Wireless computing, 330
Withdrawing, coping strategies, in conflict, 302, 303t
Women, multiple roles of, 57–58
Worker's compensation, 122
Work/family
  balance of, 52–54
  coping strategies for, 59–60
  harmony, 53
  integration, 53
Work interferes with family (WIF), 54
Work, quality of, family interference and, 56
World War II, nursing and, 25–26
World War I nursing and, 25
Writing resources, 75–76

Z
Zakrzewska, Marie, 32